The Diversity Promise

Success in Academic Surgery and Medicine Through Diversity, Equity, and Inclusion

The Diversity Promise

Success in Academic Surgery and Medicine Through Diversity, Equity, and Inclusion

Editors

Michael W. Mulholland, MD, PhD

Professor of Surgery
Executive Director, University of Michigan Medical Group
Senior Associate Dean for Clinical Affairs
Michigan Medicine – University of Michigan
Ann Arbor, Michigan

Erika Adams Newman, MD

Associate Professor of Surgery
Associate Chair for Faculty Development
Department of Surgery
Michigan Medicine – University of Michigan
Ann Arbor, Michigan

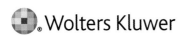 Wolters Kluwer

Philadelphia • Baltimore • New York • London
Buenos Aires • Hong Kong • Sydney • Tokyo

Acquisitions Editor: Keith Donnellan
Development Editor: Sean McGuire
Editorial Coordinator: Mary Woodman/Annette Ferran
Marketing Manager: Phyllis Hitner
Senior Production Project Manager: Alicia Jackson
Design Coordinator: Elaine Kasmer
Senior Manufacturing Coordinator: Beth Welsh
Prepress Vendor: TNQ Technologies

9 8 7 6 5 4 3 2 1

Printed in China

Library of Congress Cataloging-in-Publication Data

ISBN-13: 978-1-975135-47-8

Cataloging in Publication data available on request from publisher.

To my wife, Patricia
Michael W. Mulholland

To my mother, Gwendolyn, my bridge
To my grandmothers Allie and Millie, shoulders on which I stand
And to Robert, Grayson, and Gabriella, my light and love
Erika Adams Newman

Acknowledgments

The editors gratefully recognize the contributions of Paul D. Trombley and Erin Larowe (University of Michigan) and Sean McGuire (Wolters Kluwer) for their dedication to the visual appearance of this work. The adoption of a visual abstract style matches aesthetic appeal and intellectual content in a unique and compelling fashion. Many thanks as well to Mary Woodman for her editorial suggestions and help. Much appreciated.

Preface

The surgical treatment of human disease is inherently complex. Patients present with symptoms or disabilities that may relate to a variety of underlying causes. In evaluating those symptoms, modern medicine provides multiple diagnostic modalities that may be applied but in proper sequence and economically. Once a diagnosis is secured, treatment recommendations may include both surgical and nonsurgical therapies. In turn, when operative treatment is recommended, a variety of approaches—open, laparoscopic, robotic—are available, each with its particular efficacy, risk, and cost. In addition, surgical patients are inherently variable. Each patient has a unique set of comorbidities and an individual biological milieu. Each requires personalized treatment. These are the complexities that surgeons confront every day, and for which creativity and diversity of thought are essential. Exciting new research demonstrates that problems characterized by complexity and high variability are best solved by teams intentionally constructed to maximize diversity.

The premise of *The Diversity Promise: Success in Academic Surgery and Medicine Through Diversity, Equity, and Inclusion* is that demonstrable advantages come from the intentional mixture of talented people in a stimulating environment. Maximizing performance depends upon teamwork but teams constructed and enabled in a specific way. To be truly impactful, team members must be both talented and diverse. People have differing life experiences based upon age, race, gender, religious belief, and myriad other factors. These experiences, in turn, produce differing perspectives that create a strong competitive advantage for diverse teams. Team members must also believe that they are treated with equity and that the environment is inclusive for the full potential of talented and diverse teams to be unleashed. All elements are required—talented and diverse individuals formed into teams and an environment based upon equity that is open, supportive, and inclusive.

In *The Diversity Promise: Success in Academic Surgery and Medicine Through Diversity, Equity, and Inclusion,* the editors have convened thought leaders in the application of these ideas to the discipline of Academic Surgery. The book is organized in three sections that explore the building of a creative faculty, attracting the best and brightest medical students to the field, and training surgical residents to lead a new and different future. Emerging concepts from social science research are presented that explore the evolution of team science and interdisciplinary care as well as the effects of unconscious bias on healthcare disparities. Novel models of surgical teaching are combined with new findings on adult learning. A view emerges of a field in flux—Surgery as a new discipline defined as much by creative thinking as by technical virtuosity. A new discipline for new challenges.

MICHAEL W. MULHOLLAND, MD, PHD
ERIKA ADAMS NEWMAN, MD

Contributors

EDITORS

Michael W. Mulholland, MD, PhD
Professor of Surgery
Executive Director, University of
  Michigan Medical Group
Senior Associate Dean for Clinical Affairs
Michigan Medicine – University of
  Michigan
Ann Arbor, Michigan

Erika Adams Newman, MD
Associate Professor of Surgery
Associate Chair for Faculty Development
Department of Surgery
Michigan Medicine – University of
  Michigan
Ann Arbor, Michigan

CONTRIBUTORS

David J. Brown, MD
Associate Vice President and Associate
  Dean for Health Equity and Inclusion,
  Medical School and University of
  Michigan Hospitals and Health Centers
Associate Professor of Otolaryngology-
  Head and Neck Surgery
Michigan Medicine – University of
  Michigan
Ann Arbor, Michigan

Miles B. Cahill, PhD
Professor of Economics
Associate Health Professions Advisor
College of the Holy Cross
Worcester, Massachusetts

Clifford S. Cho, MD
C. Gardner Child Professor of Surgery
  and Professor of Surgery
Michigan Medicine – University of
  Michigan
Ann Arbor, Michigan

Mark S. Cohen, MD
Professor of Surgery and Professor of
  Pharmacology
Vice Chair in Surgery for Clinical
  Operations
Associate-Chair for Innovation and
  Entrepreneurship
Director, Medical School Pathway of
  Innovation and Entrepreneurship
Department of Surgery
Michigan Medicine – University of
  Michigan
Ann Arbor, Michigan

Dawn Coleman, MD
Marion and David Handleman Research
  Professor of Vascular Surgery
Associate Professor of Pediatrics and
  Associate Professor of Surgery
Michigan Medicine – University of
  Michigan
Ann Arbor, Michigan

Justin B. Dimick, MD, MPH
Frederick A. Coller Distinguished
  Professor
Chair, Department of Surgery
Michigan Medicine – University of
  Michigan
Professor of Health Management and
  Policy, School of Public Health
Ann Arbor, Michigan

Lesly A. Dossett, MD, MPH
Assistant Professor of Surgery
Michigan Medicine – University of
  Michigan
Ann Arbor, Michigan

Michael Englesbe, MD
Cyrenus G. Darling, Sr, MD and Cyrenus
  G. Darling, Jr, MD Professor of
  Surgery
Michigan Medicine – University of
  Michigan
Ann Arbor, Michigan

Samir K. Gadepalli, MD, MBA
Assistant Professor of Surgery
Michigan Medicine – University of
  Michigan
Ann Arbor, Michigan

Paul G. Gauger, MD
William J. Fry Professor of Surgery
George D. Zuidema Professor of
  Surgery, Professor of Surgery
Michigan Medicine – University of
  Michigan
Ann Arbor, Michigan

Brian George, MD, MAEd
Assistant Professor of Learning Health
  Sciences
Assistant Professor of Surgery
Michigan Medicine – University of
  Michigan
Ann Arbor, Michigan

Patrick Georgoff, MD
House Officer, Surgery
University of Michigan Hospitals
Ann Arbor, Michigan
Fellow in Trauma Surgery
Memorial Hermann–Texas Medical
  Center
Houston Texas

Amir A. Ghaferi, MD
Associate Professor of Surgery
Michigan Medicine – University of
  Michigan
Associate Professor of Business,
  Stephen M. Ross School of Business
University of Michigan
Ann Arbor, Michigan

Jason Hall, MD, MPH, PhD, FACS, FASCRS
Chief, Section of Colon and Rectal
  Surgery
Associate Professor of Surgery
Boston University School of Medicine
Boston, Massachusetts

Calista M. Harbaugh, MD
House Officer, Surgery
University of Michigan Hospitals
Ann Arbor, Michigan

Rian M. Hasson, MD
Assistant Professor of Surgery
Geisel School of Medicine
Dartmouth University
Lebanon, New Hampshire

Peter K. Henke, MD
Leland Ira Doan Research Professor of
  Vascular Surgery
Professor of Surgery
Michigan Medicine – University of
  Michigan
Ann Arbor, Michigan

Marion C. W. Henry, MD, MPH, FACS, FAAP
Associate Professor of Surgery and Pediatrics
University of Arizona
Banner University Medical Center – Tucson
Banner Diamond Children's Hospital
Tucson, Arizona

Megan Johnson, BS
Philadelphia College of Osteopathic Medicine
Philadelphia, Pennsylvania

Arielle E. Kanters, MD
House Officer, Surgery
University of Michigan Hospitals
Ann Arbor, Michigan

Gifty Kwakye, MD
Assistant Professor of Surgery
Michigan Medicine – University of Michigan
Ann Arbor, Michigan

Rebecca Minter, MD, FACS
A.R. Curreri Distinguished Chair
Department of Surgery
University of Wisconsin School of Medicine and Public Health
Madison, Wisconsin

Hari Nathan, MD, PhD
Assistant Professor of Surgery
Michigan Medicine – University of Michigan
Ann Arbor, Michigan

Marina Pasca di Magliano, PhD
Associate Professor of Surgery
Associate Professor of Cell and Developmental Biology
Associate Director of Cancer Biology Graduate Program
Michigan Medicine – University of Michigan
Ann Arbor, Michigan

Erin E. Perrone, MD
Assistant Professor of Surgery
Michigan Medicine – University of Michigan
CS Mott Children's Hospital
Ann Arbor, Michigan

Krishnan Raghavendran, MD
Professor of Surgery
Michigan Medicine – University of Michigan
Ann Arbor, Michigan

Rishindra M. Reddy, MD
Jose Alvarez Research Professor of Thoracic Surgery
Associate Professor of Surgery
Michigan Medicine – University of Michigan
Ann Arbor, Michigan

Gurjit Sandhu, PhD
Associate Professor of Surgery
Associate Professor of Learning Health Sciences
Vice-Chair, Resident Life
Associate Program Director General Surgery
Departments of Surgery & Learning Health Sciences
Michigan Medicine – University of Michigan
Ann Arbor, Michigan

Kyle H. Sheetz, MD
House Officer, Surgery
University of Michigan Hospitals
Ann Arbor, Michigan

Mark G. Shrime, MD, MPH, PhD, FACS
Assistant Professor of Surgery
Center for Global Surgery Evaluation
Massachusetts Eye and Ear Infirmary
Program in Global Surgery and Social Change, Harvard Medical School
Boston, Massachusetts
Center for Health and Wellbeing, Princeton University
Princeton, New Jersey

Sarah P. Shubeck, MD, MS
House Officer, Surgery
University of Michigan Hospitals
Ann Arbor, Michigan

Christopher J. Sonnenday, MD, MHS
The Darrell A. Campbell, Jr, MD,
   Collegiate Professor in Transplant
   Surgery
Associate Professor of Surgery
Associate Professor of Health
   Management & Policy
Michigan Medicine – University of
   Michigan
Ann Arbor, Michigan

Dana A. Telem, MD, MPH
Associate Professor of Surgery
Michigan Medicine – University of
   Michigan
Ann Arbor, Michigan

Jennifer F. Tseng, MD, MPH
Surgeon-in-Chief, Boston Medical
   Center
Utley Professor and Chair of Surgery
Boston University School of Medicine
Boston, Massachusetts

Joceline V. Vu, MD
House Officer, Surgery
University of Michigan Hospitals
Ann Arbor, Michigan

Thomas William Wakefield, MD
James C. Stanley Professor of Vascular
   Surgery
Professor of Surgery and Section Head,
   Vascular Surgery, Department of
   Surgery
Director, Samuel and Jean Frankel
   Cardiovascular Center
Michigan Medicine – University of
   Michigan
Ann Arbor, Michigan

Jennifer F. Waljee, MD
George D. Zuidema Professor of
   Surgery, Professor of Surgery
Associate Professor of Surgery
Associate Professor of Orthopedic
   Surgery
Michigan Medicine – University of
   Michigan
Ann Arbor, Michigan

Andrea B. Wolffing, MD
Clinical Assistant Professor of Surgery
The Dartmouth Institute
Geisel School of Medicine
Lebanon, New Hampshire

Sandra L. Wong, MD, MS
Chair and Professor of Surgery
Professor of The Dartmouth Institute
Geisel School of Medicine
Lebanon, New Hampshire

Contents

Part **2**

ATTRACTING TALENTED MEDICAL STUDENTS

Part **3**

DEVELOPING TALENT IN SURGERY RESIDENTS

Part 1

BUILDING AN OPEN AND INCLUSIVE ENVIRONMENT FOR FACULTY

Building a Creative Culture

Michael W. Mulholland

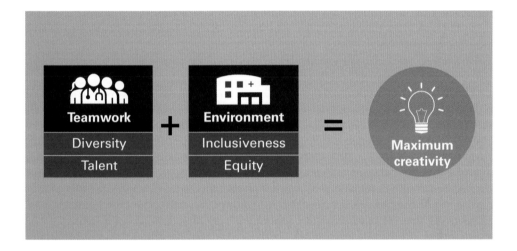

CREATIVITY

Creativity is the key to success.

Contemporary American surgery is uniquely expensive, highly scrutinized, and challenged by societal and economic expectations. In 2018, almost 52,000 surgeons across all surgical specialties practiced in the United States.[1] While surgeons comprise only 10% of specialty physicians, excluding physicians engaged in delivery of primary care, this fraction of the physician workforce has a disproportionate impact on American health care. Payments for surgical care represent fully half of all Medicare spending, and by extrapolation, half of all spending on adult medical services.[2]

Surgical care requires unique physical infrastructure. Surgical suites are prominent physical assets of every hospital, and the 24-hour nature of surgical emergencies requires 24-hour staffing with skilled, and expensive, nursing, anesthesiology, and support personnel. Modern operating rooms command greater ancillary support in the form of blood banks, pathology and radiology, and transport services than other hospital units. Construction costs for operating rooms are higher than for most other inpatient units, which are, in turn, higher than other forms of commercial real estate. For most large hospitals, surgical activity is the source of more than half of revenue.

Academic medical centers provide critical services and are subjected to additional pressures. The teaching hospital members of the Association of American Medical Colleges represent only 5% of all hospitals in the United States, yet they provide 26% of Medicare services and more than one-third of all charity care.[3] Many academic medical centers provide highly specialized services, often for entire states or regions of the country. As one measure, academic medical centers accept 38% of transfers from other hospitals that cannot provide complex care.[4] As another example, 80% of level I trauma centers and burn units are located in academic medical centers.

Academic centers provide the greatest share of graduate medical education (GME), with total federal funding for GME at $16 billion annually.[5] Postgraduate surgical training and surgical subspecialty training are longer than for most nonsurgical specialties, impacting institutional GME budgets disproportionately. In addition to patient care and education, academic departments of surgery also have a mission to improve the care of future patients through research. This mission is threatened by the clinical and economic challenges of modern practice. In 2014, only 2.3% of NIH funding in the top-funded 25 academic medical centers was awarded to surgeons.[6]

Challenges abound. The challenges of contemporary surgery require innovation and both the willingness and flexibility to change.

The pace of scientific change is both exciting and daunting. Within the past 20 years, the human genome was sequenced, and humans were joined by a long list of other sequenced organisms including dog, rat, fruit fly, mosquito, salmon, mastodon, and our cousin Neanderthals. The potential now exists to edit genes in living humans. Surgeons trained in the 20th century entered practice before the concepts of the microbiome, big data, or machine learning were developed. Many senior surgeons, trained before the deployment of word processors, now teach medical students who have never known a world without mobile phones. Teaching the next generation of learners requires adaptation to that generation's preferred modes of learning.

Scientific and technical advances which derive from these new insights are being rapidly applied to existing problems. Increasingly, caring for the sick requires an appreciation of the intersection of scientific, social, and financial factors. Fortunately, these are the areas in which academic surgeons excel—scientific discovery, teaching young doctors, and navigating societal issues. Change and innovation requires creativity. Seen in this way, creative change is an enduring competitive advantage for academic surgeons. If this is true, how can creativity be maximized?

TEAMS

The Wisdom of the Crowd

A large body of evidence supports the concept that groups of people make better decisions than individuals. This idea has become known as the wisdom of the crowd. The power of crowds to make accurate predictions has been recognized for almost 100 years in the form of prediction markets. Prediction markets have that name because that is precisely what they do—make predictions. In its most common form, a prediction market is incredibly simple. The market creates a security (takes a bet) that a future event will occur. The security pays $1 if the event takes place, $0 if it does not. Through the wisdom of the crowd, the price of the security reflects the market's assessment of the probability of that future event.

For example, a prediction market security might pay $1 if the New England Patriots win the upcoming Super Bowl and pay nothing if they do not. The Super Bowl occurs each year, and the winner is determined with absolute certainty. In this example, the price of the security during the NFL regular season is the collective assessment of the investing (betting) crowd that the Patriots will win. A price of $1 means that victory in the Super Bowl is guaranteed, and a price of $0 means that winning is impossible, for example, by being eliminated from the playoffs. Any price between $0 and $1 reflects the market's current assessment of the likelihood of a Super Bowl win by the Patriots.

These sorts of crowd-sourced markets have been used to predict outcomes of events that are highly complex, even those that are fluid day-to-day. Prediction markets have been used to predict outcomes of political elections since the presidential race between Charles Evans Hughes and Woodrow Wilson in 1916. The Iowa Electronic Market is a well-known research prediction market, in existence since the 1988 presidential election. *Figure 1.1* demonstrates the likelihood that the 2008 presidential election would be won by the Democratic or the Republican candidate, as forecast by the Iowa Electronic Market.

Prediction markets reflect the power of one form of cognitive diversity. Accurate forecasting occurs because very large numbers of individuals, with correspondingly very diverse perspectives, are actively engaged in solving a complex problem related to a future event. Predictive power occurs when individuals with varied perspectives consider a common set of facts. In the example of the 2008 election, millions of individuals were aware of the domestic and international events depicted in the timeline of *Figure 1.1* (and many other events not noted). Each individual (investor)

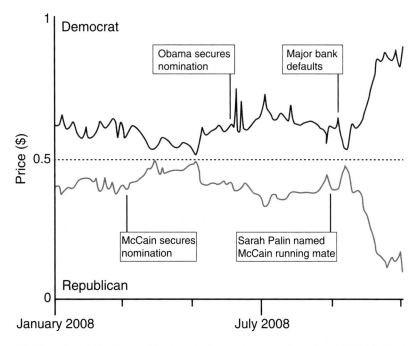

Figure 1.1 Results of the Iowa Electronic Market regarding the 2008 United States presidential election.

received the same information. Each judged the events as relevant or irrelevant to the upcoming election, important or trivial, of lasting importance or transient. Each applied a different perspective based upon his or her own personal experiences in making these judgments. No two individuals have identical life experiences, and no two are likely to process these complex inputs identically or to predict the impending election results identically. Yet the collective assessment of the crowd proved to be remarkably prescient. Predictive power comes from differences, not similarities.

Predictive markets have lessons to teach that are relevant to the practice of surgery. A multidisciplinary tumor board convenes a much smaller group of decision-makers and provides treatment recommendations in the moment. Optimizing clinical rotations for a surgical residency, crucial for the involved trainees, is performed by a committee of faculty members and house staff. While it is not possible to enlist thousands (millions) of decision-makers, intentional efforts to welcome differing perspectives can lead to more accurate treatment or teaching recommendations.

Science as a Team Endeavor

The reordering of scientific discovery from an area of individual brilliance to a team endeavor over the past several decades is striking. Large-scale collaborative projects have become increasingly common in fields ranging from medicine to high-energy physics, and entirely new fields of science have developed as a result, with genomics and bioinformatics as examples.

The rise of larger scientific teams can be quantified using authorship of scientific papers. The number of co-authors per paper has increased steadily for most of the past century, growing by 25% from 1997 through 2016.[7] The evolution of team science has also increased scientific impact. When primary manuscripts are considered, increased co-authorship is associated with an increased citation index. The positive effect of co-author number on citations has been demonstrated for both biomedical and physical sciences. A recent study mapped collaborative scientific dynamics on a mass scale. Parish, Boyack, and Ioannidis examined 249,054 investigators using the Scopus database (https://www.scopus.com/) for the period 2006 to 2015 in order to construct a collaboration index.[8] In medicine and health sciences, greater collaboration was associated with a higher citation index (h-index).

When individual investigators are examined, those with larger numbers of collaborators demonstrate greater scientific productivity. Recent studies have ascribed the positive effects of co-authorship to the establishment of collaboration networks. Collaboration networks represent scientific communities with investigators connected by ideas (*Figure 1.2*). Positive network effects have been demonstrated in fields ranging from statistics to pharmacology and informatics. Increased network effects are associated with greater scientific productivity. Not surprisingly, the correlations between collaboration, networking, and scientific productivity increase as investigators progress professionally as more time spent as part of a scientific team permits relationships to persist and deepen. International collaborations are also very strongly correlated with scientific productivity.

Recent evidence suggests that networks that provide greater ethnic diversity offer competitive advantage, allowing teams to publish more frequently cited papers. Freeman and Huang used bibliometric techniques to examine 2.5 million papers, all written by American authors.[9] Ethnicity was implied by analysis of surnames. For example, Smith was assigned English ethnicity; Chang was assigned Chinese ethnicity. Manuscripts with four or more authors in which authors had multiple ethnicities were cited more frequently than those written by authors of the same ethnicity.

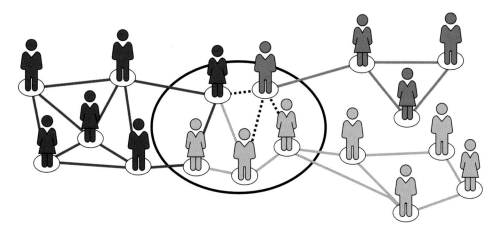

Figure 1.2 Collaboration networks represent communities of individuals, each with unique perspectives, connected by ideas.

The advantage of ethnic diversity represented a difference of 5% to 10% additional citations per publication. Ethnic homogeneity was associated with publication in lower-impact journals and fewer citations. Freeman and Huang believe that more ethnically diverse research groups benefit from different, richer networks and perhaps a greater variety of perspectives.

The effects of sex and gender diversity are also emerging in science. Female authorship in high-impact medical journals increased from 27% to 37% in the years 1994 to 2014.[10] Biological sex and gender (behaviors and social attitudes associated with being a man or woman) are crucial factors in human health. Biological sex and gender also clearly shape life experiences, with effects on cognition and perspective that are relevant to the scientific workplace.

In spite of direct relevance, the effects of biological sex and gender on disease risk and health outcomes have been widely neglected in the medical literature. Attention to gender and sex in clinical trial design is an essential element of scientific quality. In a recent study, a global sample of more than 1.5 million medical research publications examined the effects of women's authorship on gender and sex analysis as a means of improving scientific validity of health studies.[11] Women's participation as first or last author was strongly correlated with use of gender and sex analysis. The effect attributable to women's participation was strongest when women served as senior authors.

The benefits of scientific teams are also apparent in corporate research and development. Reagans and Zuckerman analyzed 224 research and development teams in 29 corporations across seven industries: automotive, chemicals, electronics, aerospace, pharmaceuticals, biotechnology, and energy.[12] Some teams were productive, others less so. Teams that demonstrated both demographic heterogeneity and strong communication exhibited enhanced learning capabilities and high productivity. Homogeneous teams or those that were unable to develop strong connections among team members were underproductive. Greater demographic diversity brings together people with different skills, information, life experiences, and perspectives. These attributes enhance creative problem solving if team members allocate time to activities that cross the bounds of individual expertise. However, crossing boundaries is inherently uncomfortable and requires trust and strong communication.

The Science of Team Science

While scientific collaboration is unquestionably more prevalent today than in past years, not all scientific teams are equally productive. The most successful teams are characterized by high levels of integration and interaction.

Recent research has examined the elements of productive scientific teams. The foundation of a successful team is a compelling scientific question. To address the question, the productive team brings together members with specific, different, and complementary scientific expertise. Regular team meetings are crucial. Scheduled meetings are obviously important to discuss the overall scientific goal, to highlight the different objectives of the individuals composing the team, to share and critique data, and to plan next steps. Less obvious but more important, regular meetings serve a socialization purpose, helping team members form bonds with each other. These bonds promote trust, which is the single most important factor in team science. Trust permits scientific teams to engage in disagreement while limiting conflict. Trust enables the equitable sharing of credit and authorship. Often, successful scientific teams have an overall lead, but other members have key leadership roles that are relevant to achieving the overall goal. Leadership is participatory.

The National Cancer Institute has examined the science of team science. The major influences on successful team science are not technological, rather interpersonal and organizational. Stokols et al. cite interpersonal factors to include team members' familiarity, informality, and social cohesiveness; diversity of members' perspectives and abilities; regular and effective communication among members to develop consensus and shared goals; and establishment of a hospitable conversational environment through mutual respect among team members.[13] Organizations that are nonhierarchical facilitate autonomy and participatory goal setting. Spatial proximity allows frequent opportunities for face-to-face communication and informal information exchange. To be sure, technological resources are important. But social factors trump technological prowess every time.

The National High Magnetic Field Laboratory is the world's largest and most powerful magnet laboratory, funded by the United States National Science Foundation. The national laboratory provides highly specialized scientific instruments, unusual technologies, and the expertise of resident scientists. Scientific teams apply to use the facilities, and subject matter experts approve proposals. Scientific teams do not pay to use the facilities. The laboratory hosts over 900 scientists each year who use the magnets for a wide variety of projects.

Each year, there are more applicants than can be accommodated, so maximizing productivity of teams is crucial. The National High Magnetic Field Laboratory examined 1415 experiments performed from 2005 through 2008 with productivity measured in the form of publications. Eighty-nine teams were examined to determine whether team diversity and network characteristics impacted productivity. The most highly productive teams were associated with the highest disciplinary diversity, combining physicists from different scientific backgrounds or different institutions. Team cohesion was also positively associated with productivity.[14]

Scientific Synthesis

Many scientific disciplines now face a problem that was unimaginable in the past—too much data. A new form of scientific work is emerging to cope with this bounty, termed scientific synthesis. As used here, scientific synthesis refers to the process of integration of diverse research by teams to create new knowledge. In this mode of collaboration, teams are convened to synthesize existing data rather than to create new data.

In 1995, the National Science Foundation created the National Center for Ecological Analysis and Synthesis. This center undertook a radical new approach to science. No new data were collected. Rather, new knowledge was created by the synthesis of existing data. The Center's primary function was to be convener of environmental scientists, providing a creative environment for immersive collaboration. At the center, working groups are provided the time, physical environment, and monetary resources to synthesize existing data in novel ways.

The idea worked. In terms of scientific publishing and impact factor, the National Center for Ecological Analysis and Synthesis ranked in the top 1% of 38,000 institutions worldwide in 2005, just 10 years after its inception.[15] The social milieu of the center has attracted new talent. As the years have passed, the proportion of women and non-US scientists has increased. The numbers of collaborating authors have risen dramatically, from an average of 4 in 1996 to an average of 10 in 2006.

The center has examined the working groups extensively via interviews, surveys, social network analysis, and direct ethnographic observation. The success of the center is grounded in microsocial interactions, not technological resources: focused face-to-face meetings, effective communication, and freedom from outside distractions. In turn, these conditions engender trust, limit conflict, and stimulate creativity. The benefits of face-to-face meetings are not just the exchange of scientific findings but also the fostering of interpersonal relationships.

Multidisciplinary Clinical Care

Multidisciplinary teams have become the model for contemporary clinical care worldwide. First introduced for the care of cancer patients, multidisciplinary teams are ubiquitous in fields as diverse as organ transplantation, critical care, neonatology, cardiovascular disease, and gastrointestinal disorders. The goals of multidisciplinary care include optimizing the patient experience as gauged by patient safety and satisfaction. Hospital systems that embrace multidisciplinary approaches have been reported to benefit from reduced inpatient length of stay, reduced costs, and improved clinical endpoints. Additional reported benefits include increased job satisfaction of involved healthcare workers.

Multidisciplinary care developed first in oncology, with breast cancer clinics the initial foray of most medical centers. The goal of most multidisciplinary breast care clinics is to provide patients with exposure to multiple medical and surgical specialists, a full array of diagnostic modalities, sophisticated decision-making, and an individualized treatment plan, all in 1 day. Similar clinics are now available for virtually every tumor type. Exposure to multiple specialists has been reported to refine treatment options. One recent analysis included 37 separate studies of multidisciplinary cancer programs.[16] Cancer treatment options developed by individual physicians were altered in up to 52% of cases through review by a multidisciplinary tumor board. This approach is attractive to cancer patients. In a separate report, 98% of patients rated the overall experience as "excellent."[17]

The effect of multidisciplinary care teams has been examined extensively in intensive care units. A recent report examined 112 hospitals and 107,324 patients.[18] Overall 30-day mortality was 18.3%, but multidisciplinary care was associated with a significant reduction in the odds of dying. The beneficial effects of multidisciplinary care were observed for a variety of patients, including those with sepsis, patients needing mechanical ventilation, and those with the highest severity of illness.

Sepsis is the leading cause of death in ICUs. The involvement of a multidisciplinary sepsis response team has been shown to reduce ICU deaths due to sepsis.[19] Compliance with a sepsis resuscitation bundle increased from a baseline of 12.7% to 37.7% with weekly feedback and to 53.7% when feedback was combined with activation of a multidisciplinary sepsis response team. Mortality declined from 30.3% at baseline to 28.3% and 22.0% when feedback and feedback plus sepsis response team activation were combined. Multidisciplinary care allows for better performance through the beneficial effects of improved decision-making. In one study, when a pharmacist was added to the ICU team, adverse drug events decreased 66%. The pharmacist made 366 recommendations related to drug ordering, with 99% accepted by attending physicians.[20]

DIVERSITY

Scott Page has pioneered the idea that for problems of high complexity, diverse perspectives improve collective understanding and lead to superior problem solving.[21] Diverse teams outperform more homogeneous teams in part because they provide an influx of novel ideas, but also because more careful processing of information occurs in diverse groups. This performance advantage arises from "cognitive diversity." The uplift of cognitive diversity comes from the ability of diverse groups to apply differing perspectives to unsolved problems. The competitive advantage of cognitive diversity is well demonstrated in the corporate world with measurable superiority in predictive ability, innovation, efficiency, and financial return.

If cognitive diversity provides such a crucial competitive advantage, how might it be measured? Unfortunately, there is no test for cognitive diversity, nothing analogous to the MCAT, or the American Board of Surgery In-Service Examination. The key to cognitive diversity lies in identity diversity. Talent is evenly distributed across sexes, genders, ethnicities, and religions. But experiences are not. The life experiences of individuals are markedly different based upon these characteristics, among many others, and those experiences lead to differing perspectives and variable approaches to problem solving, termed heuristics. Cognitive diversity provides collective advantage, realized as groups of individuals with varied perspectives and heuristics work together to solve complex problems.

Corporate Performance and Diversity

The business case for diversity is strong. Companies that are more diverse—defined as a greater proportion of women and more varied ethnic and cultural composition—have higher financial performance. A recent study of more than 1000 companies in 12 countries found that profitability (earnings before interest and taxes) and long-term value creation were greater in more diverse companies.[22] For companies in the top quartile for gender diversity in executive leadership, profitability was 21% greater than for corporations in the lowest quartile. Firms with the greatest ethnic and cultural diversity outperformed less diverse firms by 35% in terms of operating margin.

Conversely, companies that ignore diversity do so at their own peril. Firms in the lowest quartile with regard to gender and ethnic diversity underperformed industry peers by 29%. In the United States, ethnic and racial diversity in executive leadership are related to financial performance. For every 10% increase in leadership diversity, earnings before interest and taxes increase by 0.8%.[23] As another example, for every percentage increase in gender and racial diversity, sales revenue increases by 3% and 9%, respectively.[24]

Business studies suggest that diversity is a competitive advantage because it stimulates greater creativity and innovation and also because diverse groups process complex information more carefully. Homogeneous groups have fewer perspectives to draw upon and are more often wrong (although more certain) in their conclusions. Clear evidence demonstrates that gender, ethnic, and cultural diversity make companies more attractive to top talent, increase customer orientation, and are associated with greater employee satisfaction.

Diversity in American Health Care

American health professions have lagged behind corporate American in recognizing the benefits of diversity. According to the most recent US Census data, 30% of the American population are African-Americans, Hispanic Americans, or American Indians, yet in 2007 these groups composed only 9% of physicians, 7% of dentists, 10% of pharmacists, and 6% of registered nurses.[25] Minorities are underrepresented on faculties of American medical schools, with only 1% of full professors being African-American. Minorities are underrepresented among federally funded investigators and are less likely to have leadership positions in American medical institutions.

In a landmark study in 2000, Nonnemaker demonstrated that women were significantly more likely than male physicians to hold faculty positions after graduation.[26] However, a significantly smaller proportion of women advanced from assistant professor to associate professor. In the two decades following this report, female enrollment in medical schools has topped 50%, but senior academic ranks and administrative leadership positions are still disproportionately male.

Cognitive Diversity in Surgical Practice

The Critical View of Safety

In 1985, general surgery was in the doldrums. Virtually all abdominal operations were performed through open laparotomy incisions, using techniques that had been developed decades earlier. Operative maneuvers and instruments in common use—Kocher maneuver, Billroth I anastomosis, Metzenbaum scissors—carried the names of surgical pioneers long dead.

Everything changed on September 12, 1985 when Dr. Erich Muhe of Boblinger, Germany, performed the first laparoscopic cholecystectomy. The minimally invasive surgical revolution of the next three decades utterly changed the operative experience for patients—smaller incisions, less operative trauma, shorter hospitalizations, and faster recovery with return to normal activities.

The revolution had a rocky start. Initial series of laparoscopic cholecystectomy reported injury to bile ducts in excess of 1%. Many injuries were serious and occurred because of the misidentification of the common bile duct as the cystic duct. Reoperation and biliary reconstruction were almost always required in such cases. At the same time, Clavien reported 1252 open cholecystectomies with no ductal injury.[27] Morgenstern reported two injuries (0.17%) in a series of 1200 patients.[28] It was hard for laparoscopic pioneers to make the case that this new approach was superior to long-established technique if complication rates were so dissimilar.

Initially, it was believed that the rash bile duct injuries were a result of inexperience or poor preparation or just inadequate effort. For example, many injuries occurred during a surgeon's first 100 cases and were attributed to a "learning curve." The premise was that injuries would decline as each surgeon became more experienced, as they passed beyond the learning curve, but woe to the patient operated upon during the first 100 cases. And every surgeon must necessarily have a first 100 cases. Injuries were also thought to be avoidable by training more diligently; a period of preceptorship of 20 cases was a common recommendation. Perhaps injuries could be avoided by being more careful. Surgeons were cautioned to be judicious in the use of cautery in the portal area, to be wary of acute or chronic inflammation, and to readily convert to open cholecystectomy. In essence, the problem could be solved if surgeons just tried harder or were more careful.

A major advance was provided in 2002 by Lawrence Way and John Hunter.[29] These surgeons used the tools of human factors research and the science of human error processing to reframe the injury problem as one of misperception. They postulated that perceptual errors, not inadequate practice or knowledge, or deficiencies in manual skill were the root causes of biliary injury. Unconscious decision-making processes, termed heuristics, provided rapid, but incorrect, processing of visual information because the three-dimensional world of human anatomy had been converted to a two-dimensional video screen. They wrote, "Our conscious minds are at the mercy of the subconscious heuristics."

Millions of years of human evolution have equipped the unconscious part of the human mind with the ability to detect patterns incredibly rapidly and to promote immediate action. Humans are superb at detecting fleeting visual cues. Consider how readily humans detect tiny changes in facial expression. A blink, a tiny grimace, a flicker of a smile, the smallest pursing of the lips, all detected and interpreted hundreds of times a day, and all without conscious effort.

In laparoscopic surgery, this great talent can become a great handicap. The unconscious mind rushes to provide an explanation of the world we encounter (in this case, the operative field). The surgeon sees a duct, and the unconscious mind "knows" it is the cystic duct. And it usually is, unless the common bile duct is misidentified.

The work of Way and Hunter began a paradigm shift in laparoscopic surgery, designing operations with a "brake" to cognitive momentum and an opportunity to examine the reality of the environment more objectively. This insight led directly to the now-ubiquitous "critical view of safety" as the means to identify the cystic duct. The triangle of Calot is dissected so that it is bounded by a duct emanating from the tapering neck of the gallbladder with the liver surface seen behind. Only one structure passes through this triangular view, the cystic artery. With this scenario, the cystic duct is identified by criteria that require engagement of the conscious mind, not pattern recognition by the subconscious. It requires time for the conscious mind to check off these criteria: tapering neck of gallbladder, one duct emanating from that tapering neck, liver seen through a triangular opening, only one structure passing through that triangle.

More than video camera design or new cautery devices, the contributions of these surgeons unleashed the revolution in minimally invasive surgery. The contribution was not in instruments or suture material. The true advance by Way and Hunter was to bring the perspectives of two fields then unknown in operative surgery—human factors research and the psychology of pattern recognition—to bear on an operative problem, cognitive diversity.

Kidney Donor Chains

Renal transplantation has the largest treatment effect in modern medicine, eliminating the need for intermittent dialysis and extending life expectancy for all causes of end-stage renal disease. However, the current state of deceased and living donation has not met the demand for transplant kidneys. In 2016, 19,062 renal transplants were performed, while 100,000 individuals were listed for transplantation.[30] Demand greatly exceeds supply, and demand is growing.

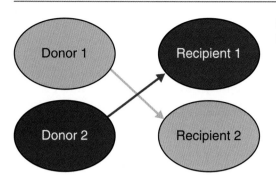

Figure 1.3 Two-way swap involved in paired kidney donation.

Living related kidney donation is a long-standing practice in which A/B blood type–compatible individuals donate a kidney, most often to a relative or close friend. Unfortunately, blood type incompatibility and immunologic barriers prohibit many motivated donors from kidney donation. Kidney paired donation was developed as a two-way swap between A/B and B/A incompatible pairs. In this schema, donor 1 provides the kidney for recipient 2 while donor 2 provides the kidney for recipient 1 (*Figure 1.3*). Paired donation was originally performed concurrently to prevent donors from withdrawing after their paired recipient had received an organ. Kidney paired donation programs now encourage compatible pairs to enter the match, permitting some recipients to receive an even better-matched or younger kidney. Adding compatible pairs to the program increases the number of matches for incompatible pairs, improving the matching potential of the waiting list as a whole.

Kidney chains developed from the demonstrated success of paired swaps, but chains differ in fundamental aspects from swaps. Kidney chains are composed of a series of donations and transplants that are not concurrent. In essence, an altruistic individual donates a kidney to provide a voucher for a kidney in the future for a loved one.

The kidney chain is initiated by a nondirected donor (Donor 0, *Figure 1.4*). Donor 0 donates to Recipient 1 whose living donor (Donor 1) then donates to Recipient 2. Donor 2 donates to Recipient 3. Donor 3 donates to Recipient 4 and so on until Donor N donates to a recipient without a living donor. Recipient Z, the final recipient, is a patient on the waiting list. Kidney chains now comprise 12% of all living donations in the United States.[31] Graft function has been excellent.

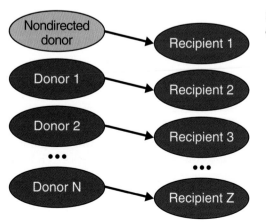

Figure 1.4 Schema of organ chain donation.

Kidney chains presented novel mathematical, legal, and ethical challenges. Initial paired swaps used algorithms to match the optimal donor-recipient pairs. A radically different mathematical challenge was presented with the advent of kidney chains, and the programming solutions used for paired swaps were inadequate as the number of potential pairings increased exponentially. Kidney chains became possible because a matching algorithm was imported from the New York Stock Exchange, applying technology employed by capital market exchange systems to medical decision-making.

The concept of kidney chains also faced legal hurdles in the United States. Initially, the voucher concept utilized by kidney chains appeared to violate the "valuable consideration" provision of the National Organ Transplantation Act. This law prohibits exchange of organs for valuable consideration (money). This legal barrier was erased by the federal government in 2007 when new legislation specifically excluded paired organ exchange as "valuable consideration."

The final barriers were ethical. As the chain is initiated, Donor 0 provides a kidney to a stranger (Recipient 1). In turn, a loved one of Donor 0 receives a "voucher" that may be exchanged for a kidney in the future. Who can be listed as the voucher holder? Does that person "own" the voucher? When many voucher holders exist, how are they prioritized when a single desirable kidney becomes available? These and many related ethical questions have been addressed by transplant stakeholders—physicians, ethicists, patients.

New math, new legislation, new ethics, drawing on new and different perspectives—cognitive diversity.

EQUITY

A central tenet of high-reliability teams is that team members are engaged and enthusiastic about their work and that all feel they are treated fairly and rewarded equitably. Perceptions of equity strongly and positively reinforce the culture of high-reliability organizations.

However, the traditional hierarchical nature of academic medicine can lead to inequity, with women affected more negatively than men. Compensation has been used as a quantitative measure of equity. In 2004, Ash reported a salary deficit among women physicians of $11,691 relative to male colleagues.[32] A wide array of other professional characteristics such as publication rates, seniority, hours per week worked, specialty, and school were controlled. Greater seniority was associated with larger salary discrepancy. Perceptions of unequal treatment negatively affect work culture. In a qualitative study of academic medical culture, lack of female achievement and feelings of inequity led to malalignment between personal values and institutional goals.[33,34]

INCLUSION

High-performing organizations embrace the power of diversity and distribute opportunity and rewards equitably. The highest-performing organizations move to another level, also focusing on inclusion. Superior creative performance = Diversity + Equity + Inclusion.

In a recent study of retail, manufacturing, and healthcare industries, business performance was examined in relationship to diversity and inclusion. Business performance was improved by 80% when both conditions were high.[35] Employees who felt their organization supported diversity and was also inclusive were more likely to view their employer as a high-performance organization.

The study identified two elements of inclusion: a process of change and integration and an outcome, a feeling of belonging. Belonging is tightly linked to concepts of fairness and equality of treatment. Fairness and equality of treatment are, in turn, perceived on the basis of employee experiences over time that demonstrate similar opportunities, compensation, and evaluation. When these conditions exist, individuals are able to express their uniqueness while still being part of a group. Individual team members become more than isolated subject matter experts and are able to speak up with confidence, to share their unique perspectives. The ability to share ideas with confidence and with mutual support allows a full range of ideas to be explored, and a wider range of solutions to be developed. Cognitive diversity is the seed, inclusion the sunshine.

The premise of this book is that creativity comes from the intentional mixture of talented people in a stimulating environment. Maximizing creativity depends upon teamwork. Teams win! But teams constructed and enabled in a specific way. To be truly impactful, team members must be both talented and cognitively diverse. In addition, team members must believe that they are treated with equity and that the environment is inclusive for the full creativity of talented and diverse teams to be unleashed. All elements are required—talented and diverse individuals formed into teams and an environment based upon equity that is open, supportive, and inclusive.

REFERENCES

1. U.S. Bureau of Labor Statistics 2018. Available at http://www.bls.gov/oes/current. Accessed 6, 2019.
2. Kaye DR, Min HS, Herrel LA, et al. Costs of cancer care across the disease continuum. *Oncologist.* 2018;23:798-805.
3. Grover A, Slavin PL, Willson P. The economics of academic medical centers. *N Engl J Med.* 2014;370:2360-2361.
4. Huderson A, Habermann M, Conroy J. *Medicare Patient Hospital Transfers in the Era of Health Care Reform.* Washington, DC: Association of American Medical Colleges; 2013. Available at https://www.aamc.org/download/333654. Accessed 6, 2019.
5. Chandra A, Khullar D, Wilensky G. The economics of graduate medical education. *N Engl J Med.* 2014;370:2357-2360.
6. Keswani SG, Moles CM, Morowitz M, et al. The future of basic science in academic surgery: identifying barriers to success for surgeon-scientists. *Ann Surg.* 2017;265:1053-1059.
7. Fanelli D, Larivière V. Researchers' individual publication rate has not increased in a century. *PLoS One.* 2016;11:e0149504.
8. Parish AJ, Boyack KW, Ioannidis JPA. Dynamics of co-authorship and productivity across different fields of scientific research. *PLoS One.* 2018;13:e0189742.
9. Freeman RB, Huang W. Strength in diversity. *Nature.* 2014;513:305.
10. Filardo G, da Graca B, Sass DM, et al. Trends and comparison of female first authorship in high impact medical journals: observational study (1994-2014). *BMJ.* 2016;352:1-8.
11. Nielsen MW, Andersen JP, Schiebinger L, Schneider JW. One and a half million medical papers reveal a link between author gender and attention to gender and sex analysis. *Nature.* 2017;1:791-796.
12. Reagans R, Zuckerman EW. Networks, diversity, and productivity: the social capital of corporate R&D teams. *Organ Sci.* 2001;12:502-517.
13. Stokols D, Taylor B, Hall K, Moser R. The science of team science: an overview of the field. NCI Conference on the Science of Team Science: Assessing the Value of Transdisciplinary Research. Bethesda, MD, October 30-31, 2006.

14. Stvilla B, Hinnant C, Schindler K, et al. Composition of scientific teams and publication productivity. *J Am Soc Inform Sci Tech.* 2011;62:270-283.

15. Hampton SE, Parker JN. Collaboration and productivity in scientific synthesis. *BioScience.* 2011;61:900-908.

16. Lamb BW, Brown KF, Nagpal K, et al. Quality of care management decisions by multidisciplinary cancer teams: a systematic review. *Ann Surg Oncol.* 2011;18:2116-2125.

17. Litton G, Kane D, Clay G, et al. Multidisciplinary cancer care with a patient and physician satisfaction focus. *J Oncol Pract.* 2010;6:e35-e37.

18. Kim MM, Barnato AE, Angus DC, et al. The effect of multidisciplinary care teams on intensive care unit mortality. *Arch Int Med.* 2010;170:369-376.

19. Schramm GE, Kashyap R, Mullon JJ, et al. Septic shock: a multidisciplinary response team and weekly feedback to clinicians improve the process of care and mortality. *Crit Care Med.* 2011;39:252-258.

20. Leape LL, Cullen DJ, Clapp MD, et al. Pharmacist participation on physician rounds and adverse drug events in the intensive care unit. *JAMA.* 1999;282:267-270.

21. Hong L, Page S. Groups of diverse problem solvers can outperform groups of high-ability problem solvers. *Proc Natl Acad Sci USA.* 2004;101:16385-16389.

22. Hunt V, Layton D, Prince S. *Why Diversity Matters.* New York: McKinsey & Co; 2015.

23. Hunt V, Yee L, Prince S, Dixon-Fyle S. *Delivering Through Diversity.* New York: McKinsey & Co; 2018.

24. Herring C. Does diversity pay? Race, gender, and the business case for diversity. *Am Soc Rev.* 2009;74(2):208-224.

25. Sullivan LW, Suez Mittman I. The state of diversity in the health professions a century after Flexner. *Acad Med.* 2010;85:246-253.

26. Nonnemaker L. Women physicians in academic medicine. *New Eng J Med.* 2000;342:399-405.

27. Clavien PA, Sanabria JR, Mentha G, et al. Recent results of elective open cholecystectomy in a North American and a European center. *Ann Surg.* 1992;216:618-626.

28. Morgenstern L, Wong L, Berci G. Twelve hundred open cholecystectomies before the laparoscopic era. A standard for comparison. *Ann Surg.* 1992;127:400-403.

29. Way LW, Stewart L, Gantert W, et al. Causes and prevention of laparoscopic bile duct injuries: analysis of 252 cases from a human factors and cognitive psychology perspective. *Ann Surg.* 2003;237:460-469.

30. Organ Procurement and Transplantation Network 2017. Available at https://opth.transplant.hrsa.gov/data/view-data-reports/national data/#. Accessed 6, 2019.

31. Wall AE, Veale JL, Melcher ML, et al. Advanced donation programs and deceased donor-initiated chains-2 innovations in kidney paired donation. *Transplantation.* 2017;101:2818-2824.

32. Ash AS, Carr PL, Goldstein R, Friedman RH. Compensation and advancement for women in academic medicine: is there equity? *Ann Int Med.* 2004;141:205-214.

33. Wright AL, Ryan K, St Germain P, et al. Compensation in academic medicine: progress toward gender equity. *J Gen Intern Med.* 2007;22:1398-1402.

34. Pololi LH, Civian JT, Brennan RT, Dottolo AL, Krupat E. Experiencing the culture of academic medicine: gender matters, a national survey. *J Gen Intern Med.* 2012;28:201-207.

35. Swiegers G, Toohey K. Waiter, is that inclusion in my soup? www.deloitte.com.au.

2

Women in Surgery

Dawn Coleman
Dana A. Telem

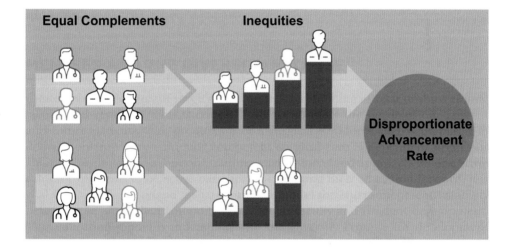

For the past 15 years, near-equal complements of men and women have entered American medical schools. Despite this, considerable gender-based inequities persist in academic advancement across medicine.[1-4] While some argue this is reflective of demographic inertia and the expected time lag before the full effects of the gender workforce change are seen, the rate of advancement for women still remains disproportionately slower than expected.[5-7] Data from the Association of American Medical Colleges (AAMC) comparing trends from 1989 to 2018 support this finding. Over the past 30 years, the percent of women department chairs has risen slowly from 4% of all academic departments to 18%. This growth trend has remained relatively flat over the past 5 years, which has seen a nominal 3% growth. These statistics parallel other upper echelon leadership positions such as dean of a medical school. As of 2018, only 19% of medical school deans were women, with only a 3% increase since 2015.[3] These findings suggest gender-based differences play a significant role, and time alone will not correct this inequity.

These data fare worse for woman in academic surgery, who may face additional challenges, given the traditional male-dominated hierarchical culture.[8,9] Similar to other disciplines within academic medicine, over the past decade, nearly 40% of general surgery trainees are women. Despite the robust pipeline, the achievement gap between men and women in academic surgery is more pronounced as compared with the aggregated AAMC data. As of 2014, only 19% of Associate Professors, 10% of Full Professors, and less than 5% of Department Chairs in Surgery were women.[8,9] Data also suggest that women faculty have increased attrition rates from both academic surgery and the practice of surgery overall compared with men in surgery and women in other fields of academic medicine.

DRIVERS OF GENDER INEQUITY

In recent years, the lay press, surgical societies, and leaders within academic surgery have given considerable attention to closing the gender achievement gap. This attention, coupled with a robust pipeline, begs the question of "*Why aren't there more women in the upper ranks of academic surgery?*" Available data suggest multifactorial drivers that perpetuate the gender achievement gap (*Figure 2.1*).

Explicit Bias

Explicit bias refers to the conscious attitudes and beliefs one has about a person or a group. Historical bias against women in surgery is well documented, and women were discouraged and often not permitted to pursue surgical training. For instance, it was not until 1940 when the first woman attained board certification in surgery. At that time, women who graduated surgery residencies were not permitted to sit for the boards.[10] While explicit bias is no longer overtly tolerated within the United States, elements of explicit bias still exist. A recent cross-sectional study assessing explicit bias related to gender and surgery demonstrated the persistence

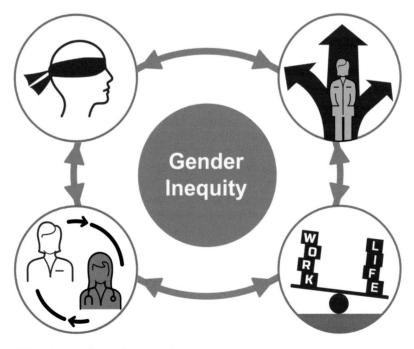

Figure 2.1 Drivers of gender inequity.

of certain fixed beliefs.[11] Assessment of almost 1 million records from persons who took the Gender-Career Implicit Association Test (IAT) demonstrated a significant association of men with career and women with family. Persons taking the Gender-Career IAT who self-identified as healthcare professionals exhibited more explicit bias than non–healthcare professionals, and all categories of healthcare professionals exhibited this bias. Interestingly, comparison of categories of healthcare professionals demonstrated that those professionals who were diagnosing and treating patients were more likely to explicitly associate men with career and women with family than were nursing and home healthcare assistants and other healthcare support.

Another mechanism by which explicit bias persists is in revelations of the persistence of sexual harassment in the workplace and within academic settings. A recent report by the National Academies of Sciences, Engineering and Medicine demonstrated the persistence of sexual harassment and its extent on negatively impacting recruitment, retention, and advancement of women within STEM (Science, Technology, Engineering, and Mathematics) fields.[12] Other data corroborate this finding. In a sample of 1719 K-award recipient clinician–researchers, 30% of women reported having experienced sexual harassment as compared with 4% of men.[13] Moreover, women who experienced harassment reported that these experiences negatively impacted their career advancement.

Challenges of Work–Life Integration

Women in surgical fields are more likely than men to have a partner who is employed full-time and bear family responsibilities such as disruption in childcare disproportionately.[14,15] While not specific to surgery, studies reveal high-achieving women in academic medicine on average spend 8.5 hours more per week on domestic activities than male counterparts.[14] These hours are often at the expense of academic development time and may account for differential achievement. Work–life challenges may also be perpetuated in nonwhite women (e.g., black American, Latino American) who are often alone within their social networks to achieve high socioeconomic status and more likely to rely on network caregiving and economic care.[16]

Unconscious Bias and Prescriptive Gender Norms

Unconscious assumptions (bias) of traits and behaviors men and women are expected to display form prescriptive gender norms that impact career advancement.[17] Behaviors such as assertiveness and confidence that are traditionally associated with the "model surgeon" and leader are often incongruent with gender role expectations of women and can have significant consequences. For instance, assertive behavior in a woman often has a paradoxical effect where she is perceived to be unlikeable, hostile, and "not leadership material." Gender norm biases are also believed to perpetuate well-known disparities in salary, start-up packages for new hires, retention packages, and service expectations.[18-20] The impact of prescriptive expectations associated with race/ethnicity on gender is largely unexplored in academic surgery but likely very significant. Studies demonstrate that belonging to a group subject to racialization increases the exposure one has to distal stressors such as prejudice, discrimination, and rejection that are then internalized into proximal stressors that may interfere with achievement.[21]

Variable Academic Opportunities

Career advancement in academic surgery is highly dependent on publications, citations, and external research funding, especially from the National Institutes of Health (NIH). Studies demonstrate gender disparity in applicant award probability for R01 external research funding, which is accentuated in minority women.[22] When success is achieved, women on average receive less funding and are underrepresented among the top 1% of award winners. In surgery, even when controlling for achievement, gender gaps remain in academic opportunities needed for promotion including editorial board positions and authorship.[23-25]

Differential Mentorship and Sponsorship

There is clear benefit of mentorship on career advancement, yet a lack of same-sex mentors and role models exists for women in academic surgery, and gender–race/ethnicity group matches are likely rare.[26,27] While many women find male mentors within the field, data suggest women may be hesitant to discuss gender-specific issues impeding their advancement with mentors of the opposite gender. Moreover, women in academic medicine are less likely than men to benefit from sponsorship. While mentors provide advice, feedback, and coaching, sponsors advocate in positions of authority and use their influence to help others advance. Studies demonstrate that sponsorship is critical to academic success and to the development of future leaders in academic medicine.

STRATEGIES TO ADDRESS THE GENDER ACHIEVEMENT GAP

Diverse teams produce better health science with broader impact. To eradicate the gender achievement gap, change is required at multiple levels including departmental, institutional, academic community, and beyond. Currently, most strategies for faculty advancement target the individual via training, mentoring, and networking or the institution, with search committee training and child- or elder care programs as examples.[28] Organizational climate is defined as an organization's policies, practices, and procedures that should reflect organizational culture, defined as the shared values and beliefs that influence workplace and employee behavior.[29,30] Both climate and culture changes are necessary to disrupt the self-reinforcing systems of bias that perpetuate disparities in achievement by gender and ensure that women feel welcome, safe, supported, successful, and respected in surgery.

The Development of Inclusive Leadership

Organizational change toward gender equality in surgery, science, and medicine, broadly, is only part of the broader societal challenge of reducing gender stereotyping of girls and boys and empowering men to embrace gender equality as a goal that also serves their interests.[29] Leaders, policy makers, and male colleagues are critical to affecting this change. Inclusive leaders attempt to normalize diversity, not limited to gender.[31] Consider the following strategies:

1. Make women's contributions visible

2. Create safe spaces for conversations about diversity in surgery

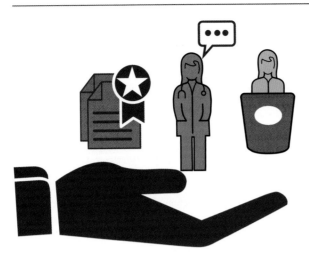

Figure 2.2 Inclusive leadership.

3. Recognize and celebrate the contributions of diverse women to surgery at all levels as the positive representations of women scientists have been shown to positively influence how younger women view their future professional identities[32] (*Figure 2.2*)

Inclusive leaders will drive higher organizational change in academic surgery, with caution taken to avoid placing the burden of this work on women or those most motivated to seek cultural change (i.e., the "minority tax").[33] It is critically important that members of the dominant group (typically white men) take a visibly active and positive role in developing equity, diversity, and inclusion program.[29] Inclusive leaders engage in thoughtful self-reflection and commit resources to recruiting, establishing, and training core competencies that include culture intelligence, self-awareness of implicit bias, and gender stereotypes.[31] Importantly, inclusive leaders prioritize equity and core competency training with action plans that have measurable outcomes holding individuals accountable to "performance indicators." Intense effort should be placed on identifying and documenting process- or institutional-based issues that are supporting inequities, often through implicit bias. Incentivizing competencies as essential components for hiring, merit, and promotion are preferred to the introduction of such training as a "checkbox" initiative.

Gender bias (implicit bias) functions like a habit as an ingrained pattern of thoughts and behaviors; changing a habit is a multistep process.[34] Authors from the University of Wisconsin implemented a pair-matched, single-blind, cluster-randomized, controlled study of a gender-bias habit-changing intervention at a large public university.[35] Faculty participants crossed 92 departments or divisions, and experimental departments were offered a gender-bias habit-changing intervention as a 2.5-hour workshop designed to increase faculty's awareness of gender bias in academic medicine, science, and engineering, and then to promote motivation, self-efficacy, and positive outcome expectations for habitually acting in ways consistent with gender equity. Linear mixed-effects models showed significantly greater changes in self-efficacy to engage gender equity–promoting behaviors, greater perceptions of fit, valuing of their research, and comfort in raising personal and professional conflicts.

Allyship is an important tool for those leading from the middle, as traditional "leaders" only comprise a small proportion of the surgical workforce and communities. This approach has proved useful to combat school and workplace bullying.[29,36] Effective allyship can similarly be coached and requires self-awareness, diligence, commitment, humility, respect, and accountability. Consider the following examples:

1. Speak up in support of women

2. Amplify women's voices in a group

3. Call out discrimination when it happens, rather than remaining silent

The NIH-funded TAC (Transforming Academic Culture) Trial evaluated the impact of a 3-year cluster-randomized intervention designed to improve key indicators of academic success among women assistant professors as well as to drive broader changes in culture at the department and institutional level of a research-intensive medical school.[37] Twenty-seven departments/divisions were randomly assigned to intervention or control groups. The three-tiered intervention included components that were aimed at: (1) the professional development of women assistant professors (inclusive of a manuscript writing program and a total leadership program), (2) changes at the department/division level through faculty-led task forces, and (3) engagement of institutional leaders.[38,39] Significant improvements in academic productivity and work self-efficacy occurred in both intervention and control groups, potentially due to school-wide intervention effects. A greater decline in work hours in the intervention group despite similar increases in academic productivity may reflect learning to "work smarter" or reveal efficiencies brought about as a result of the multifaceted intervention. The intervention appeared to benefit the academic productivity of faculty with PhDs, but not MDs, suggesting that interventions should be more intense or tailored to specific faculty groups. With full engagement of all eligible departments and divisions, the major improvements in both groups were proposed to have resulted from the trial itself (i.e., the Hawthorne effect). Specifically, the trial was highly visible, and the authors hypothesize that it was likely that extensive knowledge of the trial and strong support of the senior leadership at multiple levels affected both control and intervention departments/divisions and the women assistant professors in those departments/divisions.

Recruitment and Retention

Intentional recruitment and retention of underrepresented groups, including women, will achieve a high-performance and diverse team. Procedure can enhance effective recruitment and counter implicit bias and ensure open announcements and hiring for faculty positions and those of leadership. Institutions should consider a selection committee receptive of implicit bias training and coached with awareness tools that are diverse in thought, clinical practice, research interests, sex, and ethnic background to follow process in compiling candidate pools, interviewing, conducting campus visits, and evaluating candidates.[40] Standard behavioral interviewing and a standardized objective assessment tool reduce implicit bias of candidate evaluation at all ranks.[41]

Leadership must establish equality in compensation for comparable work. They should explicitly state that salary is negotiable, which improves women's negotiating position and salary equity, and create written compensation plans to inform faculty how compensation is determined and conduct audits of initial job offers and start-up packages to ensure equality.[41] For physicians, compensation goes beyond pay to include bonuses, incentives, and professional reimbursement for continuing medical education. Onboarding, as an example, is accompanied by moving expenses, signing bonuses, and start-up packages. Additional resources to consider include clinical support staff (including scribes), space (clinic examination rooms and operating room block time), and administrative support for academic or nonclinical efforts. An example of policy-level change was the 2018 update to the 1954 Massachusetts Equal Pay Act (MEPA) to address gender pay disparity.[42] Among other provisions, this law defines comparable work, makes it illegal to ask about current salary during compensation negotiations, and makes it illegal to penalize or retaliate against employees for discussing their salaries. The provisions do, however, allow for differential pay based on seniority, merit, geographic location, quantity or quality of sales/revenue, education or training, and travel.

Change requires establishment of institutional support for family responsibilities. Social norms for such require improvement, for example, offering family leave for maternity/paternity care and elder care. Leave policies should offer pay and sufficient time to ensure their utility for young families, and leaves should be structured to provide incentive for men to take them. Institutions should subsidize onsite childcare and implement policies that support breastfeeding and lactation.[43]

Mentoring and Professional Development

Given the insufficient representation of women in academic medical leadership and research positions, providing women faculty with effective, well-fitting mentorship becomes a critical feature of the work culture. While commonly an unfunded mandate for academic faculty, policies rarely prioritize the mentoring of female faculty. A number of medical schools already have programs that support the professional development of female faculty, but the nature and extent of such support varies substantially. The University of California Davis School of Medicine established the Women in Medicine and Health Science (WIMHS) program in 2000 to ensure the full participation and success of women in all roles within academic medicine.[44] Two senior faculty members developed the program during their tenure as faculty assistants to the dean, as part of their Executive Leadership in Academic Medicine (ELAM) fellowship, and in concert with the school of medicine's faculty development, diversity, and mentoring programs. Since 2000, the WIMHS directors have served as the Women Liaison Officers, now the Group on Women in Medicine and Science, to the AAMC. The WIMHS program provides an inclusive and supportive climate and unique opportunities for female faculty to network, interact, and collaborate with each other. A multipronged approach to career development was employed that encompassed: (1) advocating for women's advancement and leadership in education, research, clinical practice, and administration; (2) promoting sustainable strategies to enhance an institutional climate of inclusion, equity, and opportunity; (3) collecting, analyzing, and applying data to inform institutional and individual decisions and actions; (4) developing and disseminating initiatives, resources, and mentoring and professional career development programs; (5) recognizing and celebrating women's accomplishments; (6) creating opportunities for networking; and (7) working with the AAMC and other medical schools to advance women in medicine and science nationally. A subsequent and steady increase in the number and percentage of female faculty and department chairs, as well as a relatively low departure rate for female faculty, strong and growing internal partnerships, and enthusiastic support from faculty and the school of medicine leadership, support that the WIMHS program has had a positive influence on recruitment and retention, career satisfaction, and institutional climate to provide a more inclusive and supportive culture for women.

A recent review builds on extensive literature regarding the contributors to gender inequality in academic medicine and other disciplines and synthesizes current evidence regarding interventions to address this inequality.[16] Included studies were limited to those reporting quantitative outcomes only, with a focus on tangible outcomes such as retention, promotion, research grant success, and salary. Of 18 eligible studies that evaluated a range of structured programs inclusive of peer mentoring, education and skill development and networking opportunities revealed that overall study quality was low to moderate and all studies reported positive outcomes on at least one indicator. This review suggests that targeted programs have the potential to improve some outcomes for women in academia. However, the success of an intervention appears to be undermined when it relies on the additional labor of those it is intending to support (i.e., "bottom-up" approaches). As such, the authors propose that academic institutions should consider and evaluate the efficacy of "top-down" interventions that start with change in practice of higher-level faculty.

Although mentoring, networking, and leadership training programs at the academic community level (i.e., the Hedwig van Ameringen ELAM Program and the AAMC early and midcareer faculty development programs) have been shown to be effective in advancing the careers of women, many institutions are not held accountable for not having programs to support their women faculty, suggesting a missed opportunity.[28] ELAM is an American 1-year leadership training program for senior academic women with coaching, networking, and mentoring opportunities. The curriculum aims to improve skills in paradigms of leadership, financial management, strategic planning, emerging issues in academic medicine, communication, personal dimensions of leadership, and career advancement strategies.[45-47] ELAM has a positive effect on the rank, retention, and/or self-rated capabilities of women faculty in all studies with specific attributes over other programs cited as greater length and intensity and intentional community building with other female staff. Additional larger-scale programs like the ADVANCE grants of the National Science Foundation focus on institution-wide change to promote the careers of women.

Academic Community

There are growing examples of higher-level academic community accountability. The AAMC's Increasing Women's Leadership Project Implementation Committee recommended in 2002 that medical schools, teaching hospitals, and academic societies: (1) emphasize faculty diversity in departmental reviews, evaluating department chairs on their development of women faculty; (2) target women's professional development needs within the context of helping all faculty maximize their faculty appointments, including helping men become more effective mentors of women; (3) assess which institutional practices tend to favor men's over women's professional development, such as defining "academic success" as largely an independent act and rewarding unrestricted availability to work (i.e., neglect of personal life); (4) enhance the effectiveness of search committees to attract women candidates, including assessment of group process and of how candidates' qualifications are defined and evaluated; and (5) financially support institutional Women in Medicine programs and the AAMC Women Liaison Officer and regularly monitor the representation of women at senior ranks.[1]

Recognizing that publication is a chief currency within science, medicine, and public health and key to the ability of women and others to contribute, receive recognition, and accrue the experience, visibility, and achievement to compete for advancement, *The Lancet* issued in 2019 a *Diversity Pledge* and *No All-Male Panel Policy* as part of the Lancet Group's commitment to increasing gender equity, diversity, and inclusion in research and publishing.[48] The *Diversity Pledge* expresses a particular commitment to increasing the representation of women and colleagues from low-income and middle-income countries among editorial advisers, peer reviewers, and authors. The new *No All-Male Panel Policy* acknowledges the traditional predominance of male speakers, which excludes the full breadth of available expertise and opinion. The policy states that Lancet Group editors will not serve as panelists at a public conference or event when there are no women on the panel ("manels"), and it commits to gender balance in events the Lancet Group sponsors or organizes. The preference is for women to be included as panelists, not only as chairs or moderators.

THE ROLE OF SOCIAL MEDIA

More than 2 billion people engage with social media, which enables near instantaneous interactions with a global community providing opportunities for networking, learning, and dissemination of knowledge.[49] Social media has allowed for the breaking down of barriers in the healthcare field related to communication, geography, culture, specialties, and practice tools and is a powerful tool used to build and maintain communities.[50] The #ILookLikeASurgeon and parallel #HeForShe campaign dramatically symbolize the ability of social media to unite surgeons across continents and cultures in a call for diversity and equality in the surgical workforce challenging stereotypes and celebrating differences.[50] Closed Facebook communities like "Surgeons Mom Group" and "Women in Surgery Support Group" facilitate global networking and the free exchange of motivation and support, dissemination of opportunity and sponsorship, and crowd sourcing assistance to aid with clinical, professional, or personal challenges. Survey data have supported that social media serves as a valuable tool to enhance the networking and mentorship of surgeons, particularly for women in surgical specialties that may lack exposure to same-sex mentors at their home institution.[49]

Social media can also be used strategically to increase the dissemination of research articles and collect solution-focused feedback. A strategic online social media approach employing a tweet chat has been shown to increase the dissemination of the selected research, amplifying the authors' works and driving active discussion about gender equity issues and accumulate potential solutions.[31] This tactic has widespread potential for accelerating awareness (advocacy) as well as more rapid development and implementation of potential solutions to a variety of problems in medicine (*Figure 2.3*).

CURRENT KNOWLEDGE GAPS AND FUTURE DIRECTIONS

Medicine has made relatively slow progress in achieving gender equity, particularly at the highest levels of executive leadership, academic promotion, and compensation. In the ground breaking 2007 report from the National Academies, *Beyond Biases and Barriers: Fulfilling the Potential of Women in Academic Science and Engineering,*

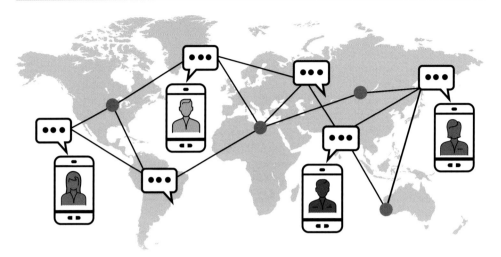

Figure 2.3 The role of social media.

the authors note that "the problem is not old style, overt sex discrimination, but rather unrecognized features of the organizational culture that affect men and women differently" and they made two key recommendations to use research: (1) to deepen the academic medicine community's understanding of the culture of the work environment and (2) to identify those salient cultural aspects that impact women's careers. Research is urgently needed to drive evidence-based best practices to eliminate barriers to career advancement for diverse surgical faculty. In this regard, gender equality can be posed as an innovation challenge, with an open-minded yet scientific attitude, given the complex and multifaceted challenge. Behavioral and systemic changes that focus on climate and culture change, as aforementioned, hold promise. Importantly, diversity training programs often challenge an individual's sense of autonomy and self-determination and control risk of failure. Rather, successful diversity programs support individual autonomy and engagement and create a culture in which people feel personally responsible for change.[51] Consider the following examples:

1. Mentoring programs that effectively increase representation among minority women

2. The establishment of diversity task forces

3. Sponsorship programs in which sponsors become personally invested in their protégé's career success, take risks to champion their recognition and advancement, and ultimately embed them in powerful networks

As strategized, goals must then be translated into action plans and organizations held accountable for change. This requires ongoing data collection, transparency, and the allowance for failure as part of the experimental process. A construct of a culture conducive to women's academic success (CCWAS) has recently been defined, and a tool created to evaluate it.[52] A CCWAS consists of four distinct but related dimensions: equal access, work–life balance, freedom from gender biases, and supportive leadership. The authors found evidence that women within departments/divisions agree on the supportiveness of their units, but that substantial differences among units exist. The analyses provided strong evidence for the reliability and validity of their measure.

In 2018, to intentionally build an equitable and inclusive environment, targeted faculty development programs were integrated within the organizational structure of the University of Michigan's Department of Surgery.[40] New policies and procedures were implemented to ensure that each faculty member has a clear and equal opportunity for career advancement in an open and inclusive environment (*The Michigan Promise*), efforts since established as a critical component of the departmental mission. The Michigan Promise is centered around six domains: environment, achievement, recruitment, leadership development, innovation, and outreach. While each element was developed by teams of volunteer faculty within the Department of Surgery, the Department Chair and Executive Committee were fully engaged in strategic planning and have made a 10-year financial commitment to long-term creativity and program growth. For long-term sustainability, each programmatic initiative is executed in a newly established Office of Faculty and Resident Life and the departmental governance structure reorganized to include a Vice Chair of Faculty Life and an Associate Chair of Faculty Development with responsibilities to advance the work described. To broaden impact and reach, work is now focused on building national academic partnerships (The Promise Coalition) that will bring surgical departments together to assess measurable metrics and establish best practices. Together, these efforts represent major steps toward achieving equity and are a full and longitudinal commitment to professional fulfillment and career success for all surgeons.

REFERENCES

1. Bickel J, Wara D, Atkinson BF, et al. Increasing women's leadership in academic medicine: report of the AAMC Project Implementation Committee. *Acad Med.* 2002;77(10):1043-1061.
2. Yedidia MJ, Bickel J. Why aren't there more women leaders in academic medicine? the views of clinical department chairs. *Acad Med.* 2001;76(5):453-465.
3. McGuire LK, Bergen MR, Polan ML. Career advancement for women faculty in a U.S. school of medicine: perceived needs. *Acad Med.* 2004;79(4):319-325.
4. Abelson JS, Chartrand G, Moo TA, Moore M, Yeo H. The climb to break the glass ceiling in surgery: trends in women progressing from medical school to surgical training and academic leadership from 1994 to 2015. *Am J Surg.* 2016;212(4):566-572.e1.
5. Zhuge Y, Kaufman J, Simeone DM, Chen H, Velazquez OC. Is there still a glass ceiling for women in academic surgery?. *Ann Surg.* 2011;253(4):637-643.
6. Levine RB, Lin F, Kern DE, Wright SM, Carrese J. Stories from early-career women physicians who have left academic medicine: a qualitative study at a single institution. *Acad Med.* 2011;86(6):752-758.
7. Bickel J. What can be done to improve the retention of clinical faculty?. *J Womens Health (Larchmt).* 2012;21(10):1028-1030.
8. Yeo HL, Abelson JS, Mao J, et al. Who makes it to the end?: a novel predictive model for identifying surgical residents at risk for attrition. *Ann Surg.* 2017;266(3):499-507.
9. Cochran A, Elder WB, Crandall M, Brasel K, Hauschild T, Neumayer L. Barriers to advancement in academic surgery: views of senior residents and early career faculty. *Am J Surg.* 2013;206(5):661-666.
10. McLemore EC, Ramamoorthy S, Peterson CY, Bass BL. Women in surgery: bright, sharp, brave, and temperate. *Perm J.* 2012;16(3):54-59.
11. Salles A, Awad M, Goldin L, et al. Estimating implicit and explicit gender bias among health care professionals and surgeons. *JAMA Netw Open.* 2019;2(7):e196545.
12. National Academies of Sciences E, and Medicine. *Sexual Harassment of Women: Climate, Culture, and Consequences in Academic Sciences, Engineering, and Medicine.* Washington, DC: The National Academies Press; 2018.

13. Jagsi R, Griffith KA, Jones R, Perumalswami CR, Ubel P, Stewart A. Sexual harassment and discrimination experiences of academic medical faculty. *J Am Med Assoc.* 2016;315(19):2120-2121.

14. Jagsi R, Griffith KA, Jones RD, Stewart A, Ubel PA. Factors associated with success of clinician-researchers receiving career development awards from the National Institutes of Health: a longitudinal cohort study. *Acad Med.* 2017;92(10):1429-1439.

15. Colletti LM, Mulholland MW, Sonnad SS. Perceived obstacles to career success for women in academic surgery. *Arch Surg.* 2000;135(8):972-977.

16. Pattillo M. *Black Picket Fences: Privilege and Peril Amonth the Black Middle Class.* Chicago, IL: University of Chicago Press; 1999.

17. Burgess DJ, Joseph A, van Ryn M, Carnes M. Does stereotype threat affect women in academic medicine?. *Acad Med.* 2012;87(4):506-512.

18. Holliday E, Griffith KA, De Castro R, Stewart A, Ubel P, Jagsi R. Gender differences in resources and negotiation among highly motivated physician-scientists. *J Gen Intern Med.* 2015;30(4):401-407.

19. Merluzzi J, Dobrev SD. Unequal on top: gender profiling and the income gap among high earner male and female professionals. *Soc Sci Res.* 2015;53:45-58.

20. Sanfey H, Crandall M, Shaughnessy E, et al. Strategies for identifying and closing the gender salary gap in surgery. *J Am Coll Surg.* 2017;225(2):333-338.

21. Williams DR. Race, socioeconomic status, and health. The added effects of racism and discrimination. *Ann N Y Acad Sci.* 1999;896:173-188.

22. Ginther DK, Kahn S, Schaffer WT. Gender, race/ethnicity, and National Institutes of Health R01 research awards: is there evidence of a double bind for women of color?. *Acad Med.* 2016;91(8):1098-1107.

23. Harris CA, Banerjee T, Cramer M, et al. Editorial (spring) board? Gender composition in high-impact general surgery journals over 20 years. *Ann Surg.* 2019;269(3):582-588.

24. Waljee JF. Discussion: gender authorship trends of plastic surgery research in the United States. *Plast Reconstr Surg.* 2016;138(1):143e-144e.

25. Waljee JF, Chang KW, Kim HM, et al. Gender disparities in academic practice. *Plast Reconstr Surg.* 2015;136(3):380e-387e.

26. Kaderli R, Muff B, Stefenelli U, Businger A. Female surgeons' mentoring experiences and success in an academic career in Switzerland. *Swiss Med Wkly.* 2011;141:w13233.

27. Patton EW, Griffith KA, Jones RD, Stewart A, Ubel PA, Jagsi R. Differences in mentor-mentee sponsorship in male vs female recipients of National Institutes of Health Grants. *JAMA Intern Med.* 2017;177(4):580-582.

28. Carr PL, Gunn C, Raj A, Kaplan S, Freund KM. Recruitment, promotion, and retention of women in academic medicine: how institutions are addressing gender disparities. *Womens Health Issues.* 2017;27(3):374-381.

29. Coe IR, Wiley R, Bekker LG. Organisational best practices towards gender equality in science and medicine. *Lancet.* 2019;393(10171):587-593.

30. Schneider B, Ehrhart MG, Macey WH. Organizational climate and culture. *Annu Rev Psychol.* 2013;64:361-388.

31. Cawcutt KA, Erdahl LM, Englander MJ, et al. Use of a coordinated social media strategy to improve dissemination of research and collect solutions related to workforce gender equity. *J Womens Health (Larchmt).* 2019;28(6):849-862.

32. Steinke J. Adolescent girls' STEM identity formation and media images of STEM professionals: considering the influence of contextual cues. *Front Psychol.* 2017;8:716.

33. Rodriguez JE, Campbell KM, Pololi LH. Addressing disparities in academic medicine: what of the minority tax?. *BMC Med Educ.* 2015;15:6.

34. Carnes M, Devine PG, Isaac C, et al. Promoting institutional change through bias literacy. *J Divers High Educ.* 2012;5(2):63-77.

35. Carnes M, Devine PG, Baier Manwell L, et al. The effect of an intervention to break the gender bias habit for faculty at one institution: a cluster randomized, controlled trial. *Acad Med.* 2015;90(2):221-230.

36. Wagner KC, Yates D, Walcott Q. Engaging men and women as allies: a workplace curriculum module to challenge gender norms about domestic violence, male bullying and workplace violence and encourage ally behavior. *Work.* 2012;42(1):107-113.

37. Grisso JA, Sammel MD, Rubenstein AH, et al. A randomized controlled trial to improve the success of women assistant professors. *J Womens Health (Larchmt).* 2017;26(5):571-579.

38. Sonnad SS, Goldsack J, McGowan KL. A writing group for female assistant professors. *J Natl Med Assoc.* 2011;103(9-10):811-815.

39. Friedman SD. Be a better leader, have a richer life. *Harv Bus Rev.* 2008;86(4):112-118, 38.

40. Newman EA, Waljee J, Dimick JB, Mulholland MW. Eliminating institutional barriers to career advancement for diverse faculty in academic surgery. *Ann Surg.* 2019;270(1):23-25.

41. Raj A, Kumra T, Darmstadt GL, Freund KM. Achieving gender and social equality: more than gender parity is needed. *Acad Med.* 2019;94(11):1658-1664.

42. Asgari MM, Carr PL, Bates CK. Closing the gender wage gap and achieving professional equity in medicine. *J Am Med Assoc.* 2019;321(17):1665-1666.

43. Newman C, Ng C, Pacque-Margolis S, Frymus D. Integration of gender-transformative interventions into health professional education reform for the 21st century: implications of an expert review. *Hum Resour Health.* 2016;14:14.

44. Bauman MD, Howell LP, Villablanca AC. The Women in Medicine and Health Science program: an innovative initiative to support female faculty at the University of California Davis School of Medicine. *Acad Med.* 2014;89(11):1462-1466.

45. Dannels SA, Yamagata H, McDade SA, et al. Evaluating a leadership program: a comparative, longitudinal study to assess the impact of the Executive Leadership in Academic Medicine (ELAM) Program for Women. *Acad Med.* 2008;83(5):488-495.

46. Richman RC, Morahan PS, Cohen DW, McDade SA. Advancing women and closing the leadership gap: the Executive Leadership in Academic Medicine (ELAM) program experience. *J Womens Health Gend Based Med.* 2001;10(3):271-277.

47. Helitzer DL, Newbill SL, Morahan PS, et al. Perceptions of skill development of participants in three national career development programs for women faculty in academic medicine. *Acad Med.* 2014;89(6):896-903.

48. Clark J, Horton R. What is The Lancet doing about gender and diversity?. *Lancet.* 2019;393(10171):508-510.

49. Luc JGY, Stamp NL, Antonoff MB. Social media in the mentorship and networking of physicians: important role for women in surgical specialties. *Am J Surg.* 2018;215(4):752-760.

50. Hughes KA. #ILookLikeASurgeon goes viral: how it happened. *Bull Am Coll Surg.* 2015;100(11):10-16.

51. Kang SK, Kaplan S. Working toward gender diversity and inclusion in medicine: myths and solutions. *Lancet.* 2019;393(10171):579-586.

52. Westring AF, Speck RM, Sammel MD, et al. A culture conducive to women's academic success: development of a measure. *Acad Med.* 2012;87(11):1622-1631.

3

Underrepresented Minorities in Surgery

Erika Adams Newman
David J. Brown

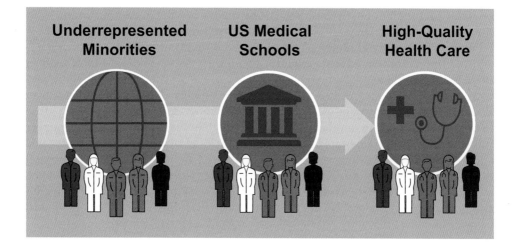

CATALYSTS FOR DIVERSITY

Medical school enrollment of ethnic minority groups continues to decline, and underrepresented minorities (URMs: African American, Mexican American, mainland Puerto Rican Hispanic, American Indian, and Alaskan Native)—make up only 4% of full-time medical faculty.[1] This underrepresentation in academic medicine is important to address because disproportionate representation is thought to account for major disparities in health care. Inclusion of URM faculty improves the ability of US medical schools to fulfill their missions of providing high-quality health care to multicultural populations.[2] Diversity within academic medicine also propels all aspects of medical education and research.

Underrepresented minorities are more likely to leave academic medicine, are less satisfied with their career trajectories, and advance more slowly compared with majority groups. These are large long-standing racial and ethnic inequities in career success of URMs in medicine. In a landmark study, Palepu and colleagues found that minority faculty were less likely than white faculty to hold senior academic rank.[3] The authors concluded that this discrepancy was not explained by potential confounders like number of years on faculty or academic productivity. Faculty of color, particularly women faculty, are absent from department chair, medical school executive positions, and decanal roles.

Underrepresented faculty experience unique identity-related barriers that impair success. Although many constraints are the same as those faced by majority groups, there are critical environmental and cultural barriers that account for large achievement gaps for ethnic minorities. Faculty of color report that they experience explicit and implicit racism, bias, devaluing of work, and a complex social isolation (being the "only one") within academic medical centers.[4] Nearly half of URM faculty report personally experiencing racial discrimination by a peer or superior compared with 7% of majority faculty.[4] Many also report encountering racial or disparaging ethnic remarks at work. Beyond self-reported analyses, little else is known about faculty of color experiences within predominantly white academic medical centers.

Social isolation, exclusion, and subtle unequal treatment are known barriers that URMs navigate in academic medical centers that cannot be understated. Unequal treatment is complex and multifactorial because inequities may not be clear or can be easily reasoned away. In fact, few URMs report or openly discuss instances in which they may have been socially isolated or treated unequally because of fear of retaliation or career derailment. It may also be difficult to pinpoint covert racism and discrimination, and URMs may not be empowered to address topics such as these in the workplace.

To overcome these constraints, it is the responsibility of department leaders to acknowledge and maintain awareness of the unique experiences of URMs. It is important for leaders to develop a skill set that enables them to identify and counter subtle acts of bias and unequal treatment. This includes being able to recognize and address racial achievement gaps, acknowledging that unique barriers exist, and putting systemic processes into place that eliminate inequities. Success is not appropriately achieved by lowering metrics or performance expectations but by recognizing and working to eliminate the unique barriers that URMs face in academic fields and in medical education.

PROFESSIONAL IDENTITY

Although progress has been made in providing an inclusive culture for URMs in Academic Medicine, professional identity is often at odds with cultural, social, and personal identities and with traditions of the academy. Recently, education researchers have begun to understand more about the connection between professional identity and academic success.[5] Specifically, URMs that develop a positive professional identity may buffer negative stereotypes associated with their social identities. For example, a woman scientist struggling with negative stereotypes about women in Science, Technology, Engineering, and Mathematics (STEM) may try to minimize her social identity in science classes by developing a strong professional identify as an excellent scientist and in turn tend to perform higher on science examinations and be more accepted by her peers.[5] A similar line of research found that the development of strong professional identity predicted success for first-generation college women.[6] Professional identity may be difficult to develop because social norms of academic medicine do not align URMs with positions of leadership or with successful rank advancement:

> I am struck by my lived contradiction: To be a professor is to be an anglo; to be a latina is not to be an anglo. So how can I be both a Latina and a professor? To be a Latina professor, I conclude, means to be unlike and like me. Que locura! What madness! … As Latina professors, we are newcomers to a world defined and controlled by discourses that do not address our realities, that do not affirm our intellectual contributions, that do not seriously examine our worlds. Can I be both Latina and professor without compromise?
> (Ana M. Martinez Aleman in Padilla & Chavez, *The Leaning Ivory Tower*, 1995:74-75).

It is beneficial for URMs to develop professional identities that are recognized and supported by peers and department leaders. This will require insight into the impact of negative social norms and how URMs in the academy are initially perceived and placed into categories based on these norms. For example, stereotyping and images that ethnic minorities generally represent, men with dark skin may not initially be considered honest and upstanding, based on current national police-related events or the environment in the US criminal justice system. It is up to mentors, sponsors, and department leaders to facilitate URMs in developing professional identities based on individual talent, passion, and strengths and not based on societal norms or historical standards. This requires an intentionality that is prioritized by[2]:

- acknowledging that societal norms highly impact professional identities

- helping URM faculty determine and develop a positive professional identity matching their clinical, research, and educational passions and interests

- ushering an open culture in which professional paths are not outlined or driven by social norms and common ethnic stereotypes

Another important aspect of professional identity is the avoidance of labeling research focused on underserved populations, health equity, or community-based activities as "soft" research.[2] URMs in academic medicine report that a career that is community-based is not valued or highly promoted among their peers in the same supportive ways as traditional laboratory or clinical research. This is a significant threat to the success of research programs focused on eliminating health disparities or tackling social determinants of health, many of which are driven by and led by URM researchers. On the other hand, if departments are able to maintain a broad slate of diverse research goals, particularly for underserved populations, URMs may perceive the environment as more favorable and are likely to succeed. Academic departments that value community-based research as "real science" will have improved opportunities to develop and maintain URM faculty.

SOCIAL CAPITAL

The underlying causes for the achievement gap in URMs in medical education and at the faculty level are unclear and not explained by discrimination alone. Organizational science and medical educators have determined that there are multifaceted and complex reasons for disparities between URMs and majority peers. An example of this is "stereotype threat," which suggests that work achievements are impaired by societal expectations of performance. Because certain societal expectations of URMs are negative, studies have suggested that this results in a constant awareness that affects URM performance and underachievement.[7] Another study found that rather than stereotype threat, lack of social interventions that bolster self-affirmation and debunk negative stereotypes accounts for achievement gaps.[8]

Researchers are paying closer attention to the role of social capital in overall health and professional well-being. The idea that a sense of community and group interactions can have positive impact on individuals is well known by sociologists. Social capital is a core principle in social sciences including economics, political science, and public health. There is increasing understanding of the value of social networks and meaningful connections, particularly in underrepresented communities.[9] For example, students report that they are more likely to be friends with others from the same gender and ethnicity.[10] Network analysis examines how individuals are situated socially within a network. Such knowledge informs the ways in which access or limitations of opportunities and resources differ among social groups.[9] The term social capital, coined by Pierre Bourdieu in 1971, expands "capital" to include social and cultural resources. These are resources linked to a supportive network of organizational relationships and acquaintances. Coleman et al. studied social capital and found that peer and community networks influenced students' academic performances, outweighing school quality or policy.[11] In *Bowling Alone: The Collapse and Revival of American Community* (Putnam 2000), the author described social capital as a collective resource possessed by communities and organizations. The message was that civic participation is decreasing in the United States, reducing opportunities for positive social interconnections, thereby reducing national social capital. Even more compelling is the notion that social capital has a link to health and wellness.

While human capital reflects knowledge—an individual's thoughts and abilities—and economic capital is measured as wealth or bank accounts, social capital is defined by the structure of relationships.[12] Portes explains that in order to have social capital, an individual must be related to others, and it is others, not self, who are the sources of advantages.[12] Social factors and positive relationships have been found to improve the achievement gap for URMs in the medical school.[10] Positive relationships are significant in the success of URMs in academics because they provide a close circle, bonding, flow of knowledge, and sharing of educational resources. In most medical school environments, such positive relationships are most frequently observed among homogeneous groups and among individuals connected to the same social identity groups. There is compelling evidence for homophily by ethnicity.[10] These networks are important for URM students' success. In the study by Vaughan and colleagues, naming a tutor or being in a personal academic support network was significantly linked to higher achievement.[10] Relationships with senior colleagues and bridging social capital with successful peers may also impact success (*Figure 3.1*).

THE HIDDEN CURRICULUM

Now there is no question at all that the education in attitude and skill that the physician obtains in medical school and in the hospital… is an absolute source of much of his performance as a practitioner…Nonetheless, I argue that education is a less important variable than work environment. There is some very persuasive evidence that 'socialization' does not explain some important elements of professional performance half so well as does the organization of the immediate work environment.

(Freidson, 1970a:88-89).

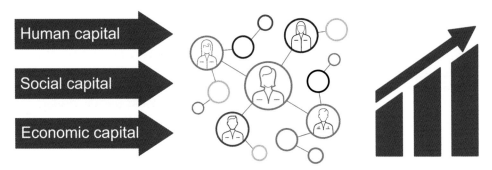

Figure 3.1 Social capital.

Social capital is a component of the broader "*hidden curriculum*" in medical education. The hidden curriculum has been defined as the culture, accepted behaviors, and beliefs that are not taught in the classroom but are passed on to students who enact them.[13] Much of what is learned about medicine takes place outside of formal courses and within the hidden curriculum. Such knowledge transfer is selectively passed on from senior colleagues and students and influences students' enactment of professionalism and professional identity.[14] URM students and faculty have described the hidden curriculum in careers such as surgery and have a clear sense of the difficulty navigating and uncovering steps to succeed. It is critically important to account for a set of rules in an environment that are not clearly stated or formalized. It is also critically important to not assume that individuals from marginalized groups are included in and have access to curriculum specifics.

Specialty-specific hidden curricula exist and shape how students and faculty excel. In a field such as surgery, there is evidence of differing access and negative experiences of the hidden curriculum for women and URMs. Surgical professional culture has been used to explore negative issues of the hidden curriculum. These include unequal access, engagement, and exclusion.[14] Building strong and trusting relationships is the main priority and challenge of navigating the hidden curriculum, and this is easier for majority groups. Access to the hidden curriculum is not equal, and URMs may have difficulty accessing and enacting practical elements. This will exclude many URMs from success in academic medicine. Such exclusion may be overcome by opening social networks and effective mentoring and sponsorship.

MENTORING AND CAREER NETWORKING

Disparities in career achievement for URMs are not only a threat to the ability of US medical schools to fulfill their social missions of providing quality health care to all populations but also limit the number of qualified senior mentors and role models for URM trainees and junior faculty. While there are focused programs for URM learners, there is not intentional focus at the faculty level at most institutions. Achievement in medicine is not a simple process of clinical learning, practicing, and teaching. When surveyed, many faculty of color acknowledge that they lack role models for themselves and yet feel obligated to serve as role models for URM trainees and other faculty.[2] Many URMs are first-generation higher education graduates and have not had as much academic guidance as the majority of faculty. In a survey conducted by Pololi and colleagues, a URM woman leader pointed out:

> When you're the first person in your family to reach this point, you are clueless. I was not receiving any counseling at all about what the next move was... A lot of people of color don't know that.
>
> (URM female, leader).[2]

In "Don't Leave Us Behind: The Importance of Mentoring for Underrepresented Minority Faculty," the authors examined mentoring experiences of 58 URM faculty at 22 research-extensive institutions.[15] Participants engaged in interviews and focus groups that discussed the attributes of mentoring relationships and the role of political guidance for their careers. The data found common themes: (1) social capital is critical, (2) barriers are linked to undervaluing of faculty research in healthcare disparities and community engagement, and (3) connections with mentors who understand struggles specific to URMs at predominantly white institutions can boost retention and success.[15] One study participant commented:

> At each of our institutions there's clearly a culture that exists there that is very informal, and you don't know about it unless you have these very informal personal conversations with people that are senior to tell you this is what you should do in this situation. These aren't the written rules, but these are the understood norms of what's going on...But, I'm a little bit jaded about what African American faculty, junior faculty particularly, miss out on because they don't have those kinds of relationships with senior faculty because the senior faculty of color just aren't there.
>
> (African American, male).[15]

Many of these obstacles may be addressed by effective and intentional mentoring and sponsorship from peers, department leaders, and deans. Effective knowledge transfer is critical for URMs to gain insight into institutional norms and patterns of success. Access to meaningful mentoring relationships is more limited for URM faculty and trainees, and URMs report lower levels of satisfaction with tenured professors and fewer opportunities to collaborate. Several qualitative research projects have sought to identify the sociocultural experiences that influence success of URMs. Although the solutions are complex with multifaceted variables, meaningful mentorship and sponsorship is always at the forefront as a critical component of academic success. Mentoring relationships for URMs require bidirectional trust and engagement.

An effective mentor works to elevate the mentee's academic progress, sponsors leadership potential, provides social capital, and ensures access to the hidden curriculum.

THE ROLE OF LEADERSHIP IN THE SUCCESS OF URMS

Department and medical school leaders can drive a culture for success of URMs in academic medicine and in surgery. For URMs to be successful, the leadership must embrace, value, articulate, and actively engage in behaviors that foster an open and inclusive culture for all individuals to thrive. Successful diversity missions are emphasized as part of the core values of the organization and not a side tagline. The most authentic and equitable cultures are those in which leaders openly value diversity as much as grants, publications, teaching, revenue, and patient care. This also includes treating all members with fairness and valuing the unique contributions that each person brings to the team. Leaders have unconscious biases that they need to be aware of, so that they don't influence important decisions. Strong active listening skills, curiosity, and humility are important to hear different points of view and actively seek contributions from others with differing, and often valid, perspectives.

The most effective leaders also place high value on diverse cognitive repertoires, understanding the complex relationships between identity diversity and cognitive diversity. It is important to assure equal access and voice of all individuals no matter their personal identity or position within the organization. Strong leaders have the courage to challenge the organization's status quo and encourage the entire team to think of new directions that support the current and future diversity of the organization.

Conscious leaders also understand and strive to learn as much as possible about the negative impact of stereotyping and social norms that URM trainees and faculty navigate daily. Aspects of this can be addressed by broad focus and educational initiatives to lower implicit bias, though bias is not the only factor to consider. Leaders have a pivotal role of advancing qualified URMs as leaders and for executive roles. This is not and should never be about lowering a metric bar or "putting" individuals into positions in which they are not qualified or have not demonstrated excellence. Respondents in the study by Pololi also described their experience:

> ...leaders rarely selected people of color for leadership positions as doing so would detract from their sense of comfort interacting with people like themselves.[2]

The advancement of URMs into leadership roles has to be a priority of the institution and of department leaders; this often takes courage and being willing to take a stand in decisions that may not be the most popular or that challenge social norms. Not until there are more URMs in positions of leadership who can reinforce their commitment to excellence will the stereotyping and social categories begin to soften and not be driven by gender or race. Furthermore, issues around social capital and the hidden curriculum may be more accessible to URMs.

CONCLUSION

Ultimately, the topics presented above require broad accountability and ownership for the success of all individuals. Accountability is multidirectional and not top-down. Effective diversity goals are established and then evaluated regularly. A leadership team that empowers the entire team to hold each other accountable for achieving the goals, including holding leadership accountable, can achieve broad equity and inclusion. This can be challenging with power differentials; though leaders can level the playing field by reinforcing that in diversity, we are all learners. For example, we have found that groups that do unconscious bias trainings together, i.e., learning together, are able to hold each other accountable for their biases, despite power differences. Shared learning experiences lead to shared accountability.

REFERENCES

1. Merchant JL, Omary MB. Underrepresentation of underrepresented minorities in academic medicine: the need to enhance the pipeline and the pipe. *Gastroenterology.* 2010;138:19-26.e3. doi:10.1053/j.gastro.2009.11.017.

2. Pololi L, Cooper LA, Carr P. Race, disadvantage and faculty experiences in academic medicine. *J Gen Intern Med.* 2010;25:1363-1369. doi:10.1007/s11606-010-1478-7.

3. Palepu A, Carr PL, Friedman RH, Amos H, Ash AS, Moskowitz MA. Minority faculty and academic rank in medicine. *J Am Med Assoc.* 1998;280:767-771. doi:10.1001/jama.280.9.767.

4. Peterson NB, Friedman RH, Ash AS, Franco S, Carr PL. Faculty self-reported experience with racial and ethnic discrimination in academic medicine. *J Gen Intern Med.* 2004;19:259-265. doi:10.1111/j.1525-1497.2004.20409.x.

5. Prieto CK, Copeland HL, Hopson R, Simmons T, Leibowitz MJ. The role of professional identity in graduate school success for under-represented minority students. *Biochem Mol Biol Educ.* 2013;41:70-75. doi:10.1002/bmb.20673.

6. Neumeister KLS, Rinker J. An emerging professional identity: influences on the achievement of high-ability first-generation college females. *J Educ Gift.* 2006;29:305-338. doi:10.1177/016235320602900304.

7. Woolf K, Cave J, Greenhalgh T, Dacre J. Ethnic stereotypes and the underachievement of UK medical students from ethnic minorities: qualitative study. *Br Med J.* 2008;337:a1220. doi:10.1136/bmj.a1220.

8. Woolf K, McManus IC, Gill D, Dacre J. The effect of a brief social intervention on the examination results of UK medical students: a cluster randomised controlled trial. *BMC Med Educ.* 2009;9:1-15. doi:10.1186/1472-6920-9-35.

9. Domínguez S, Arford T. It is all about who you know: social capital and health in low-income communities. *Health Sociol Rev.* 2014;19:114-129. doi:10.5172/hesr.2010.19.1.114.

10. Vaughan S, Sanders T, Crossley N, O'Neill P, Wass V. Bridging the gap: the roles of social capital and ethnicity in medical student achievement. *Med Educ.* 2015;49:114-123. doi:10.1111/medu.12597.

11. Coleman JS. Social capital in the creation of human capital. *Am J Sociol* 2015;94:S95-S120. doi:10.1086/228943.

12. Portes A. Social capital: its origins and applications in modern sociology. *Ann Rev Sociol.* 2003;24:1-24. doi:10.1146/annurev.soc.24.1.1.

13. Hafferty FW, Hafler JP. *The hidden curriculum, structural disconnects, and the socialization of new professionals.* In: *Extraordinary Learning in the Workplace.* Vol 136. 2nd ed. Dordrecht: Springer; 2011:17-35. doi:10.1007/978-94-007-0271-4_2.

14. Hill E, Bowman K, Stalmeijer R, Hart J. You've got to know the rules to play the game: how medical students negotiate the hidden curriculum of surgical careers. *Med Educ.* 2014;48:884-894. doi:10.1111/medu.12488.

15. Zambrana RE, Ray R, Espino MM, Castro C, Cohen BD, Eliason J. "Don't leave us behind": the importance of mentoring for underrepresented minority faculty. *Am Educ Res J.* 2015;52:40-72. doi:10.3102/0002831214563063.

4

Unconscious Bias

Samir K. Gadepalli
Erin E. Perrone
Erika Adams Newman

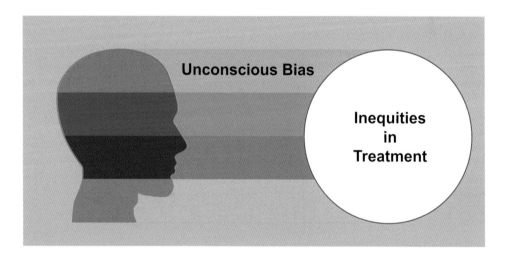

Unconscious and implicit biases are the immediate and rapid thoughts carried beneath conscious awareness. Such thoughts form stereotypes and "gut feelings" that shape discriminatory behaviors. Although the term implicit bias may carry negative connotations or provoke uncomfortable emotions, they should not be looked upon the same as an explicit bias or prejudice. Implicit biases are instinctive thoughts utilized daily, an instinctive and immediate system of awareness that shapes fast responses and intuitions. They have evolutionary benefits in circumstances that allow us to process and think rapidly when necessary. Such categorizing into social norms can lead to harmful judgments and inequities in treatment when based on characteristics such as race, gender, or sexuality.

IMPLICIT BIAS MEDIATES INEQUITY

The quality of health care in the United States varies by race and ethnicity.[1] Numerous studies have consistently found that black and Hispanic patients receive lower quality of care than white patients, not all explained by financial or socioeconomic barriers.[2] The Institute of Medicine's (IOM) report "Unequal Treatment" states that disparities in health care emerge from bias against minorities, greater clinical uncertainty when interacting with minority patients, and stereotypes held by clinicians about the health of racial minorities.[3] There is growing evidence that healthcare providers' attitudes toward black patients are more negative than white patients and include stereotypes about noncompliance. When surveyed, ethnic minority patients rate interpersonal quality of care from physicians and trust factors[4] more negatively than white patients.[5] Negative associations and implicit racial biases mediate racial disparities in physician treatment decisions. Clinicians' implicit biases affect communication, overall ratings of care, and trust relationships.[6]

Bias may also be at the core of achievement gaps and inequities in advancement of underrepresented groups in academic medicine. The Implicit Association Test (IAT) was developed in 1998 and is the most broadly utilized tool for measuring implicit bias. The IAT connects thoughts and reaction times to mental concepts. It provides insight into unconscious mindsets. For example, participants who demonstrated implicit racial bias in the assessment rapidly associated black faces with words such as bad and white faces with words such as good. Salles et al. examined data from health professionals taking the gender-based IAT.[7] The study found that both men and women have explicit and implicit biases in mental models of women with families and men with careers. This was further explored for biases that specifically exist within surgery, finding that surgeons perceived men with surgical careers and women with careers in family medicine. This is important because women are underrepresented in surgical fields, and implicit bias may affect their success and the contexts in which they are perceived. The IAT is not perfect because it is not known if higher bias scores translate into discriminatory behaviors and low scores may be falsely reassuring. Other studies have shown that when participants are presented with identical job resumes for hypothetical jobs in Science, Technology, Engineering, and Mathematics (STEM) fields, male candidates were considered more competent, offered greater mentoring, given higher salaries, and offered more career mentoring.[8] Preexisting subtle bias against women is associated with less support in general[8] (*Figure 4.1*).

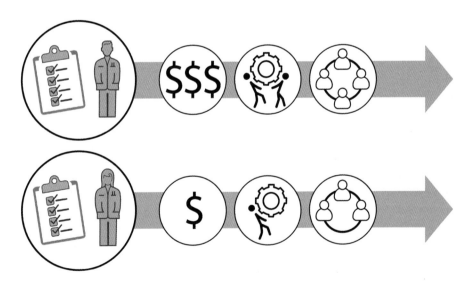

Figure 4.1 Selection and support barriers for women in Science, Technology, Engineering, and Mathematics (STEM) fields.

Understanding and addressing such bias is complex because it occurs beneath consciousness and is difficult to measure. Best practices or proven approaches do not currently exist. It is important that academic leaders begin to acknowledge and decrease the influences of implicit bias in order to achieve equity for all. This will require implementing innovative processes for career advancement that are specifically aimed at eliminating unequal barriers to achievement for women and underrepresented ethnic groups.

#WHATADOCTORLOOKSLIKE

Tamika Cross, MD, was a resident in obstetrics and gynecology when she volunteered her services on an airplane when another passenger required medical attention. She describes that she rose her hand when asked if there were any doctors on the plane only to be met with skepticism and told that "we are looking for actual physicians."[9] Dr. Cross then shared her experience on social media and explained that a white man offered his assistance and was allowed to help without questioning. She wrote "I'm sure many of my fellow young, corporate America working women of color can understand my frustration when I say I'm sick of being disrespected."[9,10] Dr. Cross is a black, female physician who didn't fit the picture of a doctor in the eyes of those requesting help. This is just one example of the implicit bias in medicine faced by anyone who doesn't "look the part." The post that Dr. Cross shared went viral and #WhatADoctorLooksLike was born. This hashtag has been used by anyone whose physician identity has been questioned because of race or gender, and the numbers are overwhelming.[10]

It would be easy for the profession to blame society and perceive this issue as one that is external to medicine. However, despite the fact that women make up approximately half of the medical school admissions and residency spots, the percent of women in advanced faculty positions and leadership roles plummets.[11] Reasons for this are multifactorial. In 2013, a survey of academic surgeons revealed that 54% of women had experienced being treated differently due to their gender, and 36% of women reported experiencing negative comments about gender, significantly more than male respondents (16% and 4%, respectively, $P < .001$ for both).[12] In 2017, a retrospective study of milestone achievement among 359 emergency medicine residents at eight different residencies showed that although female residents were equivalent to male residents in the first year of training, male residents had a nearly 13% higher rate of milestone attainment by graduation.[13] This gender gap in evaluations was seen in men and women faculty evaluations, leading the authors to suggest that implicit gender bias was present and that it should be recognized as a potential factor limiting advancement of women.[13] The same authors reviewed the quality of comments made by attending physicians in the resident evaluations in a follow-up publication. They showed that ideal residents had more stereotypically masculine traits and that male residents were more likely to receive clear and consistent feedback for areas of improvement than women residents.[14] These are all examples of gender inequity ingrained in academic medicine that spans disciplines. Implicit bias is a systemic limitation with opportunities to recognize, discuss, and address openly, without shame or fear of career hindrance at all ranks.

Limitations in advancement and inequity in evaluations are the tip of the iceberg when it comes to gender bias in academic medicine. Dr. Caprice Greenberg addressed the Association for Academic Surgery (AAS) in her 2017 presidential address regarding the many obstacles facing women surgeons.[10] She presented that women earn fewer grants from the National Institutes of Health (NIH), those that do earn grants are awarded lower dollar amounts, and that qualitative analysis of the reviewer's comments suggested that gender bias may play a role. She also presented the pay gap present in medicine with women earning, on average, thousands of dollars per year less than male counterparts.[10] The reasons for these differences are not simple or solitary, but implicit bias is an underlying theme.

RACIAL AND ETHNIC INEQUITIES IN ACADEMIC AWARDS

There is evidence of racial bias in the receipt of academic awards in medicine. The majority of ethnic minority faculty aggregate at the assistant professor ranks in US medical schools, and men are more likely to hold associate and full professor ranks. These achievement gaps also include lower success rates in obtaining NIH research grants, slower promotion rates, lower career satisfaction, and subtle work environment discrimination.[15]

The Alpha Omega Alpha (AOA) honor society is a prestigious organization thought to predict success in academic medicine, and members are more likely to match into their chosen subspecialties, particularly surgical subspecialties. AOA members have a track record of excellence and are also more likely to attain the rank of full professor, dean, or departmental chair.[16] Studies have shown that the honors medical society's members scored higher on the medical school admissions test, had a higher proportion of parents attending college, and were disproportionately white students.[17] A landmark study in 2017 by Boatwright and colleagues found that black and Asian students were less likely than their white peers to be members of AOA, which may be a result of selection bias at a single academic medical school.[18] These data may prompt local and national chapters of the society to examine membership characteristics and to develop benchmark trends in member selection. Taken together, studies such as these suggest that processes that utilize both subjective and objective evaluation criteria are vulnerable to bias. Residency program directors and faculty recruitment committees can intervene and potentially prevent systemic bias by utilizing multifaceted and holistic recruitment criteria that deemphasize achievements and mediate racial disparities.

BIAS AND BARRIERS AGAINST LGBTQ GROUPS

Public views on equality and the societal role of lesbian, gay, bisexual, transgender, and queer (LGBTQ) individuals in the United States have changed dramatically over the last decade. In some communities and work settings, attitudes have changed to be more accepting and inclusive. Despite this, there remains substantial evidence that sexual minority patients perceive discrimination in healthcare environments. Moreover, the IOM has also reported that gay and lesbian individuals "face discrimination in the healthcare system that can lead to an outright denial of care or to the delivery of inadequate care."[19] Bias among clinicians may explain disparities faced by sexual minority groups such as risk for cancer, HIV/AIDS, eating disorders, and depression. To begin to address these inequities, medical schools and health systems have highlighted the need for more research on the root causes and addressing physician bias.[19]

Academic health centers are poised to examine and improve both the healthcare experience and work environment for LGBTQ physicians. Little is known about the experiences of physicians from identity groups such as LGBTQ. In a 2011 study of 427 LGBTQ physicians, the majority of respondents reported discrimination, harassment, social rejection, and witnessing substandard or denial of care to LGBTQ patients.[20] In this study, 65% had heard derogatory comments about LGBTQ individuals, 34% had seen discriminatory treatment of an LGBTQ patient, 27% had witnessed discriminatory treatment of an LGBTQ coworker, 22% felt socially ostracized, and 15% reported being harassed by a colleague. Few medical schools or residencies have formal education on bias or care of LGBTQ priorities and issues.

Sexual and gender diversity are important aspects of physicians in workplace environments. In many cases, individuals hide their identity due to fear of discrimination and exclusion. A study by Burke and colleagues examined both explicit and implicit biases against lesbian women and gay men among medical students.[21] In this study, almost half of the respondents expressed explicit bias, and most exhibited at least some implicit bias against gay and lesbian individuals. Cognitive and emotional empathy predicted positive explicit attitudes but did not predict implicit bias.

These data present an exciting opportunity for medical schools and residency programs to begin to incorporate curricula-based interventions that educate and raise consciousness on intergroup contact and empathy in health care. Broad educational initiatives that include curricula with empathy teaching and more positive intergroup contact such as that described by Burke et al. may not only address bias for sexual minority groups but also be of benefit for all marginalized groups that include equity for individuals with disabilities and mental health disorders.

IMPACT OF BIAS IN PATIENT CARE AND OUTCOMES

Healthcare professionals exhibit the same levels of bias as the overall population.[22] Interactions between physicians and their patients create multiple opportunities for miscommunication and misunderstanding. Correlating IAT with other metrics shows influence on diagnosis and treatment decisions, the quality of treatment, and patient outcomes and satisfaction. Though patients should not receive a lower standard of care due to race, gender, or other characteristics, studies have shown that medical trainees hold and use false beliefs about biological differences to inform medical judgments.[23]

In the 2002 report by the IOM, there was evidence that "bias, prejudice, and stereotyping on the part of healthcare providers" may impact healthcare disparities. Using studies of clinical vignettes to examine clinical decision-making, there was an implicit preference favoring white people across providers, regardless of specialty.[24] Black patients are less likely to receive pain medication for abdominal pain, have longer wait times in the emergency room, are less likely to be admitted for their pain, and are less likely to receive laboratory evaluations or percutaneous interventions or thrombolysis for acute coronary syndromes (*Figure 4.2*).[24-26]

These disparities are striking and are not clearly explained by implicit and explicit biases. For example, though total knee replacement (TKR) is a cost-effective treatment for severe osteoarthritis, which is more prevalent among blacks, TKR rates are lower among blacks. Assessment of family and internal medicine physicians via web-based survey using clinical vignettes demonstrates the disparities are not fully

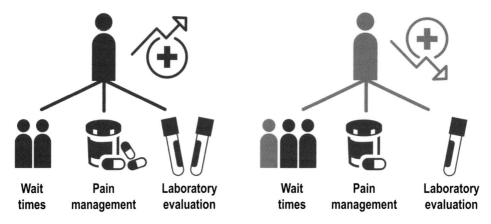

| Wait | Pain | Laboratory | Wait | Pain | Laboratory |
| times | management | evaluation | times | management | evaluation |

Figure 4.2 Examples of disparities in health care related to race.

explained by the strong implicit preference for white patients among physicians.[27] Perhaps some of these disparities are secondary to the patient's neighborhood, insurance status, and access to care, impacting the quality of care received.[28,29] All of these interrelated phenomena lead to implicit biases in physician–patient relationships and eventually the quality of care provided. In the 2018 National Healthcare Quality and Disparity Report (AHRQ), of 250 quality measures, there were improvements in only four measures for blacks, who with American Indians, Alaska Natives, and Native Hawaiians/Pacific Islanders, received worse care than whites for approximately 40% of the measures.[30]

Discussions of race and gender in clinical practice and in academic career achievement are uncomfortable but necessary to limit bias and inequities. Education should use evidence-based approaches that do not reinforce gender- or race-based discrepancies in outcomes or advancement. Awareness and education is enhanced by open engagement of colleagues, peers, and trainees in discussions and change initiatives. This requires leaders that promote understanding the impact of language and the development of innovative policies that eliminate disparities and barriers. Examples include intentional practices around informed consent and pain management that target "cultural humility, not competence."[31] Such processes can lead to sustained improvements. Strategies to reduce implicit bias such as stereotype replacement, counterstereotype imaging, individuation, perspective taking, increasing opportunities for contact with individuals from different groups, and partnership building have been described in the Institute of Health's white paper.[32]

REFERENCES

1. Saha S, Arbelaez JJ, Cooper LA. Patient-physician relationships and racial disparities in the quality of health care. *Am J Public Health*. 2003;93(10):1713-1719.
2. Ayanian JZ, Weissman JS, Chasan-Taber S, Epstein AM. Quality of care by race and gender for congestive heart failure and pneumonia. *Med Care*. 1999;37:1260-1269. doi:10.1097/00005650-199912000-00009.
3. Smedley BD, Stith AY, Nelson AR, Institute of Medicine (US) Committee on Understanding and Eliminating Racial and Ethnic Disparities in Health Care. *Unequal Treatment: Confronting Racial and Ethnic Disparities in Health Care*. Washington, DC: The National Academies Press; 2003. doi:10.17226/12875.

4. Horn IB, Mitchell SJ, Wang J, Joseph JG, Wissow LS. African-American parents" trust in their child"s primary care provider. *Acad Pediatr* 2012;12:399-404. doi:10.1016/j.acap.2012.06.003.

5. Racial and Ethnic Disparities in Perceptions of Physician Style and Trust. Racial and ethnic disparities in perceptions of physician style and trust. 2000;9(10):1156-1163. doi:10.1001/archfami.9.10.1156.

6. Cooper LA, Roter DL, Carson KA, et al. The associations of clinicians' implicit attitudes about race with medical visit communication and patient ratings of interpersonal care. *Am J Public Health.* 2012;102:979-987. doi:10.2105/AJPH.2011.300558.

7. Salles A, Awad M, Goldin L, et al. Estimating implicit and explicit gender bias among health care professionals and surgeons. *JAMA Netw Open.* 2019;2:e196545. doi:10.1001/jamanetworkopen.2019.6545.

8. Moss-Racusin CA, Dovidio JF, Brescoll VL, Graham MJ, Handelsman J. Science faculty's subtle gender biases favor male students. *Proc Natl Acad Sci U S A.* 2012;109:16474-16479. doi:10.1073/pnas.1211286109.

9. Hauser C. *Black Doctor Says Delta Flight Attendant Rejected Her; Sought 'Actual Physician'.* The New York Times; 2016.

10. Greenberg CC. Association for Academic Surgery presidential address: sticky floors and glass ceilings. *J Surg Res.* 2017;219:ix-xviii.

11. Cooke M. Implicit bias in academic medicine: #WhatADoctorLooksLike. *JAMA Intern Med.* 2017;177(5):657-658.

12. Cochran A, Hauschild T, Elder WB, et al. Perceived gender-based barriers to careers in academic surgery. *Am J Surg.* 2013;206(2):263-268.

13. Dayal A, O'Connor DM, Qadri U, Arora VM. Comparison of male vs female resident milestone evaluations by faculty during emergency medicine residency training. *JAMA Intern Med.* 2017;177(5):651-657.

14. Mueller AS, Jenkins TM, Osborne M, Dayal A, O'Connor DM, Arora VM. Gender differences in attending physicians' feedback to residents: a qualitative analysis. *J Grad Med Educ.* 2017;9(5):577-585.

15. Nunez-Smith M, Ciarleglio MM, Sandoval-Schaefer T, et al. Institutional variation in the promotion of racial/ethnic minority faculty at U.S medical schools. *Am J Public Health.* 2012;102:852-858. doi:10.2105/AJPH.2011.300552.

16. Brancati FL, Mead LA, Levine DM, Martin D, Margolis S, Klag MJ. Early predictors of career achievement in academic medicine. *J Am Med Assoc.* 1992;267:1372-1376.

17. Babbott D, Weaver SO, Baldwin DC. Personal characteristics, career plans, and specialty choices of medical students elected to Alpha Omega Alpha. *Arch Intern Med.* 1989;149:576-580.

18. Boatright D, Ross D, O'Connor P, Moore E, Nunez-Smith M. Racial disparities in medical student membership in the Alpha Omega Alpha Honor Society. *JAMA Intern Med.* 2017;177:659-665. doi:10.1001/jamainternmed.2016.9623.

19. The National Academies Collection: Reports funded by National Institutes of Health. *The health of lesbian, gay, bisexual, and transgender people: building a foundation for better understanding.* In: *Institute of Medicine (US) Committee on Lesbian, Gay, Bisexual, and Transgender Health Issues and Research Gaps and Opportunities.* Washington, DC: National Academies Press; 2011.

20. Eliason MJ, Dibble S, Robertson PA. Lesbian, gay, bisexual, and transgender (LGBT) physicians' experiences in the workplace. *J Homosexuality.* 2011;58(10):1355-1371. doi:10.1080/00918369.2011.614902.

21. Burke SE, Dovidio JF, Przedworski JM, et al. Do contact and empathy Mitigate bias against gay and lesbian people among Heterosexual medical students? A report from medical student changes. *Acad Med.* 2015;90:645-651. doi:10.1097/ACM.0000000000000661.

22. Fitzgerald C, Hurst S. Implicit Bias in healthcare professionals: a systematic review. *BMC Med Ethics.* 2017;18:19.

23. Hoffman KM, Trawalter S, Axt JR, Oliver MN. Racial bias in pain assessment and treatment recommendations, and false beliefs about biological differences between blacks and whites. *Proc Natl Acad Sci U S A.* 2016;113(16):4296-4301. doi:10.1073/pnas.1516047113.

24. Dehon E, Weiss N, Jones J, et al. A systematic review of the impact of physician implicit racial bias on clinical decision making. *Acad Emerg Med.* 2017;24(8):895-904.

25. Shah AA, Zogg CK, Zafar SN, et al. Analgesic access for acute abdominal pain in the emergency department among racial/ethnic minority patients: a nationwide examination. *Med Care.* 2015;53:1000-1009.

26. Pezzin LE, Keyl PM, Green GB, et al. Disparities in the emergency department evaluation of chest pain patients. *Acad Emerg Med.* 2007;14:149-156.

27. Oliver MN, Wells KM, Joy-Gaba JA, et al. Do physicians' implicit views of African Americans affect clinical decision making? *J Am Board Fam Med.* 2014;27(2):177-188.

28. Kahn KL, Pearson ML, Harrison ER, et al. Health care for black and poor hospitalized Medicare patients. *J Am Med Assoc.* 1994;271(15):1169-1174.

29. Leigh WA, Lillie-Blanton M, Martinez RM, Collins KS. Managed care in three states: experiences of low-income African Americans and Hispanics. *Inquiry.* 1999;36(3):318-331.

30. Agency for Healthcare Research and Quality. *2018 National Healthcare Quality and Disparities Report.* Content last reviewed September 2019. Rockville, MD: Agency for Healthcare Research and Quality. Available at https://www.ahrq.gov/research/findings/nhqrdr/nhqdr18/index.html.

31. Tsai J, Brooks K, DeAndrade S, et al. Addressing racial bias in wards. *Adv Med Educ Pract.* 2018;9:691-696.

32. Wyatt R, Laderman M, Botwinick L, Mate K, Whittington J. *Achieving Health Equity: A Guide for Health Care Organizations.* IHI White Paper. Cambridge, MA: Institute for Health Improvement; 2016. Available at ihi.org.

5

Faculty Recruitment

Erika Adams Newman
David J. Brown

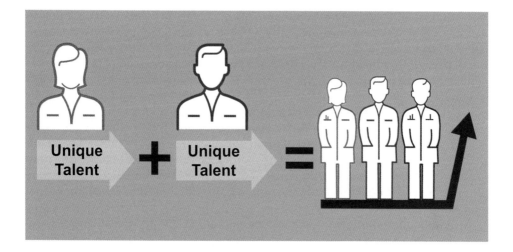

BENEFITS OF TEAM DIVERSITY

The faculty makeup at academic institutions does not represent modern society. Women and faculty of color are underrepresented in the higher echelons of academics. According to the Association of American Medical Colleges (AAMC), women represent only 34% of associate professors and 21% of full professors.[1] These numbers are much lower for medical school deans (16%) and for department chairs (15%). Given the current rate of advancement, it has been predicted that parity will not be achieved at the current rates. These gaps are thought to account for ongoing health disparities and for achievement gaps for women and faculty of color.

It has been well demonstrated that the highest performing teams reflect the globalization of society and the communities in which they serve. The AAMC has stated that increasing diversity of academic health centers is a significant component of the strategy to reduce health disparities in the United States. Importantly, a representative faculty and leadership team are critical to achieve highest excellence in clinical care, research, and education. The benefits of diversity and representation are strong and reach well beyond demographics and social justice causes. Organizational effectiveness is optimized by diverse talents that span abilities, background, thought, and identity. This concept has been researched by organizational scholars and is put into perspective by Scott Page in his book, *The Diversity Bonus*. The foundational element of the model connects cognitive repertoires and identity diversity to produce bonuses for teams with high stakes and complex tasks: *one* talent plus a *different* talent equals *more than two* and leads to higher performance.

In terms of great team building in medicine, this concept creates an exciting opportunity to leverage unique differences for performance strength. For example, consider a strategy on how a team of surgeons is assembled to establish a new specialty division within a department of surgery. The Chair, in drafting successful teammates, will first need to soundly put forth and demonstrate the value of creating the most inclusive culture of individuals with diverse cognitive repertoires. Bonus is added when surgeons with different skill sets from different backgrounds and experiences work together to solve complex problems. Based on what we will call the *"academic surgery case"* for diversity, a high-performing team would consist of a surgeon that has the experience to drive the busy clinical enterprise and has also spent time studying implementation of novel surgical techniques in urban environments. This surgeon also obtained a master's degree in public health and is interested in addressing social determinants of health and disparities; a clinician scientist is added to the team, one that is working out the technical details of a translational surgical model in the laboratory. The two doctors are paired with a surgeon with a background in education who has experience teaching complex procedures and has plans to integrate an innovative simulation series for the residents and medical students. The three doctors with their unique identities and talents produce bonuses for the team that are predicted to increase creativity and revenue as well as improve outcomes. These bonuses drive excellence and advance team performance *more than* if the team had consisted of three doctors with a background in health disparities or if all were translational scientists, for example. Cognitive diversity within healthcare teams leverages the full benefit of teams working together to solve complex problems, more than can be accomplished by any individual and more than teams that lack diversity.

An additional component is that its members are able to serve as mentors, sponsors, and role models for learners with diverse backgrounds and interests. This is critically important to allow students and trainees from underrepresented groups to connect with mentors from similar backgrounds, to share experiences, and to minimize identity isolation. Mentors and sponsors are critical for career success and knowledge transfer of successful norms.

A diverse team is also more culturally competent with the knowledge and skills to serve patients from different cultural and ethnic backgrounds. To effectively care for patients with diverse backgrounds, healthcare teams must have an understanding of how belief systems, cultural biases, and family structure may influence health and medical decision-making.[2] A culturally competent team transcends the effects that language barriers, religion, unconventional beliefs, or alternative medicine may have on patients and families (*Figure 5.1*).

BARRIERS TO INCLUSIVE RECRUITMENT

Broadening representation requires an intentional shift in the traditional recruitment mindset; standard procedures will not work. This is not entirely a pipeline issue. There have been long-standing inequities and exclusion in academia, particularly for women and faculty of color. Only organizations that recognize this can

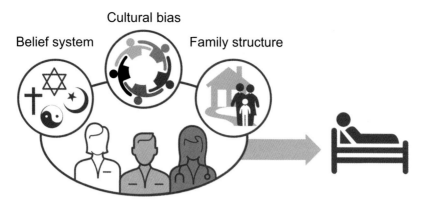

Cultural bias

Belief system

Family structure

Figure 5.1 Healthcare teams must be culturally competent.

directly address it. Leaders that cultivate a culture of building high-performing teams with intellectual (and identity) diversity can successfully recruit and retain the best talent. Approaching faculty recruitment utilizing these principles provides an exciting growth opportunity for healthcare systems. Challenges are high because national standards or best practices have not been established.

Influence of Implicit Bias

At the forefront is the influence of implicit bias in the recruitment process. Inclusive recruitment procedures are severely limited by individual biases and associations that exist outside of conscious awareness. These biases are not intentional but can be harmful and may hinder recruitment and retention of diverse faculty.

People are treated differently based on the social and identity groups to which they belong. Stereotyping and schemas—the "unconscious hypothesis" about who people are, their motives, and what they are about—are rapid and many times inaccurate. It is important to consider and acknowledge that subtle negative biases contribute to negative evaluations and attitudes toward women and faculty of color. Gender and racial disparities in the science fields can be closely linked to bias and is responsible, at least in part, for large achievement gaps. This stereotyping must be validated and understood by department leaders and search teams in order to decrease, and perhaps account for, the major influence of bias on hiring decisions.

It has been well documented that both male and female faculty judge a female student to be *less* competent and *less* worthy of being hired in the biological sciences than an identical male student and offered less direct mentoring and sponsorship. Even more negative schemas around competency and integrity are tied to students and faculty of color. Studies on hiring suggest that men and women tend to have stronger preferences for male candidates even with identical qualifications.[3] Men are favored leaders among both men and women faculty.[4] Analysis of large numbers of studies comparing male and female leaders shows that when women carry a directive and autocratic leadership style, they receive the lowest ratings. This is thought to reflect a violation of social norms for women. Men, on the other hand, are rated higher with this form of leadership style. These biases are real, pervasive, and difficult to overcome. Academic leaders should be able to recognize and stand against such bias.

Bias in Recommendations

Note should also be made of gender bias in recommendation letters for surgical residency candidates and for faculty hiring. Although letters of recommendation are influential in the match and hiring processes, the subjective descriptions found in letters are gender biased. Qualitative text analysis, quantitative text mining, and topic modeling methods have been used to assess letters of recommendations for applicants in surgery.[5] This study found gendered differences in word count—higher for male compared with female applicants; and standout adjectives such as exceptional as well as references to awards, achievements, ability, hardship, leadership, and scholarship were most often applied to men. Positive general terms such as delightful and hard working, as well as physical descriptions and doubt-raisers, were most often applied to women. Topic modeling revealed that words such as *care* and *support* were used more commonly with women applicants. These biases held up even when applicants had the same accomplishments and standardized test scores. Given the broad use of letters of recommendation, search teams should look for biased, subjective descriptions and avoid making hiring decisions based on them. Similarly, subjective assessments and "word on the street" about candidates are often negatively biased. Such details are often confusing and difficult to understand how to incorporate into candidate evaluations. This is particularly true for surgical skill assessment and interpersonal skills, which may be difficult to assess objectively.

Bias of Cognitive-Based and Standardized Tests

The majority of US residency programs utilize the United States Medical Licensing Examination (USMLE) Step 1 examination to determine which medical students to offer interviews and for ranking candidates.[6] The USMLE and other standardized testing are also thought to predict success on future licensing tests. Given this, program directors most often rely on test scores as an indicator of how students will perform on licensing examinations, an important metric for training programs. Black students' USMLE and MCAT scores have been shown to be lower than those of their white peers and have a negative impact on access to residency interviews and selection. The racial gap has widened over the last several decades for nearly all standardized tests and is not explained by socioeconomic class. Such gaps are complex and involve racial inequities in US education and society in general. Because of this, many elite colleges no longer require standardized testing (SAT or ACT) for admissions. Medical schools, residency programs, and faculty recruitment teams should not ignore the bias of standardized test scores, and consideration should be given to how these are utilized in evaluating and selecting candidates.

Lack of Meaningful Mentorship

The AAMC percentages of tenure-track faculty of color remain less than 2% in most American departments of surgery and less than 4% of total faculty (including non–tenure-track). This has not improved in the last 5 decades and has led to keen competition for highly creative and talented diverse faculty of color. Barrett and Smith[7] analyzed reasons universities are successful in recruiting talented faculty of color and found that mentoring relationships with senior faculty was critically important. Mentoring as a form of cultural capital to students and faculty of color is linked to the number of professors of color at predominantly white institutions to serve as role models.[8] Lack of access to mentors and professional networks who understand struggles specific to navigating and advancing in academia is a significant barrier to recruitment and retention. Studies have shown that access to effective mentoring relationships that enhance faculty success is exceptionally limited for faculty of color. Zambrana et al. conducted in-depth, semistructured interviews and focus groups to obtain information from diverse faculty of color on their perceptions of mentoring and academic career path in predominantly white institutions.[8] A student described his lack of effective mentorship as:

> It's not like you're held down... it's just that, wow, it would be a whole lot easier if I could just pick up the phone and call someone. There's no senior Black male in my department. So, there's literally not any person that could tell me what the experience is going to be like to try to get tenure in [this department]. There's nobody. If I had a million dollars, there's nobody that could tell me how to do that, whereas everybody else has someone that they could ask.[8]

Another student responded:

> I think a lot of mentoring relationships don't do enough to explain all of those invisible things that make success possible, especially for people of color... In my family no one had gone to graduate school before me. I think that's true for a lot of people of color in the academy, that you don't come from a place of prior knowledge (Mexican American, female).[8]

Subtle Inequities and Discrimination

Additional barriers that lead to an absence of a critical mass and recruitment of diverse talent are inequities in training, lack of program support, and perceptions of a lack of environmental support.[9] Nearly half of faculty of color report experiencing racial/ethnic bias in academic medicine and have lower career satisfaction in US medical schools, while majority faculty infrequently perceive such bias.[10] Women and faculty of color report experiencing personalized devaluing that transcends rank.[9] This may lead to loss of confidence and disengagement. Marginalized groups report that they sense an intentional lack of trust that contributes to environmental stressors.[9] These obstacles may seem insurmountable to promising talent and lead women and faculty of color to frequently change organizations or leave academics altogether.

SUCCESSFUL RECRUITMENT OF DIVERSE FACULTY

Visionary leaders recognize the benefits of building diverse teams and work to integrate an academic environment that is welcoming and inclusive. Aligning representation and diversity of thought in faculty recruitment is a critical leadership priority and requires institutional will. Academic institutions must level the playing field by directly addressing microinequities and implicit bias along with providing intentional strategies to broaden reach. This includes putting processes into place that directly work to eliminate structural inequalities such as subjective assessments and unstructured interviews. This also includes intentional efforts to decrease the influence of implicit bias during the interview and evaluation process. Assuring effective mentoring practices and onboarding is also critical. In order to address these issues broadly, leadership teams require a clear and intentional plan for process change.

A study that consisted of interviews of faculty of color with questions about what influenced their acceptance of positions at an academic institution found that the most influential recruitment factors were[7] research opportunities and funding, career advancement and mentoring opportunities, reputations of associates, congeniality of associates, teaching opportunities, influence in the department, and rapport with department leaders. These findings may be used as a starting point and road map for strategic recruitment processes.

Best Practice Models

Rooney Rule

Since 2003, the National Football League (NFL) has required that teams interview at least one or more ethnic minority candidates for all coaching and senior football operations jobs. In 2009, the rule was expanded to include general manager and front office positions. The NFL has implemented strong accountability measures and major fines to track and maintain compliance. The Rooney Rule has had a significant impact, including the overall increase of black coaches from 6% to 22%. The rule has been adopted across many business sectors and is now considered a best practice to increase diversity within organizations.

UM STRIDE

Beginning in 2002, the University of Michigan, through the Strategies and Tactics for Recruiting to Improve Diversity and Excellence (STRIDE) Committee, has prepared search teams, faculty, and administrators to recruit women and underrepresented groups. The committee utilizes hiring practices that have been identified nationally as effective and open and updates a handbook yearly based on topical research on best practices for recruitment. Additional aspects include strategies to broaden the applicant pool and ways to assure positive candidate experiences while on campus. The STRIDE Committee spans all schools and colleges in the university, offering workshops and online presentations. There has been success in the recruitment of women in each of the colleges including the medical school. This is exemplified by the increase in proportion of new women faculty in Science, Technology, Engineering, and Mathematics (STEM) fields from 13% in 2002 to 33% in 2016.

An intentional effort to address bias in hiring, STRIDE provides ideas and tools to aid in fair and inclusive recruitment. For example, the course teaches about how social categories beyond gender and race, such as sexual identity, can also affect candidate evaluations. Applicants who are members of minority groups may be perceived as less credible and rated lower. Search teams should work to avoid such biases and implement processes to avoid this. The same holds true for parental status, where mothers are rated less competent and less committed to paid work, while fathers are rated more competent and more committed to work.[3] Mothers are less likely to be recommended for hiring and promotion and offered lower starting salaries than nonmothers.

There are also harmful stereotypes in the leadership capacity of women and faculty of color. This is exemplified in studies that have shown that race affects leadership perceptions by implicit leadership theories, e.g., being male and/or being white is positively associated with leadership functions.[10] While these microinequities and perceptions alone or one by one may seem minor, the accumulation of advantages and disadvantages is harmful and hinders diversity in recruitment and advancement.

Academic Surgery Department Pilot

Since 2017, in an intentional effort to increase diversity in hiring, the Department of Surgery at the University of Michigan expanded all recruiting procedures to implement aspects of STRIDE and open search practices.[11] The major procedural components of the department-wide policy included the following.

Education and Mandatory Training

Department-wide participation in implicit bias training was implemented. All faculty, staff, and residents attended a STRIDE workshop and were provided opportunities to understand the impact of bias in the search and recruitment process.

Department Recruitment Committee

A standing committee was established with faculty members of diverse backgrounds, academic rank, and subspecialty to assist and participate in departmental recruitment at all levels. The committee's role is to review relevant documents, provide guidance during the recruitment process, and attest that all faculty job descriptions, postings, and selections meet the best practices set forth by STRIDE and University procedures. Committee members are required to participate in ongoing training and educational activities that raise awareness and decrease bias in hiring.

A Modified "Rooney Rule"

Modifications of the rule require inclusion of at least two qualified candidates representing diversity in the applicant pool (a woman or an underrepresented minority candidate) for each position and inviting at least one of the candidates to participate in an on-campus interview (*Figure 5.2*).

Mandatory Group Interview With Attribute-Based Questions

The departmental recruitment committee conducts 60- to 90-minute group interviews of all faculty candidates at all ranks during the initial visits. For each group interview, candidates were asked standard, behavior-based questions on topics

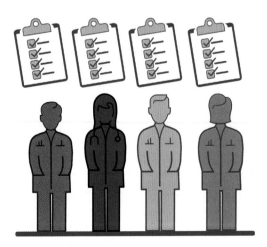

Figure 5.2 A modified Rooney Rule.

related to clinical care, research goals, education, and views on diversity and inclusion. The questions are tailored to academic rank. Candidates are evaluated utilizing an evaluation tool aimed to decrease subjective details and comments. A written summary and ranking of the candidates are delivered to the division chief and chair.

Implementation of these strategies resulted in immediate measurable benefits that have increased the diversity of the applicant pool and new hires throughout the department. The numbers of women and faculty of color both interviewed and hired have significantly increased. Both applicants and committee participants viewed the new procedures to have a positive impact on the search and recruitment process.[11] The leaders of the department considered the use of new procedures and the input of the standing committee to be insightful, accurate, and valuable to the hiring process, as job offers have aligned with rankings of the committee.

Challenges have included the significant amount of time that the committee members and administrative assistants spend in coordinating schedules and interview dates. Committee members are also expected to participate in continuous learning in strategies to decrease implicit bias, broadening reach, and objective evaluations. This may lead to potential delays in hiring decisions. These are opportunities for further growth and metric setting. This intentional recruitment strategy is expected to intentionally eliminate underrepresentation in surgery over the next 10 years and beyond.

CONCLUSIONS

In order to improve diversity in faculty recruitment, new and innovative approaches are required. Department leaders and hiring teams that thoughtfully evaluate their practices and hiring protocols will advance a diverse workforce, one that is inclusive, higher performing, and representative of the communities in which we serve.

REFERENCES

1. Zhou MJ, Doral MY, DuBois SG, Villablanca JG, Yanik GA, Matthaya KK. Different outcomes for relapsed versus refractory neuroblastoma after therapy with 131I-metaiodobenzylguanidine (131I-MIBG). *Eur J Cancer.* 2015;51(16):2465-2472.
2. Cohen JJ, Gabriel BA, Terrell C. The case for diversity in the health care workforce. *Health Aff.* 2017;21:90-102. doi:10.1377/hlthaff.21.5.90.
3. Correll SJ, Benard S, Paik I. Getting a job: is there a motherhood penalty?. *Am J Sociol* 2015;112:1297-1339. doi:10.1086/511799.
4. Girod S, Fassiotto M, Grewal D, et al. Reducing implicit gender leadership bias in academic medicine with an educational intervention. *Acad Med.* 2016;91:1143-1150. doi:10.1097/ACM.0000000000001099.
5. Turrentine FE, Dreisbach CN, St Ivany AR, Hanks JB, Schroen AT. Influence of gender on surgical residency applicants' recommendation letters. *J Am Coll Surg* 2019;228:356-365.e3. doi:10.1016/j.jamcollsurg.2018.12.020.
6. Edmond MB, Deschenes JL, Eckler M, Wenzel RP. Racial bias in using USMLE step 1 scores to grant internal medicine residency interviews. *Acad Med.* 2001;76:1253.
7. Barrett TG, Smith T. Southern coup: recruiting African American faculty members at an Elite Private Southern Research University. *Am Educ Res J.* 2017;45:946-973. doi:10.3102/0002831208321445.
8. Zambrana RE, Ray R, Espino MM, Castro C, Cohen BD, Eliason J. "Don't leave us behind": the importance of mentoring for underrepresented minority faculty. *Am Educ Res J.* 2015;52:40-72. doi:10.3102/0002831214563063.

9. Whittaker JA, Montgomery BL, Martinez Acosta VG. Retention of underrepresented minority faculty: strategic initiatives for institutional value proposition based on perspectives from a range of academic institutions. *J Undergrad Neurosci Educ.* 2015;13:A136-A145. doi:10.1093/biosci/biu199.

10. Peterson NB, Friedman RH, Ash AS, Franco S, Carr PL. Faculty self-reported experience with racial and ethnic discrimination in academic medicine. *J Gen Intern Med.* 2004;19:259-265. doi:10.1111/j.1525-1497.2004.20409.x.

11. Dossett LA, Mulholland MW, Newman EA, Michigan Promise Working Group for Faculty Life Research. Building high-performing teams in academic surgery: the opportunities and challenges of inclusive recruitment strategies. *Acad Med.* 2019;94:1142-1145. doi:10.1097/ACM.0000000000002647.

6

Mentorship and Sponsorship

Jennifer F. Waljee

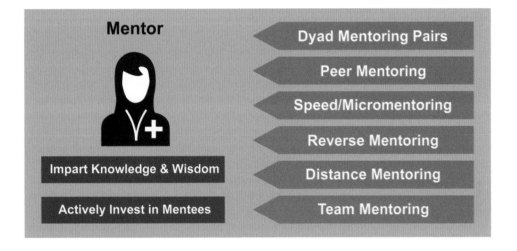

INTRODUCTION

Mentorship is defined as a professional partnership in which knowledge, skills, and wisdom are imparted between individuals for the purpose of career development and advancement. Substantial research has demonstrated the positive effect of successful mentoring relationships on professional achievement and satisfaction in many occupational sectors.[1,2] In medical and surgical disciplines, ensuring a strong and vibrant physician workforce is paramount, given the projected shortages in upcoming years among the physician workforce in the United States. For example, recent reports from the American Association of Medical Colleges suggest a lack of over 120,000 physicians within 20 years, with notable and rising differences in supply and demand for surgical specialties.[3,4] Moreover, the projected gaps in the physician workforce may be even more pronounced for individuals entering academic practice.[5,6] As such, mentorship remains the cornerstone of ensuring a vibrant, diverse, successful, and engaged workforce in academic medicine and surgery.[7]

Mentorship has been consistently cited as a successful strategy to increase the pipeline of individuals entering careers as physician scientists, as well as reducing attrition from the academic community. Successful mentorship models have been shown to enhance the professional advancement of women and underrepresented minorities, for whom substantial gaps in achievement persist and attrition is high.[8-13] For example, studies examining the career aspirations of underrepresented minority high-school, college, and medical school students reveal that few have mentorship from physician scientists, but early exposure to mentors and role models is correlated with a student's decision to pursue a career as a physician scientist.[5,8,14] In addition, studies of early career faculty members consistently demonstrate that faculty with successful mentoring relationships are more likely to have successful research portfolios and academic clinical practices.[15-17] Faculty development initiatives that explicitly emphasize mentoring have been shown to be of the most effective strategies to recruit, promote, and retain academic faculty in underrepresented minority groups.[18] Nonetheless, the penetration of structured mentorship models into academic specialties remains variable, and understanding the mentorship archetypes and challenges is important to identify best practices for achieving successful mentoring relationships.[19]

MENTORSHIP

A mentor is distinct from a teacher or role model. In their roles, mentors impart not only knowledge, as an educator would, but also wisdom regarding the expectations, opportunities, and norms of an academic career. Unlike role models who passively demonstrate behavioral norms, mentors actively invest in their mentees.[20] Numerous mentorship models have been described, including dyad mentoring pairs, peer mentoring, speed/micromentoring, reverse mentoring, distance mentoring, and team mentoring.[21] These mentoring paradigms are not mutually exclusive, and the needs of mentors and mentees are dynamic and fluid across the trajectory of a career. No single mentoring model has been identified as superior over another. Instead, the attributes of successful mentoring relationships are dependent on the context and individuals in the relationship, the organization, and professional development goals.

Dyad mentoring remains the most common model of mentorship.[21] Most traditionally, dyad mentorship appears in the form of a one-on-one relationship in which a more senior individual guides a junior individual along their career path. The mentor and mentee typically meet individually for periodic meetings at a cadence set by both.[22,23] The mentor provides feedback regarding aspects of professional life, such as academic productivity, clinical care, educator roles, and administrative service (*Figure 6.1*). Mentees will often present progress on projects, such as a manuscript for publication or a grant application to be reviewed. Other dyad models include coaching mentorship. In contrast to a traditional mentor who provides a holistic approach to professional growth, a coach is focused on helping the mentee acquire a specific skill or highly targeted areas of professional growth.[22,24] Coaching models often have meetings that occur in briefer intervals, as the guidance is tailored to focused topics, such as methodological techniques, writing, or oral presentations.

Peer mentoring models have been most commonly used for youth and education programs and involve joining mentors and mentees of similar age or level in an organization.[25-27] Peer mentors are well suited to guiding an individual, given their proximity in experiences, such as assembling a research grant or beginning as a faculty member in practice. Peer mentoring models have distinct advantages for both the mentor and mentee, as mentees may feel empowered to be candid regarding specific elements of support that are needed that they may not be comfortable asking of

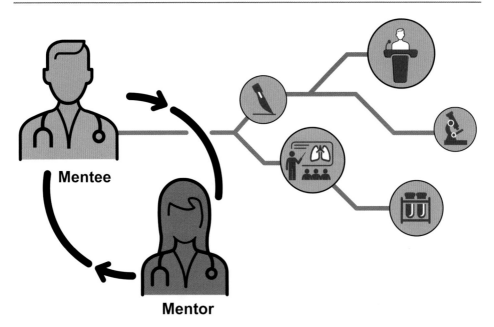

Figure 6.1 Traditional dyad mentoring relationship.

more senior mentors. In addition, peer mentorship offers an opportunity for shared resources and learning.[28] In return, peer mentors also reap tangible rewards, such as demonstrating mentorship capability that will allow them to advance for additional leadership opportunities (e.g., residency program director or medical student clerkship director), or grant programs (e.g., federally funded research mentoring awards).

Speed mentoring or micromentoring is described as mentorship that occurs in brief intervals regarding a focused topic and is often less formal than more traditional mentoring relationships.[29,30] Micromentoring models are designed for maximum efficiency and can often provide an ideal structure for mentors who have limited capacity for more in-depth mentoring relationships. Micromentoring models are best suited to specific topics, such as reviewing a curriculum vitae or personal statement, that yield tangible and pragmatic support. Micromentoring also can provide an opportunity to test out a potential mentoring relationship to determine if individuals are compatible to work together in longer-term partnerships (*Figure 6.2*).[31] Given the brevity of a micromentoring relationship, it is critical that both the mentor and mentee adhere to clear communication regarding goals, time commitment, deliverables, and expectations from the outset.

Reverse mentoring describes the process by which mentoring occurs in a bidirectional manner between the mentor and mentee and provides the mentee specific opportunities to "mentor-up."[32,33] In reverse mentoring models, mentees take ownership of learning goals to impart to a more senior mentor, which can include new techniques, methodologies, or strategies for dissemination of work (*Figure 6.3*). Reverse mentoring is advantageous in that it can allow for greater engagement of mentees in an organization. Reverse mentoring can also bridge generational gaps across mentoring relationships and provide more senior mentors unique and innovative perspectives from established norms within an organization.[22]

Although mentorship traditionally occurs in face-to-face meetings, the expansion of technology in recent decades has allowed for the evolution of distance or remote mentoring models.[34,35] These relationships can be particularly useful for mentees to

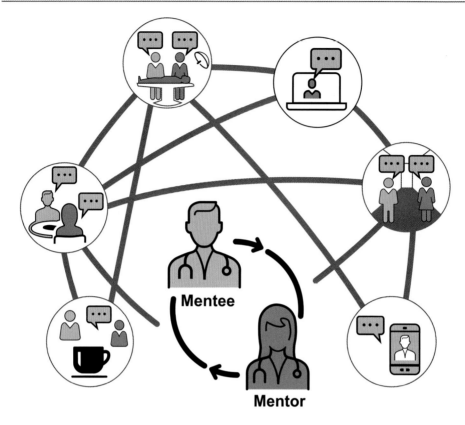

Figure 6.2 Micromentoring as a test of a potential mentoring relationship.

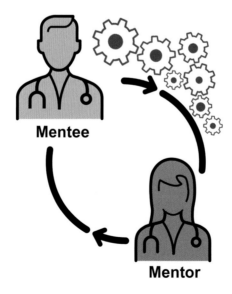

Figure 6.3 Reverse mentoring.

connect with mentors with distinct skill sets who may not be present at their institution and foster collaboration across centers. Distance mentoring is also helpful for situations in which a mentor or mentee unexpectedly transitions to a different institution, but the collaboration is expected to continue. As with other mentoring relationships, distance mentoring models function well with clear communication regarding goals and expectations and often with more regular reevaluation of progress. Explicit timelines, assigned tasks, and scheduled meetings are essential to overcome barriers due to lack of colocation.

Finally, team-based mentorship model approaches have become increasingly popular, given their ability to increase the capacity of mentorship for an individual and bring synergy across multiple phenotypes of mentors, such as traditional mentors, coaches, sponsors, and peer mentors.[28,36] Team-based models also have the advantage of engaging individuals with different areas of expertise, leveraging the power of cognitive diversity, and can allow for shared responsibility of the mentorship tasks across multiple mentors. Although mentorship teams can be challenging to coordinate logistically, they are one of the most critical strategies to provide support for individuals facing difficulty in their mentoring relationships.[36]

Mentor and Mentee Selection

Recent data suggest that identifying role models and mentors remains challenging for many early career faculty entering academic practice.[7,37] Although formal mentoring programs are increasingly prevalent, mentoring relationships most often develop organically among individuals with shared interests who meet through established academic networks.[19,23,25,27,38] For example, a recent systematic review noted that mentees most commonly prefer choosing their mentors rather than having mentors assigned.[21] Nonetheless, it may be challenging for individuals who are less visible to identify and engage mentors, such as trainees new to an academic institution or women and underrepresented minorities, and formal and intentional pathways to connect individuals in professional development remains important.[22]

The critical attributes of an effective mentor include altruism, experience, patience, and commitment.[20,36] Effective mentors are able to discern and develop an individual's talents to achieve the mentee's goals, rather than attempting to mold a mentee into a path set by the mentor. Moreover, they recognize and value potential rather than competence, and are committed to the individual rather than the tasks at hand.[2,39] As such, it is essential for mentees to recognize and select potential mentors with these attributes to develop successful relationships. Common tactics to identify potential mentors include seeking out more senior individuals with shared values and for whom the mentor's professional trajectory mirrors their goals. In addition, discussing potential mentoring relationships with current mentees and other organizational leaders (e.g., department chair or division chief) can secure recommendations for committed and effective mentors. Creating a series of introductory meetings or interactions to discuss immediate and long-term goals can illuminate the mentor's style, expectations, and commitment prior to entering a relationship.

Mentorship is defined by reciprocity, and mentors similarly derive value from mentoring relationships as well as mentees. Ideal mentee characteristics include curiosity, efficiency, accountability, engagement, and organization.[20,40] Whether relationships are initiated organically or through formal structured programs, it can be challenging to identify working and communication habits, preferences, and patterns until both mentor and mentee have invested significant time in the relationship.[39] Creating audition experiences is often advocated in order to test the compatibility of mentor/mentee relationships with small projects prior to embarking on larger projects. Examples can include tasks such as summarizing an article or writing a few paragraphs regarding a potential research topic. These opportunities provide both parties the opportunity to gauge interest, communication, and ability. Gaps, missteps, and lack of communication identified early on can provide insight and prevention for a potentially unproductive mentoring relationship.

Challenges in Mentoring Relationships and Strategies for Success

Like other partnerships, mentoring relationships evolve over time and have been described to occur in stages.[20] In the beginning, mentors and mentees are focused on understanding each other's goals and motivations in order to build the relationship.[41] In addition, trust is established during this phase in order to determine if the match is a good fit for both parties[20] (*Figure 6.4*). Most commonly, conflict arises in the second stage, in which the mentee transitions from a trainee or student to a peer. Mentors must accept the growth of the mentee and the judgment and preferences of the mentee as a colleague. Success in this transition is marked by self-awareness and generosity of both parties to respect one another's goals, ideas, and preferences, as well as honest and transparent communication.[41-43] The final stages of the relationship are marked by collaboration and advocacy, and the mentor often serves a sponsoring and coaching role for the mentee. Often, metamentorship relationships form, in which the senior mentor guides mentees in mentoring others, creating academic generations of mentees.[33]

However, mentoring relationships are vulnerable to conflict, frustration, and failure. Failure of mentoring relationships can be devastating to a career due to differences in power between individuals, the investment of resources and time, and the dissolution of collaboration between a mentor and mentee. Poor communication and lack of interpersonal connection are the primary reasons that mentoring relationships collapse. Mentee mistakes may result from conflict avoidance and/or a lack of confidence yielding communication gaps.[40] For example, mentees may be quick to commit to many projects, fearing the repercussions of saying no or due to a lack of confidence in their ability to succeed in any single project. Overcommitted mentees may be unable to deliver on products, resulting in frustration and burnout.

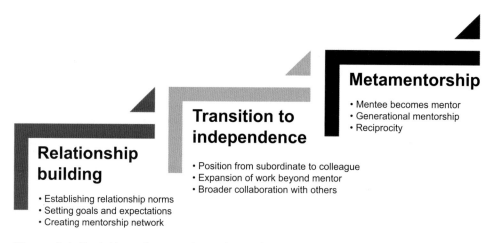

Metamentorship

• Mentee becomes mentor
• Generational mentorship
• Reciprocity

Transition to independence

• Position from subordinate to colleague
• Expansion of work beyond mentor
• Broader collaboration with others

Relationship building

• Establishing relationship norms
• Setting goals and expectations
• Creating mentorship network

Figure 6.4 Evolution of mentoring relationships.

In turn, mentors may be frustrated with mentees not recognizing their burden of work and unlikely to trust them to produce in future endeavors. Poor mentorship patterns can include both active and passive behaviors that are highly detrimental to mentees and often related to intrinsic personality and psychological attributes.[20,36] Examples include unresponsiveness, failing to acknowledge and support mentees interests and needs, isolating mentees, and failing to provide credit to mentees for their work. These maladaptive mentoring behaviors are particularly challenging, given the power differential that exists between a mentor and mentee.

As a senior or more experienced individual, mentors often set the tone of the relationship and should take the lead on conflict resolution when it arises. However, mentees should be cognizant of unhealthy behavioral patterns in mentorship, and both parties should develop active strategies to prevent the disintegration of the relationship due to misunderstanding and poor communication. Given these critical investments for both the mentor and mentee, effective communication is essential. Although conflict avoidance is common in hierarchical relationships, creating opportunities for mentees to feel empowered to speak openly regarding their goals, interests, and capacity is critical in order to avoid problematic behavior patterns.[20,36,40] In addition, it is critical that mentors create an environment in which mistakes are accepted as part of the learning process and an opportunity for growth, rather than characterized as personal failures without recourse.[42-44] At the beginning of the formal mentoring relationship, it can be helpful to document expectations and goals of both the mentor and mentee to ensure alignment. These formal agreements can also include the timing, type, and frequency for communication. Although written agreements may feel awkward to initiate, clear communication has been demonstrated as an effective practice to inform expectations for all parties and encourage accountability.[1,16,26] In addition, mentorship teams can be an important strategy to mitigate against nonproductive behaviors for both mentors and mentees.[36] Ultimately, in some cases, mentoring relationships may not be compatible, and alternate mentors may need to be considered.[42,43]

SPONSORSHIP

As distinct from mentors, sponsors serve as advocates and are typically senior individuals with sufficient connections and influence. Sponsors create opportunities for individuals, promote their work, and enhance their visibility.[45,46] Unlike mentorship, which often occurs organically and over time, sponsorship occurs episodically when individuals are noticed for their ideas and accomplishments. For example, a medical student who performs well helping gathering and organizing data will catch the eye of a more senior faculty member who then recommends the student for more prestigious opportunities. Sponsorship is explicitly different from mentorship in that it requires that a sponsor leverage his or her reputation by providing opportunities that may not otherwise be available to a protégé.[46] As such, protégés are expected to be loyal and accountable in order to deliver effectively and enhance the visibility and reputation of both parties.[47] Protégés often have a responsibility to continue to promote the mission and vision of the organization, and effective sponsorship of younger individuals can define the next generation of leaders.

Importantly, sponsors can play an active role in closing gaps in representation among women and underrepresented minorities in leadership positions by directly encouraging individuals for consideration.[45] Examples of this include recommending an individual for a speaking opportunity, a committee position, or a leadership role. Interestingly, sponsorship is often subject to implicit biases and disadvantage that perpetuate gaps in

Table 6.1 Best Practices in Mentorship and Sponsorship

	Building Relationships	Managing Conflict	Ensuring Success
Mentorship	Explicitly communicate preferences and expectations (e.g., meeting cadence, productivity, progress reporting)	Address conflict early with an open mind	Review short- and long-term career goals regularly
	Obtain references on mentor/mentee past success, productivity, and missteps	Engage a team of mentors to offer diverse perspectives and balanced feedback	Create intentional opportunities for feedback regarding preferences and experiences for both mentors and mentees
	Engage in mentorship audition experiences to test compatibility of both mentors and mentees	Develop strategies for self-awareness regarding maladaptive mentor and mentee behaviors	Prepare and embrace mentee transition to independence
	Create mentorship networks that include multiple mentoring phenotypes (e.g., coach, sponsor, peer mentor, distance mentor)	Avoid lingering in mentoring relationships marked by continued frustration	Foster generational mentoring models in which the mentee becomes mentor
Sponsorship	Seek out potential sponsors within an organization to showcase career aspirations	Create sufficient support for protégé to succeed (e.g., practice sessions for invited talks)	Create opportunities for candid feedback for sponsors and protégés
	Ascertain goals and context for sponsorship opportunities (e.g., audience at an invited talk, goals of the committee)	Communicate expectations regarding deliverables and timing to avoid unrealistic expectations	Partner with mentors to match opportunities to protégé's strengths and capacity
	Avoid overcommitment to remain accountable and deliver productively	Develop intentional sponsorship opportunities to ensure access for all potential protégés	Create awareness of opportunities for protégés to pay success forward to other individuals

academic achievement.[48] For example, sponsorship has been more commonly reported by male academic physicians than female academic physicians.[37] It is possible that female mentees have mentors with less power and opportunity to act as sponsors, especially given the propensity for same-sex mentorship dyads to occur.[49] It is also possible that implicit bias plays a role, and women are less likely to be seen as prepared or capable for sponsorship opportunities.[50] To overcome this, individuals should actively seek leaders in an organization who can serve as sponsors and share career goals, volunteer for future opportunities, and engage in projects to further the mission of the organization.

FUTURE DIRECTIONS

Given the positive effects that successful mentorship and sponsorship have on academic achievement, it is imperative to identify best practices and ensure access for all academic faculty (*Table 6.1*). Effective mentorship and menteeship are rarely explicitly taught in clinical training programs during residency or during the early years of faculty practice. Going forward, strategies to recognize the value and commitment of successful mentorship within metrics of academic promotion will be essential to foster standards of practice. In addition, formal mentor and mentee training programs can build self-awareness regarding gaps in mentoring skills to strengthen these relationships. Ensuring equitable access to strong mentorship and sponsorship for all academic faculty members can enhance the pipeline of talented individuals to pursue careers as physician scientists and create a vibrant and engaged workforce.

REFERENCES

1. Eby LT, Allen TD, Evans SC, Ng T, Dubois D. Does mentoring matter? A multidisciplinary meta-analysis comparing mentored and non-mentored individuals. *J Vocat Behav.* 2008;72(2):254-267.
2. Tjan A. *What the Best Mentors Do.* Boston, MA: Harvard Business Review; 2017.
3. American Association of Medical Colleges. *The Complexities of Physician Supply and Demand: Projections from 2017-2032.* Washington, DC: IHS Markit Ltd.; 2019.
4. Schmidt LE, Cooper CA, Guo WA. Factors influencing US medical students' decision to pursue surgery. *J Surg Res.* 2016;203(1):64-74.
5. Salata RA, Geraci MW, Rockey DC, et al. U.S. Physician-scientist workforce in the 21st century: recommendations to attract and sustain the pipeline. *Acad Med.* 2018;93(4):565-573.
6. Pololi LH, Krupat E, Civian JT, Ash AS, Brennan RT. Why are a quarter of faculty considering leaving academic medicine? A study of their perceptions of institutional culture and intentions to leave at 26 representative U.S. medical schools. *Acad Med.* 2012;87(7):859-869.
7. DeCastro R, Griffith KA, Ubel PA, Stewart A, Jagsi R. Mentoring and the career satisfaction of male and female academic medical faculty. *Acad Med.* 2014;89(2):301-311.
8. Merchant JL, Omary MB. Underrepresentation of underrepresented minorities in academic medicine: the need to enhance the pipeline and the pipe. *Gastroenterology.* 2010;138(1):19-26.e1-3.
9. Rodriguez JE, Campbell KM, Mouratidis RW. Where are the rest of us? Improving representation of minority faculty in academic medicine. *South Med J.* 2014;107(12):739-744.
10. Yu PT, Parsa PV, Hassanein O, Rogers SO, Chang DC. Minorities struggle to advance in academic medicine: a 12-y review of diversity at the highest levels of America's teaching institutions. *J Surg Res.* 2013;182(2):212-218.
11. Moyer CA, Abedini NC, Youngblood J, et al. Advancing women leaders in global health: getting to solutions. *Ann Glob Health.* 2018;84(4):743-752.
12. Abelson J, Chartrand G, Moo T, Moore M, Yeo H. The climb to break the glass ceiling in surgery: trends in women progressing from medical school to surgical training and academic leadership from 1994 to 2015. *Am J Surg.* 2016;212(4):566-572.

13. Yeo H, Viola K, Berg D, et al. Attitudes, training experiences, and professional expectations of US general surgery residents: a national survey. *J Am Med Assoc.* 2009;302(12):1301-1308.

14. Cruess SR, Cruess RL, Steinert Y. Role modelling–making the most of a powerful teaching strategy. *Br Med J.* 2008;336(7646):718-721.

15. Schoenfeld AJ. What's important: mentorship and sponsorship. *J Bone Joint Surg Am.* 2018;100(1):86-87.

16. Palepu A, Friedman RH, Barnett RC, et al. Junior faculty members' mentoring relationships and their professional development in U.S. medical schools. *Acad Med.* 1998;73(3):318-323.

17. Ries A, Wingard D, Gamst A, Larsen C, Farrell E, Reznik V. Measuring faculty retention and success in academic medicine. *Acad Med.* 2012;87(8):1046-1051.

18. Guevara JP, Adanga E, Avakame E, Carthon MB. Minority faculty development programs and underrepresented minority faculty representation at US medical schools. *J Am Med Assoc.* 2013;310(21):2297-2304.

19. Kibbe MR, Pellegrini CA, Townsend CM, Helenowski IB, Patti MG. Characterization of mentorship programs in departments of surgery in the United States. *JAMA Surg.* 2016;151(10):900-906.

20. Mulcahey MK, Waterman BR, Hart R, Daniels AH. The role of mentoring in the development of successful orthopaedic surgeons. *J Am Acad Orthop Surg.* 2018;26(13):463-471.

21. Kashiwagi DT, Varkey P, Cook DA. Mentoring programs for physicians in academic medicine: a systematic review. *Acad Med.* 2013;88(7):1029-1037.

22. Waljee JF, Chopra V, Saint S. Mentoring millennials. *J Am Med Assoc.* 2018;319(15):1547-1548.

23. Phitayakorn R, Petrusa E, Hodin RA. Development and initial results of a mandatory department of surgery faculty mentoring pilot program. *J Surg Res.* 2016;205(1):234-237.

24. McKinney CM, Mookherjee S, Fihn SD, Gallagher TH. An academic research coach: an innovative approach to increasing scholarly productivity in medicine. *J Hosp Med.* 2019;14:E1-E5.

25. Altonji SJ, Banos JH, Harada CN. Perceived benefits of a peer mentoring program for first-year medical students. *Teach Learn Med.* 2019;31(4):445-452. doi:10.1080/10401334.2019.1574579.

26. Chiu AS, Pei KY, Jean RA. Mentoring sideways-A model of resident-to-resident research mentorship. *J Surg Educ.* 2019;76(1):1-3.

27. Wiemann CM, Graham SC, Garland BH, et al. Development of a group-based, peer-mentor intervention to promote disease self-management skills among youth with chronic medical conditions. *J Pediatr Nurs.* 2019;48:1-9.

28. DeCastro R, Sambuco D, Ubel PA, Stewart A, Jagsi R. Mentor networks in academic medicine: moving beyond a dyadic conception of mentoring for junior faculty researchers. *Acad Med.* 2013;88(4):488-496.

29. Britt RC, Hildreth AN, Acker SN, Mouawad NJ, Mammen J, Moalem J. Speed mentoring: an innovative method to meet the needs of the young surgeon. *J Surg Educ.* 2017;74(6):1007-1011.

30. Wileyard K. *Engage a Mentor With a Short-Term Project.* Boston, MA: Harvard Business Review; 2014.

31. Cellini MM, Serwint JR, D'Alessandro DM, Schulte EE, Osman C. Evaluation of a speed mentoring program: achievement of short-term mentee goals and potential for longer-term relationships. *Acad Pediatr.* 2017;17(5):537-543.

32. Robinson A. Sixty seconds on… reverse mentoring. *Br Med J.* 2018;363:k4887.

33. Balmer DF, Darden A, Chandran L, D'Alessandro D, Gusic ME. How mentor identity evolves: findings from a 10-year follow-up study of a national professional development program. *Acad Med.* 2018;93(7):1085-1090.

34. Bilgic E, Turkdogan S, Watanabe Y, et al. Effectiveness of telementoring in surgery compared with on-site mentoring: a systematic review. *Surg Innov.* 2017;24(4):379-385.

35. Xu X, Schneider M, DeSorbo-Quinn AL, King AC, Allegrante JP, Nigg CR. Distance mentoring of health researchers: three case studies across the career-development trajectory. *Health Psychol Open.* 2017;4(2):2055102917734388.

36. Chopra V, Edelson DP, Saint S. A piece of my mind. Mentorship malpractice. *J Am Med Assoc.* 2016;315(14):1453-1454.

37. Patton EW, Griffith KA, Jones RD, Stewart A, Ubel PA, Jagsi R. Differences in mentor-mentee sponsorship in male vs female recipients of National Institutes of Health Grants. *JAMA Intern Med.* 2017;177(4):580-582.

38. Bussey-Jones J, Bernstein L, Higgins S, et al. Repaving the road to academic success: the IMeRGE approach to peer mentoring. *Acad Med.* 2006;81(7):674-679.
39. Chopra V, Saint S. *6 Things Every Mentor Should Do.* Boston, MA: Harvard Business Review; 2019.
40. Vaughn V, Saint S, Chopra V. Mentee missteps: tales from the academic trenches. *J Am Med Assoc.* 2017;317(5):475-476.
41. Jackson VA, Palepu A, Szalacha L, Caswell C, Carr PL, Inui T. "Having the right chemistry": a qualitative study of mentoring in academic medicine. *Acad Med.* 2003;78(3):328-334.
42. Straus SE, Johnson MO, Marquez C, Feldman MD. Characteristics of successful and failed mentoring relationships: a qualitative study across two academic health centers. *Acad Med.* 2013;88(1):82-89.
43. Straus SE, Chatur F, Taylor M. Issues in the mentor-mentee relationship in academic medicine: a qualitative study. *Acad Med.* 2009;84(1):135-139.
44. Strauss A, Corbin J. *Basics of Qualitative Research.* Thousand Oaks, CA: Sage Publications; 1998.
45. Ayyala MS, Skarupski K, Bodurtha JN, et al. Mentorship is not enough: exploring sponsorship and its role in career advancement in academic medicine. *Acad Med.* 2019;94(1):94-100.
46. Travis EL, Doty L, Helitzer DL. Sponsorship: a path to the academic medicine C-suite for women faculty?. *Acad Med.* 2013;88(10):1414-1417.
47. Hewlett SA, Marshall M, Sherbin L. *The Relationship You Need to Get Right.* Boston, MA: Harvard Business Review; 2011.
48. Hewlett SA, Marshall M, Sherbin L. *How Diversity Can Drive Innovation.* Boston, MA: Harvard Business Review; 2013.
49. Faucett EA, McCrary HC, Milinic T, Hassanzadeh T, Roward SG, Neumayer LA. The role of same-sex mentorship and organizational support in encouraging women to pursue surgery. *Am J Surg.* 2017;214(4):640-644.
50. Shakil S, Redberg RF. Gender disparities in sponsorship-how they perpetuate the glass ceiling. *JAMA Intern Med.* 2017;177(4):582.

7

Leadership Development

Justin B. Dimick

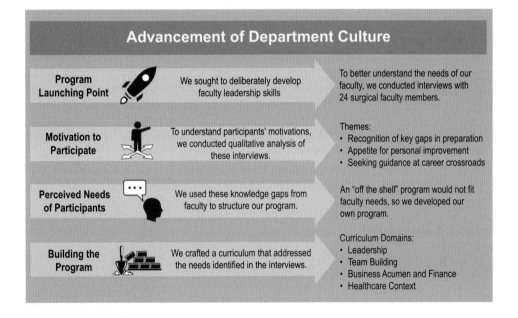

Advancement of Department Culture

| Program Launching Point | We sought to deliberately develop faculty leadership skills | To better understand the needs of our faculty, we conducted interviews with 24 surgical faculty members. |

| Motivation to Participate | To understand participants' motivations, we conducted qualitative analysis of these interviews. | Themes:
• Recognition of key gaps in preparation
• Appetite for personal improvement
• Seeking guidance at career crossroads |

| Perceived Needs of Participants | We used these knowledge gaps from faculty to structure our program. | An "off the shelf" program would not fit faculty needs, so we developed our own program. |

| Building the Program | We crafted a curriculum that addressed the needs identified in the interviews. | Curriculum Domains:
• Leadership
• Team Building
• Business Acumen and Finance
• Healthcare Context |

MOTIVATION

Leadership in academic surgery is changing. Evolving needs, structures, and sensibilities combine to create demand for a different kind of surgical leader. The hierarchical, authoritarian leadership style of many past surgical leaders will no longer (and probably never did) yield the best return on institutional resources and faculty talents.[1] At the extreme, those who exhibit the behaviors that have led to the popular characterization of surgeons as ego-driven tyrants will find themselves banished to the darkest corners of modern health systems rather than at the podium.[2]

The structures of academic health systems are also evolving rapidly. The internal structure is moving toward clinical service lines, which changes the roles of departments and their leaders.[3] This matrix structure contributes to an escalating demand for a different set of leadership skills, including collaborative goal setting, peer influence, and working as part of a team to be a good steward of the health system broadly. Moreover, as academic health systems evolve toward networks rather than hospitals, the demands for collaboration with a broader set of teammates will further accelerate these trends.[4]

The needs of leadership in science are changing as well. Investigators need to be facile in creating and leading multidisciplinary teams to be competitive in this era. True breakthroughs occur at the intersection of orthogonal fields, increasing the imperative for collaborative, interdisciplinary work. All of these changes combine to create an environment in academic surgery where a diverse set of leadership skills is required.[5]

Introduction

Despite the knowledge that more is required of surgical leaders, specific strategies to foster leadership skills among practicing surgeons are lacking. Some health systems are providing leadership development programs to develop physician leadership competencies. These programs, however, are not specifically tailored to the needs of surgeon-scientists. Given the unique demands of leading surgeon-scientists, for any such program to succeed, especially among busy clinicians, it must be designed with the specific needs of the participants in mind.[5]

This chapter tells a story of how a leadership development program was created and how it evolved over time. There were many stumbling blocks along the way, and many aspects of the program changed over the years. This process provides one path for building such a leadership development program.

Needs Assessment

In January 2011, at an annual retreat, the journey began to deliberately develop the leadership skills of faculty. All surgical faculty are leaders in their daily lives, whether conducting a complex procedure in the operating room, leading a division, or chairing a committee in a national organization. But few faculty have had the opportunity to stop, reflect, and prepare for these opportunities. Surgical training is almost entirely focused on clinical care—developing technical skills and judgment—and appropriately so. An opportunity exists to prepare faculty as leaders by addressing these gaps.

To better understand the needs of our faculty, interviews were conducted with 24 surgical faculty members who were candidates selected to participate in the first round of the program.[6] Voluntary participants were solicited for the program, including any faculty member who wanted to develop leadership skills at any rank, from Assistant to full Professor. Most had an existing leadership role or were anticipating (or hoping for) new leadership roles. All applicants were accepted, and only new faculty within 3 years of starting were not permitted to participate. These individuals should still be working on early career priorities—building clinical practices, starting research programs, and learning how to teach residents and students. These individuals did participate in a future year of the program.

Motivation to Participate

To understand the participant's motivations to participate, qualitative analysis was conducted of participant interviews.[6] These analyses demonstrated three key themes regarding faculty motivation to participate in a leadership program:

- Recognition of key gaps in preparation for leadership roles: Many participants were acutely aware that traditional medical school and residency training did not prepare them well for leadership roles.

- Appetite for personal improvement: Participants found themselves in leadership roles and were seeking opportunities to grow their skills.

- Seeking guidance while at a crossroads in their career: Participants found themselves at a point in their career where they must take on leadership responsibilities to continue to grow (*Figure 7.1*).

Perceived Needs of Participants

This qualitative analysis informed development of a competency model and curriculum.[6] There were four areas of focus for educational content:

- **Leadership and communication:** Learn effective communication and conflict resolution skills, and develop a compelling vision to motivate others.

- **Team building:** Learn to create collaborative, effective, diverse teams.

- **Business acumen/finance:** Learn about the basics of finance, marketing, strategy, and operations.

- **Understanding health care context:** Learn local context (e.g., organizational structure, and policies and procedures) and develop a greater understanding of health policy context (*Figure 7.2*).

The interviews were the basis for a competency model and guided development of the curriculum. One important insight from these interviews was that an "off the shelf" program would not fit the needs of the faculty. While there are many excellent

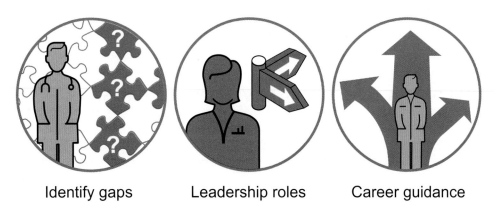

Identify gaps   Leadership roles   Career guidance

Figure 7.1 Motivation to participate in leadership development.

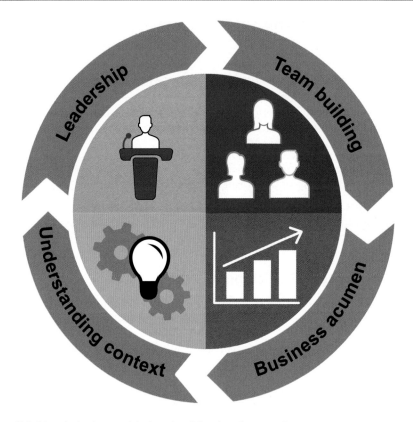

Figure 7.2 Needs to be met in leadership development.

leadership development programs offered through business schools, locally and nationally, a decision was made to develop a unique program, tailored precisely to the needs of the faculty. In particular, creating a unique program allowed substantial time in the curriculum for discussion of the local health care context, i.e., issues specific to the department and institution. To accomplish this goal, the program incorporated health system and medical school leaders to discuss granular topics, such as strategic planning, financial statements, and how the institution interfaces with national health care policies. The curriculum was also able to foster discussions with local leaders on what surgeons need to do to be active participants in health system strategy.

BUILDING A LEADERSHIP DEVELOPMENT PROGRAM

Since the needs assessment 8 years ago, the leaders have built and sustained a faculty leadership development program which has been sustained within the department of surgery. The program is repeated at intervals of 3 years, includes approximately 25 faculty, and more recently has included five to seven residents who are in their academic development time. The fourth cycle was recently completed, ushering more than half of the faculty through the program. The program became a key tool for reflection on departmental challenges and opportunities, a unique opportunity to build relationships across clinical silos, and a launching point for other faculty development initiatives. The program shows commitment to relentless development of faculty potential.

The leadership development program curriculum is shown below in *Table 7.1*.[6] The program is 8 months long and includes the following key elements:

8 Full Days of Didactics

The backbone of the program is monthly Friday sessions where the entire group is present for didactics, experiential learning, and in-person group projects.

Table 7.1 Curriculum of the University of Michigan Department of Surgery Leadership Development Program

Domain	Description	Elements in the Program
Leadership	Learn effective communication and conflict resolution skills. Develop a compelling vision to motivate others.	• 1 full day of didactics on "Leading Organizations" • Longitudinal independent reading assignments • 360-Degree evaluations completed by all participants • 2 sessions with an executive coach to debrief on 360-degree evaluations and to generate a personalized leadership action plan
Team building	Learn to foster collaborative, effective, and diverse teams.	• 2 full days of didactics on "Building Diverse Teams" and "Innovation" • Longitudinal independent reading assignments • Longitudinal team projects with an 8-mo deliverable (at program conclusion) as well as a 2-y plan to integrate the project into real-world activity within the Department of Surgery
Business acumen and finance	Learn about the basics of finance, marketing, strategy, and operations.	• 3 full days of didactics on "Understanding Financial Statements," "Capital in Healthcare Systems," and "Introduction to Operations Management" • Group exercise with hospital executive to teach how to interpret financial statements of health system and timeline for capital expenditures in the health system • Division administrators reviewing financial statements from the Department of Surgery
Healthcare context	Learn local context (e.g., organizational structure, policies, and procedures) and acquire a greater understanding of health policy context.	• 2 full days of didactics on "Healthcare Policy" and "Strategy in Healthcare" • Multiple interactive sessions with local leaders (i.e., Hospital CEO, Medical School Dean) • Reviewing Health System Strategic Plan, including Clinical Network Strategy

Prior to enrolling, faculty are required to clear their schedule and commit to attend all sessions, as it is believed that "dropping in and out" would disrupt the cohort effect. For each of the 8 days, the program makes it a priority to include high-quality didactics, engaging speakers, and content that would be valuable to the cohort. These days are designed to support learning in each of the areas of competency, including leadership, team building, business acumen, and healthcare context.

360-Degree Feedback and Coaching

Each participant undergoes a 360-degree evaluation by their direct reports, peers, and supervisors. The instrument was developed using questions from other validated sources that were combined to understand faculty performance according to the competency model. It was also thought important to expose the faculty to executive coaching as a tool for personal improvement. Each participant had two sessions with a coach to debrief and develop a personal improvement plan.

Longitudinal Group Projects

To enhance team building among the cohort, participants conducted group projects during the program. There are a broad range of group projects, but they all aim in some way to improve the department of surgery using what was learned during the program. Many of the projects have gone on to launch new faculty development programs that were designed to enhance faculty engagement and culture.

LEARNINGS

Years ago, the author was interviewing a faculty candidate and read on their CV that they had attended several leadership development seminars. As someone deeply interested in personal development, I asked the individual what they had learned from participation. They replied: "Nothing really, you know these things are mostly fluff, they just look good on your resume." Obviously, this did not reflect well on this individual's mindset about leadership development. Nonetheless, it made me reflect on my own goals in designing a leadership development program and what the learning goals should realistically be, leaving me with the question of "what can you actually learn from these programs?"

The first and foremost issue with leadership development is this: You will gain nothing if you are not open to learning. This may seem obvious, but it may be a prevalent sentiment given the anecdote shared above. It is probably worth saying that this is true for both organizations and individuals. If the culture of the organization doesn't support this type of program, then launching such a program would need to be part of a systematic attempt to shift toward a culture that intentionally fosters development. In many ways, simply organizing and running a faculty development seminar sends a strong message that department leadership is investing time, effort, and resources in the growth of faculty.

The evidence on leadership development indicates that **disciplined reflection** is the single most effective element of these programs. The design of the program and all the supporting structures should therefore be aimed at introducing new ideas (e.g., **mental models**) and providing ample space for individual and group reflection on these ideas. Physicians spend a great deal of time learning about mental

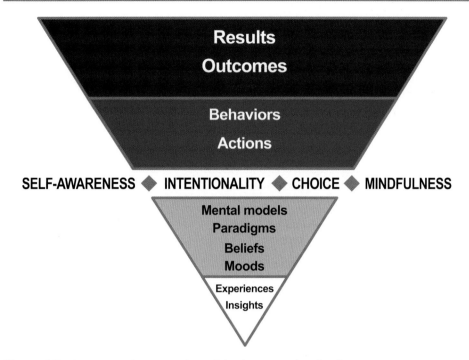

Figure 7.3 Elements of a mental model relevant to leadership.

models of molecular biology and physiology (e.g., the Krebs citric acid cycle) but spend much less time developing a deeper understanding of mental models of human interaction (*Figure 7.3*).

Disciplined reflection around mental models (e.g., conflict management, emotional intelligence, leadership, and change management) will allow individuals to see these organizational relationships in a more complex, sophisticated way. As individuals improve their ability to navigate complex organizational problems more adeptly, the organization is able to achieve more. Thus, the goal of the program was to introduce new mental models to support each of the areas of core competency, in a way that was engaging, fun, and multimodal and allowed for faculty participants to interact with, use, and discuss these new ways of seeing the world. These principles are discussed in more depth in the next section on design principles for leadership development programs.

DESIGN PRINCIPLES

This section provides several practical design principles (*Table 7.2*), which may be useful to those aiming to foster faculty leadership development through similar programs.[7]

Target the Right Participants

Selecting participants at the right time in their professional lives is important to the success of a program. First, participants need to be far enough into their faculty position, so their clinical practice and research program is fully launched. One may want to consider creating a complementary program for early career surgeons. Second, as discussed above, participants must be externally open to improving their leadership

Table 7.2 Design Principles for Building a Faculty Leadership Development Program

	Design Principle	Implementation
	Target the right participants: Faculty should be far enough along so their clinical practice and/or academic niche are defined.	We enrolled surgeons who had been on faculty at least 3 y but evaluated each individual participant's readiness.
	Ensure a high quality experience: Surgeon's time is extremely valuable and any program should be designed to use this precious resource well.	Choose high-quality speakers and facilitators. Scout for talent and evaluate by direct experience, e.g., go to the business school and watch them speak.
	Combine theory with practical information: Introducing new mental models and theory is necessary but not sufficient. Supplement didactics on theory with practical knowledge.	We combined didactics on financial management with an exercise reading department and division financial statements.
	Focus on feedback and coaching: Identifying blind spots can be essential for improving self-awareness and building leadership capabilities.	All participants engaged in 360-degree feedback and two sessions with an executive coach for debriefing and designing an action plan.
	Create leadership auditions: The best way to learn about leadership and administration is on-the-job experience. Create new roles or opportunities for emerging leaders who participate in the program.	Participants in the program were provided new roles including associate chairs (e.g., education, quality, faculty development), directors of clinical programs, and associate chief of staff with the hospital.
	Include department leadership: Active participation of department leadership allows them to role-model continuous learning and humility, participate in team building, and add their expertise.	The chair of our department was present at all sessions and participated in all program activities with other faculty.
	Rigorous evaluation: Given the amount of time allocated to these activities, it is important to evaluate their impact on growth and perceived value to participants.	We conduct evaluations at the end of each session as well as program exit. We interview participants at 1- and 5-y to formally understand the long-term career impact of the program.

Practical tips for constructing a faculty leadership development program in a department of surgery. Originally published in Dimick JB, Mulholland MW. Design principles for building a leadership development program in a Department of Surgery. *Ann Surg.* 2018;267:39-41.

skills. For the described program, all faculty who are more than 3 years out of training are invited to participate. Some but not all participants will hold leadership roles at the start of the program. It is believed that all faculty benefit from leadership training as they lead teams, run committees, and/or build clinical programs.

Ensure a High-Quality Experience

Surgeons are busy and will quickly be dismissive of any event they perceive is wasting their time. It is important to find high-quality faculty to teach and moderate the program. One must ensure that one selects the best speakers and also coordinates content to ensure it would be relevant and perceived as valuable to the enrollees. When deciding on faculty, a good idea is to visit business schools and listen to speakers in advance. Ensuring high-quality content is always a work in progress. After the first series, program evaluation guided changes to speakers and formats that were perceived as less beneficial.

Combine Theory With Practical Information

The program includes didactics on the theory of leadership, strategy, finance, and other topics. This raises the sophistication of participants' knowledge and helps them begin the process of disciplined reflection. However, it is particularly valuable to add practical context and interaction with hospital and department administrators whenever possible. Within the program, one session focuses on the theory of healthcare strategy in the morning followed by the health system CEO presenting the strategic plan in the afternoon. In the session on finance, the morning is devoted to understanding the format of financial statements. In the afternoon, department administrators walk the faculty through their own division's financial statements. The program coordinators also invite the division administrators to attend and use small group exercises for each division.

Focus on Feedback and Coaching

Learning and reflecting on new, more complex mental models is important. But the best way to accelerate learning is to help participants understand where their existing models lead them astray—i.e., help them identify their blind spots. The participants complete comprehensive 360-degree feedback evaluations. How do you help participants improve once they receive feedback? The program has found executive coaches to be extremely valuable. Each participant engages with a coach to digest the 360-degree feedback and develop a personal improvement plan. As personal coaching can be expensive, the program works with several local coaches who agreed to offer two sessions at a reduced rate, for which the department pays.

Create Leadership Auditions

It is difficult to develop more complex mental models without real-world opportunities to learn by trial and error. To provide this substrate for learning, all participants were given leadership auditions. As mentioned, some but not all of the participants held formal roles at the start of the program. For those without existing roles, the department chair created roles or opportunities that matched the needs of the individual. As with all new leadership roles, there should be clear expectations about what constitutes success.

Include Department Leadership in the Program

The program includes the department chair in all sessions of the leadership development program, including group projects, 360-degree evaluations, and coaching. It is believed that chair participation demonstrates commitment of the administration to the program. It also allows for the chair to model being externally open during the sessions—i.e., if the chair is taking it seriously and demonstrating vulnerability and learning, the other faculty should too. Finally, being present allows the chair to appreciate which faculty members need to be moved into a new leadership audition.

Rigorous Evaluation

Given the amount of time allocated to these activities by faculty, it is important to evaluate the impact of the program on personal growth and department culture. The program conducts evaluations at the end of each session to evaluate the content as well as at program exit. It also conducts semistructured interviews and subjects the transcripts to formal qualitative analysis. To date, the program has conducted interviews at 1 year and 5 years to better understand the long-term career impact of the program.

PROGRAM EVALUATION

Because program leaders were interested in the impact of the program on the organization, they engaged in methods of sociology research to explore the perspectives of the surgeon participants. To best understand what benefits the participants experienced, the program conducted semistructured interviews at 1 year and 5 years after participating in the program.[8] The transcripts were analyzed using qualitative research techniques to systematically understand the impact and room for improvement in the program.

Evaluation at 1 Year

In one-year follow-up interviews, participant comments on the effectiveness of various aspects of the program revolved around four themes: **self-empowerment, self-awareness, team building skills**, and **leadership knowledge** (*Table 7.3*).[8]

Many participants described feeling more empowered and capable of affecting change in their local environments. One participant reported, "I'm more confident about stepping up as a leader," demonstrating an empowered perspective. Participants also reported an increased self-awareness, specifically referring to their experience with the 360-degree evaluations. One surgeon commented that the program "helped me understand how others view me and my interactions." The program was broadly viewed to enhance surgeons' understanding of their own leadership strengths and weaknesses.[8]

Another theme that emerged was improved team building across the department. Participants reported a better understanding of how to foster collaborative relationships among team members.[8] Some reported specific behavioral changes, such as "giving feedback, both positive and negative," and exercising patience. Lastly, the program helped faculty surgeons become more knowledgeable regarding leadership concepts such as business acumen and organizational structure. Surgeons acknowledged a better understanding of "business/organizational issues" and "marketing and innovations concepts."

Table 7.3 **What Surgeon Participants Gained From the Leadership Development Program**

Theme	Explanation	Representative Quotes
1. Self-empowerment	Participants felt enabled and capable of affecting change locally.	"My department actually saw me as a leader." "I'm more confident about stepping up as a leader."
2. Increased self-awareness	Participants increased their understanding of how they are viewed by others. Personal blind spots were identified.	"I appear busy, frazzled. I appear unapproachable." "Didn't realize other people knew how shy I was; how valued my opinions are." "Helped me understand how others view me and my interactions."
3. Improved team building skills	Participants felt they improved their own ability to develop productive teams. The program also enhanced collegiality among surgeons enrolled in the program.	"[I can work on] giving feedback, both positive and negative." "Morale-boosting event; bringing people together to bond over a common goal." "Bonding experience; seeing, knowing colleagues better."
4. Leadership knowledge	Knowledge was gained in context of leadership definitions, business acumen, and organizational structure and purpose.	"Can now recognize leadership." "Business/organizational issues." "Marketing and innovations concepts." "Understand the higher purpose first."

Evaluation at 5 Years

To better understand the longer-term impact of the leadership development program, program leaders conducted semistructured interviews of participants at 5 years. As with the prior work, the transcripts were evaluated using qualitative research techniques with the goal of understanding important themes from the perspective of participating faculty.

This analysis demonstrated several areas of lasting impact from the curriculum of the leadership development program. Notably, the majority of participants report that the most important long-term takeaways were their personal growth and intentional reflection rather than business or technical competencies (e.g., finance or operations). Specifically, they reported the program helped develop their personal leadership skills in three ways:

Becoming More "Other-Focused"

Many participants described a shift toward a "servant-type" leadership style and improvement in leadership skills (e.g., active listening).

Opportunity for Feedback and Disciplined Reflection

Commonly, participants described that the program advanced their leadership skills by providing a structured and much-needed opportunity for reflection and personal growth (e.g., identifying and addressing blind spots).

Clarify Career Trajectory

A common theme was that the program encouraged participants to develop much greater clarity in their path to achieve their career goals, i.e., a "road map" to understand how to navigate forward (*Figure 7.4*).

Based on these qualitative data, it was concluded that at five years of follow-up, surgeons participating in the leadership development program found it to be a valuable experience with lasting impact on their personal and professional development. The dedicated time for reflection and individual development was seen as a major benefit of the program. The participants saw the program as a beneficial pause in an otherwise demanding clinical and academic schedule resulting in their ability to refocus and reprioritize personal and professional development.

IMPACT ON CULTURE

The majority of studies on leadership programs evaluate the impact on the individual surgeon. However, these programs can have a broader impact on the culture of a department. As the program advanced, leaders anecdotally noticed changes in the cultural norms that were attributed by faculty to the program. To explore this systematically, the program leaders included questions in the 5-year evaluation semistructured interviews about faculty perceptions of the impact on culture.[9]

Analysis of the interviews revealed several perceived cultural changes that were potentially attributable to the Leadership Development Program. These changes included a more participative leadership style, an increased culture of diversity, and an improved collegial environment. However, it is important to note that many participants raised the issue that it is not clear whether the program led to these changes, or the creation of a program was a part of a broader shift in these cultural values.

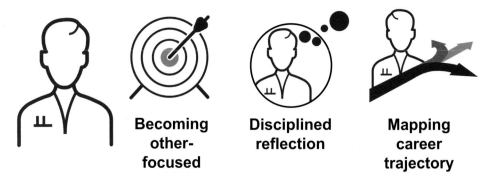

Becoming other-focused   **Disciplined reflection**   **Mapping career trajectory**

Figure 7.4 Lasting impact of leadership development.

PARTICIPATIVE LEADERSHIP

When asked to reflect on how the program impacted the prevailing leadership style in the department, many participants perceived that the norm has shifted toward being less "top-down," less hierarchical, and more collaborative. Many cited the combined personal growth of participating faculty in a variety of areas, including paying greater attention to strengths and weaknesses, improved listening skills, less agenda setting, and improved ability to delegate. This transition has contributed to a more participatory approach to how decisions are made in the department of surgery. These changes in leadership capabilities have had an impact on effectiveness within the department, and as one participant described it, when "people perform better as leaders, that translates to culture."

CULTURE OF DIVERSITY

Many participants described the department as having shifted toward being more inclusive with a more diverse range of skill sets being valued. The participants noted in particular that the increase in diversity can be seen not only in gender or race but also in the diversity of ideas being offered. These changes are reflected in how things have been done in the past, where advancement opportunities were often based on seniority. These changes were not identified as being a complete shift in hierarchal approach but rather "an awareness that we have a unique group of people and we do desire to tap into them."

COLLEGIAL ENVIRONMENT

A major prevailing theme was how the combined personal growth of participants translated to an improvement in the collegial environment, including an increase in morale and strengthened relationships. Specifically, the program helped to create opportunities to network and interact with colleagues from other clinical areas—breaking down silos of clinical specialty.

THE FUTURE

Over the last 8 years, the leadership development program has evolved in several key directions. First, its leaders are continually updating the schedule to iteratively improve the content, including both the quality of the speakers and tinkering with the recipe to find the right mix of theory and practice.

The program has added Masters Classes on years when the full program is not offered. The leaders have found that running the program every 3 years allows the program to build up a cohort of 20 to 25 faculty that are enthusiastic to participate. However, because of the ongoing appetite for faculty development, the department offers a program in Masters Classes once in the 3-year cycle. Instead of a longitudinal program, these are a la carte, allowing any faculty to sign up for any one or more of the sessions. Many faculty who sign up are alumni of the program, but others have not yet participated. These a la carte courses also allow the program to add topics that are timely and important to the department's faculty development needs at the time.

Third, the program has expanded its efforts to focus explicitly on trainee leadership development. The Leadership Development Program offers participation to residents (alongside faculty) during their academic development time. Approximately five to seven residents enroll and attend all sessions. These residents tend to be those that already have health system or department leadership in their career trajectory and want to start their learning curve earlier. However, the program leadership has noted other gaps in resident development that require addressing in a broader curriculum for house officers.[10] Namely, residents have an absolutely central role in running clinical teams within the department but receive very little training in how to do this. The program is therefore creating a curriculum for all residents to address those gaps and improve the nontechnical skills of our trainees. The program includes didactic elements, feedback on blind spots, and personal action plans to address those blind spots.[10]

CONCLUSION

Leadership development programs can be highly influential in shaping the culture of a department. Creating these programs supports a culture of relentless faculty development, sending a strong message to the faculty that the department cares about their development. Faculty engagement depends on providing tailored challenges and opportunities for growth toward individualized goals. While the challenges are everywhere in academic surgery, opportunities for growth are less common and should be intentionally created. The cadence of conducting a leadership program every few years serves as an important source of cultural rejuvenation for a department. As young leaders are developed, and opportunities for leadership auditions are created, faculty engagement increases, bringing greater levels of discretionary energy to move the department forward.

REFERENCES

1. Myers CG, Lu-Myers Y, Ghaferi AA. Excising the "surgeon ego" to accelerate progress in the culture of surgery. *Br Med J.* 2018;363:k4537.
2. Cochran A, Elder WB. A model of disruptive surgeon behavior in the perioperative environment. *J Am Coll Surg.* 2014;219:390-398.
3. Stoller JK. Recommendations and remaining questions for health care leadership training programs. *Acad Med.* 2013;88:12-15.
4. Moses H III, Matheson DH, Dorsey ER, George BP, Sadoff D, Yoshimura S. The anatomy of health care in the United States. *J Am Med Asoc.* 2013;310:1947-1963.
5. Rosengart TK, Kent KC, Bland KI, et al. Key tenets of effective surgery leadership: perspectives from the society of surgical chairs mentorship sessions. *JAMA Surg.* 2016;151:768-770.
6. Jaffe GA, Pradarelli JC, Lemak CH, Mulholland MW, Dimick JB. Designing a leadership development program for surgeons. *J Surg Res.* 2016;200:53-58.
7. Dimick JB, Mulholland MW. Design principles for building a leadership development program in a Department of Surgery. *Ann Surg.* 2018;267:39-41.
8. Pradarelli JC, Jaffe GA, Lemak CH, Mulholland MW, Dimick JB. A leadership development program for surgeons: first-year participant evaluation. *Surgery.* 2016;160:255-263.
9. Vitous CA, Shubeck SP, Kanters AE, Mulholland MW, Dimick JB. Reflections on leadership development program: impacts on culture in a surgical environment. *Surgery.* 2019;166(5):721-725.
10. Vu JV, Harbaugh CM, Dimick JB. The need for leadership training in surgical residency. *JAMA Surg.* 2019;154(7):575-576.

8

Innovation and Entrepreneurship in Surgery: Creating a Culture for Success

Mark S. Cohen

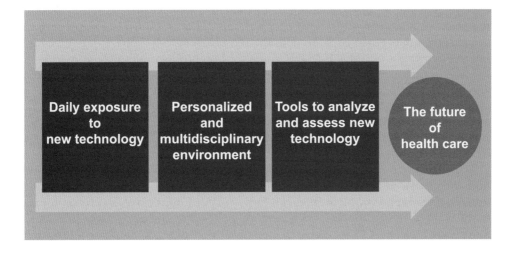

INTRODUCTION

The future of health care rides on a wave of technological advances that improve not only patients' lives but also their experience and how they can be treated in a personalized and multidisciplinary environment. Clinicians are key stakeholders in this environment where medical technology is exponentially advancing. As such, surgeons and trainees are exposed daily to new technologies being applied to their practice. More than ever, they need to have the right tools to understand how these technologies affect patient care and improve surgical diseases, but also how to decide which technologies are the safest and most impactful for their patients.

Surgeons at academic medical centers are well exposed to the missions of education, research, and clinical excellence and are continually pushing the field forward to improve care. In this role, they are commonly involved in trialing new surgical devices and are sought by industry to collaborate and develop new surgical technologies. They see problems in their practices each day that they would like to solve or improve, making them natural innovators. While identifying surgical problems is important, having the right tools to create surgical innovations that can move out of the academic environment and have meaningful impact for patients is a skill set that in the past has not been cultivated, promoted, or rewarded in academic institutions.

The goal of this chapter is to provide an overview of how building a culture in academic surgery that cultivates and rewards surgical innovation and creates multidisciplinary diverse teams can have meaningful and long-lasting success. Such efforts create value for surgeons and trainees participating in these innovative and creative endeavors, but also create meaningful impact for patients, additional sources of funding for academic departments, and build a more collaborative environment for solution implementation.

THE INNOVATIVE PROCESS

In looking at the innovation process one must start with a problem to be solved. Whether this is a need for a new device that helps with a procedure, a new drug to treat a disease, a better diagnostic tool, a new process that is more efficient, or creating a digital or virtual solution to a problem, every new innovation hinges on the problem it addresses. Therefore, as with any research effort, it is imperative to spend some quality time early on defining the problem to be solved and determining whether this is a problem that is worth solving. Problem identification, while it appears straightforward, requires a multidisciplinary approach. For every problem and solution, there are numerous stakeholders affected by both and the "value" of a solution is defined by its net positive impact across this entire map of stakeholders. Defining those stakeholders and engaging them early in the solution development process is imperative to obtaining critical feedback that can make or break an idea or solution moving forward to impact.

While there are many methods to problem identification and solution generation, the process of "design thinking" is a very effective way to create high-value solutions to meaningful problems that can move forward more easily to create impact in the market. Design thinking is an iterative process for solving complex problems. Since most problems in medicine are relatively complex, this process lends itself well to medical innovations. The common steps in design thinking include problem identification; ideation and prototype solution development; concept hardening/ prototype testing and iterative solution de-risking; and finally generating the high-impact value proposition. While these steps are often performed sequentially, they may be done out of order depending on the solution and circumstances of the problem[1] (*Figure 8.1*).

Problem Identification

The first and most important step in this innovation process is problem identification. Once a stakeholder map is generated around a problem, it is important to get feedback from as many stakeholders as possible about the impact the problem has on each of them. Empathizing with the "pain" of the problem for stakeholders is

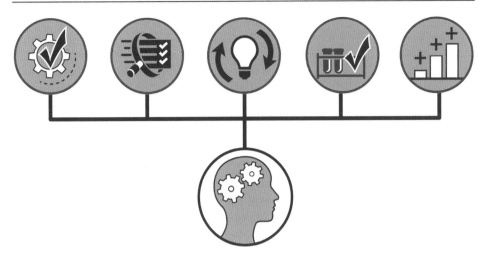

Figure 8.1 Design thinking is an iterative process for solving complex problems. Since most problems in medicine are relatively complex, this process lends itself well to medical innovations. The common steps in design thinking include problem identification; ideation and prototype solution development; concept hardening/prototype testing and iterative solution de-risking; and finally generating the high-impact value proposition.

crucial to defining the problem through a diverse lens. An example of this could be the problem of an anastomotic leak after bowel resection. Anastomotic leaks while uncommon with current anastomotic staplers can be a devastating problem for patients when they occur. This complication not only affects the patient, but also can affect their families, and prolonged hospital admissions add significant costs to the healthcare system that affects payors and insurance providers. While some surgeons create their anastomoses entirely with sutures, others use stapling devices that may be faster but have similar failure rates. Understanding the problem and impact of current solutions from each of these stakeholder lenses will be important in order to develop a new solution that best addresses each of their concerns. This stakeholder engagement is called customer discovery and is a pillar of the innovation process. Many good ideas fail in the real world due to a lack of extensive customer discovery as they either solve a problem for which customers do not need a new solution or do not adequately solve the problem the customer really has.

Scoping the Problem

Another important aspect to problem identification is scope. If the problem is only experienced by a small number of stakeholders, then it will often be very challenging to gain investors and resources to move the solution into the market unless the solution is highly impactful and one finds the right niche community to support its development and implementation. For solutions that have high value and impact millions of stakeholders, gaining investment and adoption can be much easier. An example might be the problem of postprocedural complications. While this problem affects millions of people per year globally, on root cause analysis, one would quickly determine that this problem is multifactorial and depends greatly on the type of procedure performed. As such, a single solution could never address all postprocedural complications. Instead it would be better to focus on a more solvable problem such as catheter-associated urinary tract infections after laparoscopic appendectomy procedures. Such a solution may be easier to develop and test in a group where the problem is more specifically understood. It is very important therefore to take the time to perform root cause and stakeholder analyses of what one wants to solve for the customer, and then understand the scope of how big or small the problem is for the market. This process will also help one understand the level and types of resources needed to advance the solution.

Evaluating Current Solutions and Stakeholder Feedback

After scoping and problem identification, the next step in the process is to determine what if any solutions currently exist for the problem and what are their limitations. This step will help develop the value or competitive advantage of the solution over existing technologies. Creating this competitive value is very important to gain interest not only from stakeholders who seek a better solution but also from investors who see a market advantage they can capitalize on if they provide resources to move the solution forward.

The most significant question that has to be addressed by any innovative solution is stakeholder buy-in (i.e., who will care if I solve this?) and who is affected by the solution one is proposing. As part of that identification, it is also important to determine whether that effect is positive or negative. For example, if one creates a new smartphone app that uses the camera and artificial intelligence algorithms to diagnose macular degeneration, while it may be a great potential solution and win for primary care physicians and patients, this solution may be looked at negatively by the ophthalmology community where their practice and billing would be negatively affected by such a technology. Negative influencers can have as great an impact on whether a technology makes it to the market as positive influencers so it is critical early in the solution development process to think about the effects of that solution on *all* stakeholders.

Ideation and Solution Development

Once the focused, specific problem to be solved has been defined and initial stakeholder input is obtained, the next phase of the innovation process is ideation and brainstorming potential solutions. Many successful companies and entrepreneurs advocate that the best solutions come from a diverse, team-based approach to brainstorming and problem-solving. Through the power of diversity of thought and experience, these multidisciplinary teams can create solutions that address the problem through multiple lenses and viewpoints, which often create more powerful and resilient solutions when the complexity of the problem is high. Using a diverse group to brainstorm also allows new ideas to be rapidly tested against the problem conceptually from multiple perspectives where gaps in the solution can be more quickly identified. Generating multiple solutions helps identify weaknesses in solutions as well as which ideas have the best chance at solving the problem for the most stakeholders. This helps focus solutions down more quickly to a lead innovation with which to move forward for testing.

Concept Hardening and Prototype Testing

After defining a lead solution to move forward, the idea needs to be thoroughly tested to determine how it will perform at solving the problem for stakeholders. Feedback during this period will identify additional weaknesses that can be used to update the solution to overcome and to better fit the needs of the customer. With each iterative improvement, the solution should go back to stakeholders to get more feedback to make sure the changes indeed make the solution better for them each time. This iterative process shores up weaknesses in the solution and "hardens" it to be more resilient to weather the challenges it will face in the market. Innovation concepts that have been hardened in this way are more likely to garner investors and additional stakeholder buy-in.

Creating a Compelling Value Proposition

Once a solution for a defined problem has been created and tested to make sure it solves the problem well for key stakeholders, the new innovation now needs resources, finances, and support to move forward to impact in the market. To gain these resources and support, the solution needs to be framed as a compelling value proposition. A value proposition essentially is an easily understood statement that puts forth the rationale for an innovation. In simple terms, a value proposition can be stated as: Stakeholders have a problem they would like solved, and the proposed innovation solution is better than existing alternatives, resulting in a compelling value to the customer.[2]

Defining "value" to stakeholders depends on the impact the problem has on the stakeholder as well as the limitations of current solutions being used to address or circumvent the problem. Value is often expressed in a quantifiable magnitude such as benefits of cost, time, outcomes, etc. For example, "the new solution will save $3000 per procedure," "our device will decrease operative times by an average of 35 minutes," or "this solution will result in 10% fewer wound infections than standard methods."

In the design thinking process, once a solution has gone through initial concept hardening to create a more compelling value proposition, that value proposition must then be tested further to collect enough data that the innovator and investors feel that the solution will weather market forces and create meaningful impact. This is a time for additional customer discovery with the lead product to test its value for solving the problem. Stakeholders can be separated by their level of influence on the use of the solution as well as their level of motivation for adopting the new solution. Those who pay for a product or solution typically rank higher on the axis of influence, while those who gain or lose financially as a result of adopting an innovation are typically the most motivated to promote or block implementation of the solution. Customer discovery is always better done in person and it is important for the innovation team to be prepared with the right questions to ask stakeholders to ensure they are really assessing how the solution brings value to solve the problem for the stakeholder.

A value proposition in many ways is a hypothesis that must be tested to prove its validity and meaning to stakeholders. Since this testing and validation process often has some cost associated with it, the scope of that cost may depend on the size of the problem being addressed, the invasiveness of the solution to patients, and the level of testing that was needed for current approved solutions in the market. The innovation will also need to be evaluated on how it will get into the market and how it will be adopted once in the market. This often will require understanding and navigation of its regulatory pathway, intellectual property, adoption in the market, competitive advantage, and reimbursement strategy especially if it is replacing or competing with existing solutions. All of these factors can create costs and hurdles that the innovation must clear to move forward. Identifying these hurdles early is critical in order to understand the cost, time, and process needed to overcome them. If these hurdles are too costly or too time-consuming, it may limit the viability of the innovation moving forward into the market. Defining these hurdles and failure of progression early in the process is highly important to avoid putting significant resources and time into ideas that will not ultimately succeed in the market. For each of the hurdles that can be overcome or mitigated, the technology becomes less risky from an investment standpoint and instead becomes de-risked and more likely to generate revenues or succeed in the market. As such, the more de-risked an innovation becomes, the higher the chance investors or strategic partners will be interested in putting additional resources into it to move it to the next level.

The high cost associated with moving innovations out of academia and into the market is often more than the innovator or an academic institution can bear alone and therefore partnerships with industry or investors become paramount for these technologies. Creating a compelling value proposition with early de-risking of the technology is the best way for an inventor to gain resources, partners, and investors to help move the technology through these premarket hurdles to where it can be used in the clinic.

BUILDING A CULTURE OF INNOVATION

Culture is often labeled as part of the "soul" of an organization. Culture is based on values, traditions, beliefs, and rules. For an academic surgery department, culture must also align with the institution(s) that comprise the surgeons' work environment, which often includes hospital networks and clinics, medical schools, and universities. Academic culture has long been driven by research, education, and clinical excellence. However, an integral part of those missions is to advance the field and improve the lives of patients. In this domain, innovation plays a critical role and brings together all three primary missions in a way that can leverage change and growth and adoption of new technologies in a meaningful way. Innovation, therefore, has long been an integral part of the DNA or fabric of academic medical centers, but until recently has not been a focus for developing meaningful resources to promote development and success internally. "Creating a true culture of innovation in an academic medical center has been a challenge in the past due to the rigors of academic careers, required milestones for faculty and institutions, and limitations stemming from financial concerns or mistrust of developing partnerships with Industry."[3] Fortunately, we are now in a time where new disruptive innovative technologies in health care are entering the market every week. Expansion, consumerism, and competition for patients and their healthcare dollars have created a new opportunity for hospitals to gain a competitive advantage in crowded healthcare markets. No longer can the standard academic missions be the only reason patients come to academic medical centers, but instead patients are now demanding value-based care and the most advanced, cutting-edge medical technologies and treatments. This has created a competitive atmosphere where institutions must be able to develop and disseminate innovation in order to thrive and successfully compete. This competitive culture between hospitals and institutions creates a necessity for innovation, and institutions are now realizing that putting resources into developing innovation and entrepreneurship may provide them with a competitive advantage over their peers.

In order to create a successful culture for innovation at an academic department of surgery, there are several resources that need to be made available to innovators and several traditional barriers that need to be brought down. Traditionally, academic institutions have discouraged faculty from participating in entrepreneurial activities through a number of "barriers" including lack of recognition for faculty engaging in this work, lack of opportunities for academic promotion and advancement based on innovation entrepreneurial endeavors, and lack of financial resources to help with innovation efforts. Added to this were stricter policies in the last decade regarding industry–academic relationships, conflict of interest and its management, and moving university intellectual property into startups and license deals. These barriers varied across institutions but together provided significant challenges for many surgeon-innovators and entrepreneurs to move their ideas forward or out of the university in an efficient manner.

To create culture change, one must first understand the existing local culture, the existing barriers to change, and the stakeholders affected by a change in culture. Culture change requires significant stakeholder buy-in as well as momentum from other outside efforts that allows acceptance of a new paradigm or mental model to exist and be sustainable. In the Department of Surgery at the University of Michigan, an initial stakeholder analysis was performed along with significant "customer discovery" and needs assessment. While there were a few faculty actively engaged in innovation and entrepreneurial efforts, most felt this was time spent away from the research, education, and clinical care missions upon which their academic careers and salaries were being evaluated. Additionally, there was no "extra funding" available for higher risk ideas that did not generate publications or grant applications.

As with many changes in culture, things often start with one new idea that leads to a ripple effect that then leads to several other great ideas that together build a wave of momentum that drives adoption and assimilation. In order to ensure culture change is adopted in an organization, there usually needs to be complete buy-in and often meaningful initial efforts spearheaded by leadership so that everyone within the organization feels like buy-in is acceptable and supported. In early 2014 under the leadership of Medical School Dean, a $4.35M gift from the William Davidson Foundation was awarded to the University of Michigan to support programs that accelerate the flow of U-M-generated ideas to the marketplace and spur economic activity in southeast Michigan. The medical school committed additional funds and together with $2.9M from the foundation gift created the Medical School's Fast Forward Medical Innovation (FFMI) effort to stimulate faculty innovation and entrepreneurship at the medical center. The remaining $1.45 million of the gift went for programs in the U-M Office of Technology Transfer and Center for Entrepreneurship.[4]

Over the next year, FFMI partnered with the Michigan Economic Development Corporation to create seed programs to fund promising medical innovation projects from multidisciplinary faculty teams. These awards ranged from $20,000 to $30,000 for early-stage projects to $100,000 to $200,000 awards for more advanced and de-risked innovations and covered therapeutics, devices, diagnostics, and digital health solutions. While this effort engaged faculty across the medical center, funding several projects a year and providing project management and oversight, it did not focus initially on educating faculty with tools to successfully develop their innovations and navigate them outside the university or engage more fully with industry partners. With dedicated leadership from physician-innovators and business experts, the program continued to grow. During this time the Department of Surgery developed its own Leadership Development Program (LDP) to provide senior and mid-career faculty with opportunities to learn important leadership skills to be able to take on new roles in the department and across the institution. Drawing on the success of the LDP and the Innovation programs created by FFMI, an opportunity existed to build on that momentum and synergize the two together to create the first Surgical Innovation and Entrepreneurship Development Program (SIEDP) which was run over a 9-month period in 2016.

THE SURGICAL INNOVATION AND ENTREPRENEURSHIP DEVELOPMENT PROGRAM

In 2016, the Department of Surgery in collaboration with FFMI ran the first Surgical Innovation and Entrepreneurship Development Program (SIEDP) where 13 surgery faculty (from new assistant professors to senior leadership and the department chair) participated in a 9-month training program where they had sessions 1 day per month covering the commercialization process from idea generation all the way to technology development, patent submission, customer discovery, funding, and implementation. All of the faculty participated on teams and learned this process, culminating in "final pitch" grand rounds, which were done in a *Shark Tank* style where industry experts and Venture Capital partners outside the University could evaluate the technologies more thoroughly. The program started with a departmental mission-focused ideation and brainstorming session where novel ideas around education, research, clinical excellence, and branding were put forward and voted on by the entire department at its annual retreat. Faculty teams were placed on each project and these projects were then developed in parallel with faculty-initiated individual innovation projects through the course.[5]

One of the key departmental projects produced from the SIEDP was a Department-Sponsored Contract Research Organization (CRO) (https://medicine.umich.edu/dept/surgery/news/archive/201810/surgical-innovation-prize-development-accelerator-course) to connect big industry and startup companies with faculty labs to set up contract projects that utilized the unique research tools available in the Department. This project created several new industry contracts, adding significant revenues and diversifying the Department's research funding portfolio. Currently, the CRO provides engaged faculty labs with additional support for high-risk/high-reward research.[5]

In addition to generating great surgical innovation projects, the course provided key knowledge and resources to the participating surgical faculty, allowing them the time and ability to pursue their innovation interests. Through this course and process, many have gone on to be serial innovators and have engaged other innovation resources around the campus (such as Fast Forward Medical Innovation and Coulter Funding Programs). This has created a cultural evolution in the Department where surgical innovation and entrepreneurship have become part of the academic DNA and it is seen as something worth supporting and recognizing.

Development of an innovation culture in an academic department like Surgery must start with a shared vision, mission, and buy-in from many stakeholders, from senior leadership to the most junior faculty, residents, and staff. Once a shared vision is achieved for how the department will embrace and promote innovation, there must be a meaningful mechanism and appropriate resources committed to ensure success. Just stating that a group wants more faculty to engage in innovation and entrepreneurship, without giving them time, resources, funding, and incentives for this engagement is a setup for failure. For departments of surgery these resources become challenging as time spent away from clinical productivity often has a negative impact on the operational bottom line that is needed to keep an organization financially afloat.

Given the dramatic success of the SIEDP with meaningful faculty engagement, many more faculty became interested in participating in entrepreneurial efforts or in engaging with current resources to pitch their novel innovative solutions to problems they had been working on in their research or clinical practice. Through departmental programs and initiatives from multiple faculty and departmental leadership, including the SIEDP, the LDP, efforts in Global Surgery and in faculty development, the Michigan Promise was created to provide a new culture for members of the Department of Surgery to grow and pursue their interests in a way that cultivates leadership, growth, diversity, equity, and collaboration. Innovation and Entrepreneurship became an important "spoke" in the wheel of the Michigan Promise and as part of that effort, the department created the Michigan Surgical Innovation Prize Fund and Program.

THE MICHIGAN SURGICAL INNOVATION PRIZE FUND

The University of Michigan Department of Surgery through the Michigan Promise made a commitment to foster surgical innovation and enhance its innovation culture, leading to the vision and creation of the Michigan Surgical Innovation Prize Fund. Through this fund, within the Michigan Promise, the Department created a $500,000 Michigan Surgical Innovation Prize (MSIP) to fund outstanding surgical innovations that have excelled through a department-sponsored Surgical Innovation Development Accelerator Course (SIDAC). The Michigan Surgical Innovation Prize[6] is the first of its kind in the country and its mission is to foster and accelerate the development of novel technologies that will improve surgical diseases or the care of surgical patients. The first round of the $500,000 prize was awarded in August 2018 to six outstanding surgical innovations led by core faculty in the department (*Figure 8.2*).[6,7]

THE SURGICAL INNOVATION DEVELOPMENT ACCELERATOR COURSE

In August 2017, a request for proposals for the Michigan Surgical Innovation Accelerator (MSIA) Course was sent out across the Medical School and the School of Engineering. Each proposal had to address a surgical problem or disease with an innovation or solution that improves the lives of surgical patients. These innovations could be in the form of new devices, diagnostics, therapeutics, digital health solutions, or programmatic efforts, but all had to be translatable into real patient/commercial impact. Multidisciplinary collaborative team projects were encouraged as long as a surgery faculty member was actively involved. Over 30 outstanding proposals were submitted into the competition in the form of an executive summary. Each was reviewed, discussed, and ranked by the MSIP oversight committee, made up of faculty experts in and out of the department as well as engineering, industry, and venture capital partners to assure content expertise, oversight, and expert diligence regarding funding decisions and the proper use of funds.[3,8]

From this cohort of applications, 12 finalist teams were picked to participate in the newly updated Surgical Innovation Development Accelerator Course (SIDAC), which was run by a lead instructor who was a serial entrepreneur (*Figure 8.1*). This was an 8-month course (January to August 2018) with monthly sessions set up to

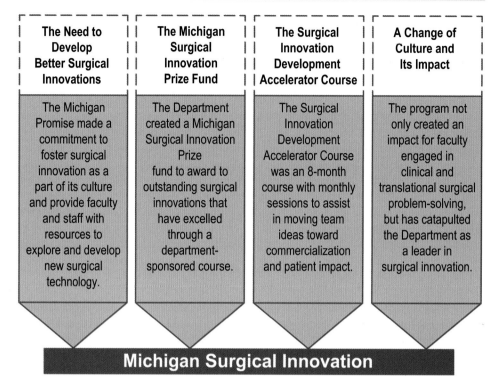

Figure 8.2 Surgical innovation prize.

assist teams in moving their ideas toward commercialization and patient impact. Each team had expert instruction, guided expert mentorship and coaching, as well as peer mentorship and coaching from others in the course, and resources for patent filing, prototyping, and customer discovery provided through the fund and supported by the Office of Technology Transfer (https://techtransfer.umich.edu) and the Fast Forward Medical Innovation group (https://innovation.medicine. umich.edu).

SIDAC taught teams the following concepts: idea generation, value proposition, intellectual property and patent submission, regulatory pathways, customer discovery, marketing and adoption, reimbursement and funding models, prototyping and pitching. The teams all worked on advancing their technologies through the course and in August 2018 they provided their updated executive summaries of their technologies and pitched their ideas to the oversight committee for questions and evaluation. Of the finalist teams presenting to the oversight committee, six of the teams had technologies advanced and de-risked enough to warrant $480,000 of funding through the Michigan Surgical Innovation Prize. The top four teams then pitched their innovations in front of the entire department and three guest Sharks (two venture capital senior partners and a physician-innovator and academic chair) at a *Shark Tank*–style grand rounds (https://www.youtube.com/ watch?v=eQzcQV6YzOs&feature=youtube).

Some thoughts from SIDAC participants include the following:

It's a real testimony to the Department of Surgery to allow their faculty to explore these interests which inherently have value to our patients, getting innovations from our brains to the bedside.

It's nice to sit in a room with a bunch of other people doing the same thing because they all have really helpful suggestions for your own idea. It's interesting to hear about the processes they have gone through and the kinds of resources that they've used because those are often helpful for your own project.

This is a fantastic program in regards to mentoring, because you have different levels and different kinds of mentorship…In this space, you really need mentorship from engineering, you need mentorship from lawyers, you need mentorship from people who understand customer exploration, people who understand prototyping.

WINNERS OF THE MICHIGAN SURGICAL INNOVATION PRIZE COMPETITION

Ferroximend—a Novel Therapeutic Device for Bone Healing

Ferroximend combines an angiogenic stimulant, deferoxamine, with an osteogenic (bone forming) tissue filler device, hyaluronic acid. This unique combination triggers the formation of blood vessels at the fracture site at the right time, leading to a remarkable ability to heal difficult fractures and accelerate that healing process.

Michigan ENdoluminal Lengthening Device

Michigan ENdoluminal Lengthening Device (MEND) is a device technology therapy that uses the well-established medical principle of mechanotrasduction to induce growth of new intestine and is intended to safely treat short bowel syndrome unlike current available therapy.

> In order for these things to move forward it goes beyond the normal skill set that we learn as a professor or as a doctor. It puts you in a different mindset and it's leading to very fruitful outcomes.

Minute Coaching System

The minute coaching system is a proprietary software product that lets medical students get real-time feedback from faculty. The goal is to sell/license this product to other medical schools, either directly from University of Michigan or via an existing company with a franchise in the medical education market.

> Part of the innovation prize is to help us figure out a way to make this applicable to a broader group of people. So can we take our feedback system, and can we make it financially viable and something that we can create into a product that could be used for other departments within the med school, other universities, other Departments of Surgery.

Surgical Asset Tracker

Surgical Asset Tracker is a University of Michigan startup that develops and commercializes software solutions for tracking temporary implantable devices, providing automated, high-fidelity device-tracking with alerts and works with any major electronic health record.

> I think it's easy to invent things, and ideas come easily to many of us, but there's a huge gap between the idea and actually making something that'll impact patients, and I think, as a physician or a scientist, we don't have a lot of knowledge about that gap, about markets and how to actually bring things to them, so this fills that gap.

Hot Spot—Using Thermochromic Material to Identify Areas at Risk for Ulcer

This technology uses thermochromic liquid crystals that change color providing an obvious, early warning sign that patients may be at risk for decubitus ulcer formation

> We were learning all about how to present a business plan, how to present our ideas, and really working closely with the innovation department here to come up with strategies of how to market our device. And this was a lot of work over the past nine months with our team but I think we learned a lot along the way and came up with a great presentation.

MULT-EYE Laparoscopic Camera

A multicamera-based integrated imaging system for improved visualization during laparoscopic surgery.

Ferroximend received additional funding in 2018-2019 from the Michigan-Pittsburgh-Wyss Regenerative Medicine Consortium through NIH. MEND received additional funding from the Michigan Coulter Program and the GI Innovation Fund as well as formed a 503c nonprofit. The device also received Breakthrough Designation from the FDA. Surgical Asset Tracker received additional funding in 2018-2019 from the M-TRAC program in partnership with Fast Forward Medical Innovation and the Michigan Economic Development Corporation and is currently in clinical trials at Michigan and University of Alabama, Birmingham.

MICHIGAN SURGICAL INNOVATION ACCELERATOR PROGRAM

Given the success of the first round of the Michigan Surgical Innovation Prize, to continue this momentum as well as develop winning team projects for the next round in 2019, an opportunity was created (during the off year between rounds of the Michigan Surgical Innovation Prize Competition) for surgical innovation teams who were early in their technology development to accelerate and de-risk their ideas through expert education/coaching/mentorship and customer discovery.[8] This accelerator funded five promising surgical technologies to move through a custom commercialization program over 6 months intended to advance these technologies to a point where they will be highly competitive for follow-on funding. Technologies needed to address a solution to a surgical problem and benefit/advance the care of surgical patients. A Department of Surgery full-time faculty must be the PI or co-PI on the project. Teams each received 14 hours of didactic education, 20 hours of one-on-one coaching and expert mentorship, and opportunities to complete 30 customer discovery interviews, a regulatory roadmap assessment from a contracted and trusted regulatory development agency, as well as funding to complete basic prototyping for devices. Funding was available for travel for additional customer discovery or experiments needed to de-risk the technology and advance it along its regulatory pathway.

Program Results

RETREVA: a Novel Specimen Retrieval Device for Laparoscopic Surgery

RETREVA is a novel device that uses a unique mechanical method to collect an organ/tumor specimen from a laparoscopic surgical procedure to more easily retrieve and extract the specimen from a tighter working space in the body to minimize trauma during extraction.

Continuous Noninvasive Monitoring of End-Organ Cellular Function with Supercontinuum Laser Spectroscopy

This project involves a novel noninvasive monitoring system that uses a transdermal laser spectroscopy system to continuously measure end-organ tissue perfusion as a means to improve resuscitation and monitor organ function following trauma, head injury, or sepsis.

Using Mobile Technology to Identify Stroke and Save Patient Lives

This project is developing an app that uses machine learning algorithms and the high functionality of an iPhone, including camera facial recognition, eye tracking, and voice recognition software to help identify patients having a stroke with the goal of getting them to treatment and better outcomes in a more timely manner.

My Weight Loss Journey: a New Digital Health App for Your Smartphone

This project is developing and validating a novel smartphone app that helps patients having bariatric surgery to better follow their pre- and postoperative instructions and connects them with resources to improve their compliance and long-term weight loss success.

A Synthetic Metastatic Niche for Early Detection of Metastatic Breast Cancer

This project involves a validation of a novel implantable synthetic scaffold that traps circulating tumor cells in breast cancer patients to create a metastatic niche of these tumor cells that can then be studied to help investigators better understand disease biology and progression as well as response to therapy.

CURRICULA

Courses offered as part of the Michigan Surgical Innovation Prize provide a unique opportunity in which novel surgical innovations and technologies at any stage are identified and moved forward to create change and impact for patients.[6] Teams participating in these courses receive expert instruction, guided expert mentorship and coaching as well as peer mentorship and coaching from others, and resources for patent filing, prototyping, and customer discovery. Each course intends to accelerate the process of bringing new technology to patients by identifying and addressing problems early in the development process.

Concepts developed throughout the SIDAC and MSIA courses include:

- Idea generation

- Value proposition

- Intellectual property and patent submission

- Regulatory pathways

- Customer discovery

- Marketing and adoption

- Reimbursement and funding models

- Prototyping and pitching

> I think the biggest challenge for innovators is making the conversion from a singular focus on technology to a broader focus on how the technology is going to fit into the larger world and how it can be commercialized.
>
> —Lead Instructor, *SIDAC*

COLLABORATION AND PARTNERSHIPS

The SIDAC and MSIA courses foster collaboration throughout the Department of Surgery and throughout the University of Michigan.[7] The program works with faculty members who specialize in different areas such as Engineering, School of Information, and departments across Michigan Medicine. Their unique perspectives encourage creativity and new ideas, leading to better technology for patients.

Courses emphasize collaboration between academia and industry. Teams benefit from the expertise of industry partners who have experience navigating the process of new technologies moving into the clinic and understand how to navigate the regulatory adoption issues that occur. The collaboration and connections help teams develop the technology effectively and provide resources beyond the course including opportunities for licensing and expansion.

- Fast Forward Medical Innovation (https://innovation.medicine.umich.edu/) provides resources for teams to conduct consumer research to better prepare their product for the market and distribution to patients.

- The Office of Tech Transfer (https://techtransfer.umich.edu/) assists teams in navigating the regulatory process and preparing to file patents.

- The Michigan Surgical Innovation Prize (https://medicine.umich.edu/dept/surgery/about-us/faculty-resident-life/our-initiatives/innovation-strategies): The Michigan Surgical Innovation Prize Oversight Committee provides expert resources for each team, including expertise outside the university from industry and venture capital. Content experts are able to give each team meaningful guidance and oversight on the development and implementation of their technologies.

- Expert Regulatory Oversight and Regulatory Roadmaps are provided to each team from Method Sense, Inc., a regulatory company from Raleigh, NC, with over 50 combined years of expertise moving technologies successfully through the FDA.

- Expert Oversight Committee is composed of members from venture capital firms, industry leadership, as well as intellectual property experts and local leaders outside of Surgery at the University.

Our physicians are in a unique space where they get to see a problem happening live. Every day. If we give them training to commercialize technology, it's also a way to look for problems and build solutions that really have an impact. This course allows you the space, the time, and the mentorship to really understand how to fail, pick yourself back up, and continue to pivot to grow and be able to make that impactful change in the future.

—Course Project Manager FFMI

THE PATH FORWARD

Through these resources deployed in Innovation and Entrepreneurship for Surgery faculty, the MSIP/SIDAC program in the Department of Surgery is one of the more advanced and tailored innovation programs on campus and is unique among Departments of Surgery in the world. Success from this program and its impact has stimulated change in other departments on the medical campus, leading other departments and centers to engage in their own innovation efforts. Together, this ripple effect has created a broader impact on the academic culture at the University of Michigan, where "Innovation" has now become one of the core values of Michigan Medicine. Through this transformative first Michigan Surgical Innovation Prize Competition and SIDAC course, over 40 surgeons, scientists, engineers, surgical residents, and medical students gained critical knowledge of the value and development of surgical technologies toward patient use and impact. These participants now understand how to navigate their ideas through the university as well as beyond into the market. The program has not only created tremendous impact within the Department for faculty engaged in clinical and translational surgical problem-solving, but has catapulted Michigan's Department of Surgery as a national leader in Surgical Innovation.[6]

In building and growing a new culture in Surgery that embraces innovation and entrepreneurship, it is imperative to expand opportunities for the future as well to continue momentum and create mechanisms of sustainability. With this in mind, several programs have recently been developed based on the curricula and engagement of clinician-innovators in the current programs through the Michigan Promise.

Training the Next Generation of Physician-Innovators

While the benefits to faculty who receive innovation training are extremely helpful to their careers, and many who have taken these courses have now gone on to become serial innovators, there is even more benefit to an academic medical center to provide the same training and resources to medical students and resident physicians. While the approach to teaching and learning can be different for this younger cohort, there are common challenges to be addressed. Programs that need to be tailored as traditional didactic-training programs will not be well attended. Significant funding sources need to exist and innovators need to be made aware of their existence to support ideas beyond the innovation phase. Physical innovation spaces are needed to allow for meetings but also to provide prototyping equipment, collaboration opportunities, and streamlined access to intellectual resources. A common challenge to innovation programs is project execution. Due to the factors discussed above, this will require unique collaborative agreements, multidisciplinary teams, and premade contracts specifying future returns and exit strategy based on longitudinal contributions. Understanding these challenges across the various groups is key to creating successful innovation programs.

MEDICAL SCHOOL PATHWAY OF EXCELLENCE IN INNOVATION AND ENTREPRENEURSHIP

Recognizing the growing need for medical students to interface with new medical technologies constantly emerging into the clinic, it becomes vital for medical schools to offer more formalized training in innovation and entrepreneurship. In order to meet the needs of a wide variety of learners, experiential learning, digital media platforms, and reversed classroom opportunities were utilized to optimize engagement and interest from such a diverse group. In addition to creating a strong foundational education that helps students identify and solve the right problems in medicine, use iterative design thinking mixed with customer discovery to de-risk, and develop a strong value proposition, medical schools wanting a sustainable effort in Innovation and Entrepreneurship must also commit financial resources toward trainee and project development. These resources are critical to establishing and sustaining the innovation culture. However, the hardest resource to allocate at major academic medical centers is time for trainees and students to engage fully in innovation efforts. For most students and trainees, time is very limited for these innovation activities, which have been marginalized as "extracurricular" at most centers. Understanding the importance of innovation in medicine for the future and resources to support trainees in this underserved mission, the department embarked on the programmatic development of an innovation and entrepreneurship curriculum for medical learners that recognizes some unique challenges for medical technologies compared to other business sectors.[3,9]

In 2015, a survey to the first-year medical school class queried whether students wished to participate in a 4-year cocurricular pathway in Innovation and Entrepreneurship. Over one-third of the class responded they would participate in such a path, and this was a big catalyst that led to the development of the first "Pathway of Excellence (PoE) in Innovation and Entrepreneurship (I&E)" being created and approved by the medical school curriculum committee for implementation that year. The PoE in I&E was approved in the fall of 2015, and in its inaugural year admitted 31 first-year medical students and 9 students from the second- or third-year medical school classes. The mission is to provide physicians-in-training the resources, perspective, and exposure they need to incorporate innovative strategies and tools that can improve the quality and equity of medical care. The goal is to develop medical students who can understand how to address real medical problems and patient needs through medical innovation and entre-preneurial solutions and explore the transformational role physician-innovators have on health care.

The I&E PoE has evolved over the last 4 years and now has a very flexible curriculum. The first part of the pathway involves a focused series of interactive sessions covering patient-focused iterative design thinking, development of diverse multidisciplinary teams, and defining an impactful value proposition with practice making a compelling investment pitch. Online modules supplement the interactive sessions and faculty as well as alumni physician-innovators are used as invited speakers to discuss navigating their ideas and learning from their failures to add real-world perspective. The second part of the pathway involves students choosing an innovation or problem to perform a deeper dive effort to create a solution, value proposition, and commercialization model through a mentored capstone experience. Students can create their own innovation, work with faculty on established projects, intern in a startup or VC firm, help with a student-run venture fund, or work collaboratively with other medical students, business graduate students, or engineering students on a multidisciplinary project. The capstone is left open-ended and supplemented with faculty mentorship and oversight. One goal is that it should seek to create meaningful impact for patients, the health system, or the community—local or abroad. Students then pitch their capstone to the group and create an executive summary of their project. Over the years the path has now engaged over 90 medical students, leading to 12 medical student startup companies, multiple patent filings, and over $2M in follow-on funding. Path students have also won prizes in several national pitch competitions. Other returns on this initial investment include a few students receiving the opportunity to take a year off from medical school to run their new company as CEO and really understand the challenges of running a startup. Also the number of medical students pursuing MD/MBA programs since initiation of the PoE has more than doubled.[3,9-11]

MEDICAL INNOVATORS PITCH CLUB

Diversity in innovation is extremely important and one of the challenges with educational curricula offered through the medical campus was that participants comprised a fairly homogenous group of medical professionals, typically either in the same specialty or training level. While this provides some diversity of thought, it is harder to generate the truly disruptive ideas that real innovation diversity can bring. Another challenge with creating courses attended by a diverse group of faculty and students from multiple fields and schools is logistical: funding of tuition differences across schools and lack of alignment with schedules. To solve this problem, a collaboration between the Medical School Path of Excellence in Innovation and Entrepreneurship, the Center for Entrepreneurship at the Engineering School, FFMI, and the Ross School of Business MBA programs helped create the Medical Innovators Pitch Club (MI-PITCH).[12]

The vision and purpose of MI-PITCH is to organically bring together medical professionals, engineers, finance and business professionals, community entrepreneurs, public health experts, scientists, and policy experts to network regularly and solve REAL MEDICAL PROBLEMS faced locally. Together in multidisciplinary teams, they brainstorm and perform design thinking to create solutions that will not only help patients locally but can translate to help patients around the country or even around the world. This inclusive and collaborative forum allows anyone with a medical problem they would like to tackle to pitch it to the audience and get feedback, build teams around a solution, and discuss best practices. Each month, one department, organization, or center sponsors the event and creates the medical design challenge for the month. For this challenge, a real medical problem is presented to the group that could be solved by a device, diagnostic, process improvement, algorithm, or digital health solution. The group sponsoring the MI-PITCH session will present the challenge to the attendees. Next, the 50-100 highly innovative people from multiple backgrounds attending the event (medical professionals, engineers, entrepreneurs, MBAs) will work in multidisciplinary teams to create a novel solution to the problem including a value proposition, a model/prototype/drawing/algorithm, and a basic cost/revenue justification for a business case. The sponsoring group can then take these creative solutions and decide if they want to invest additional resources to advance the project further and then apply for larger internal funding opportunities. This effort has brought together a large group of students and faculty on campus interested in medical innovation and has created networking and new team building opportunities for over 400 students and faculty.

FUTURE INNOVATION OPPORTUNITIES FOR RESIDENTS AND FELLOWS

Just as team science and its diversity of thought are transforming traditional research, team innovation and its diversified approach to iterative design thinking are very helpful to accelerate projects and build success. Resident trainees are encouraged to be part of the innovation process and are an integral part of innovation teams, and several have led their own teams with novel innovation strategies. Distinguishing technologies that will be impactful for patient care from those that are less useful is an important skill set for any clinician. As such, residents routinely participate in many of the educational offerings and programs in innovation offered through the department. Recently, given the interest of residents to gain additional training in Innovation and given the robust resources available on campus, the department created an approved Graduate Certificate in Innovation and Entrepreneurship in partnership with the Rackham Graduate School at the University of Michigan, the Center for Entrepreneurship, and the College of Engineering.

The Certificate in Innovation and Entrepreneurship is a 12-credit program currently open to enrolled and degree-seeking master's, PhD, and professional students at the University of Michigan's Ann Arbor campus. The Center for Entrepreneurship (CFE) manages this program jointly with Integrative Systems Design in the College of Engineering. The CFE has been working with the College of Engineering and has modified the certificate's language such that U-M medical residents will now be eligible to pursue the certificate.

The purpose of the certificate is to provide students with the opportunity to learn the tenets of innovation and entrepreneurship in a supportive and rigorous academic environment while they become experts in their fields of study. The certificate is a formal credential that will signal to employers, investors, and cofounders that the trainee has acquired the skills and knowledge to be a more versatile, well-rounded, and experienced innovator. For the certificate, 6 of the 12 credits come from core innovation courses in graduate engineering and the other 6 are electives available between the College of Engineering and Ross Business School.[13]

THE MICHIGAN PROMISE FOR INNOVATION

Any given individual will not have all of the talent required to take a project from ideation to successful execution. For example, a medical device team may need a mechanical/electrical/biomaterials engineer, whereas a process improvement team may need industrial engineers. Therefore, it is critical to create teams with the diverse intellectual resources needed for project development. It is important to consider time constraints, ability, and exit strategies when creating teams as well.[8] In addition to having the right mix of diverse talent on teams, mentorship and leadership are incredibly important to project success, and through the Michigan Promise and its commitment to mentorship, innovation, and leadership, top talent in all of these areas can be leveraged to help faculty-led teams to create impactful and successful innovations. Bringing in extramural expertise from industry leaders, the FDA, and successful surgeon-innovators from other institutions creates the right oversight and mentorship that can balance local expertise with a deeper under-standing of markets as well as provide due diligence on the novelty and benefits of the innovation outside the university.

Through the Faculty-Exchange and Mini-Sabbatical programs offered through the Michigan Promise and the Office of Faculty Life, the Department of Surgery at the University of Michigan has created meaningful partnerships with over a dozen academic institutions around the country and has provided faculty with the critical resource of time to pursue dedicated efforts around innovation and research ideas. With this in mind, the department is creating new collaborative efforts centered around surgical innovation with the goal of sharing educational resources and best practices across institutions and partnering together on bigger innovation and tech-nology development and implementation strategies.

INNOVATION TRACK FOR PROMOTION AND TENURE OF FACULTY

In academia, much effort is focused on productivity around the traditional missions of research, education, and clinical excellence as traditionally these efforts have been used to measure academic success and the ability to be promoted. This focus left little time or incentive for faculty to engage in innovation efforts. With a change in faculty culture and with more faculty engaging in innovation and entrepreneurial efforts, the University of Michigan Medical School created an "innovator portfolio" in parallel with its standard "research" and "education" portfolios as part of the promotion and tenure process. This portfolio recognizes innovation contributions such as patents and innovation funding, as well as company formation and leadership, ability to gain external investments, and educational efforts around innovations including manu-scripts, presentations, and interdisciplinary collaborations for innovation research and development. These criteria are now being evaluated and accepted as a body of work valued for promotion decisions. This process is also being evaluated at several other institutions nationally as a novel academic track for faculty.

RETURN ON INVESTMENT

From an administrative and leadership perspective, one common question around innovation programs focuses on what is the return on such an investment (ROI). How will the money spent ever be recouped? In answering this question of ROI, it is important to understand the impact of an innovation program on an academic department and its faculty, as well as the impact their innovation efforts have on the institution, patients, and society. Our investments and seed funding of projects combined with educational resources, mentorship, and accountability have impacted over 50 faculty in the Department of Surgery, creating 18 multidisciplinary teams that include senior faculty to medical students, many of which are cross-departmental and even multi-institutional projects. Faculty leading these projects have become serial entrepreneurs, developing multiple innovations in the last year. Several of the projects are in the implementation stage. The innovative faculty helped by these programs are now training residents and students in new innovation efforts and helping promote a new culture of surgical innovation that is inclusive and collegial and collaborative.

The last challenge around innovation programs and academic efforts in innovation and entrepreneurship is sustainability. In order to address this challenge, two key things need to happen: (1) the local culture must change to create support and buy-in at all levels, and (2) there need to be strategies in place to create evergreen funding and pay successes forward to the next generation. Engagement with industry, donors, and alumni are key component of promoting and maintaining the culture and support for program infrastructure. Additionally, follow-on funding and revenues generated need to flow back to the department in a meaningful way to replenish resources and create endowment for maintenance of funding. Departments should work with their technology transfer offices to create partnerships for equity investment and disbursement in faculty-generated intellectual property as well as licensing deals and startup formation. Together such efforts will provide a more impactful source of continual funding that supports critical innovation infrastructure resources (mentors, space for prototyping, engineering expertise, educational resources, expert oversight, regulatory support, etc.) and allows for sustainability and future growth of innovation efforts as surgery departments grow and adapt to future needs.

REFERENCES

1. Marshall AC. Business Insider, Primed Associates. April 10, 2013. https://www.businessinsider.com/difference-between-creativity-and-innovation-2013-4. Accessed April 10, 2013.
2. Cohen MS, Kao L, eds. *Success in Academic Surgery: Innovation and Entrepreneurship.* New York: Springer Nature; 2019:1-12:chap 1.
3. Cohen MS. Enhancing surgical innovation through a specialized medical school pathway of excellence in innovation and entrepreneurship: lessons learned and opportunities for the future. *Surgery.* 2017;162(5):989-993.
4. https://leadersandbest.umich.edu/dept/surgery/innovation.
5. Servoss J, Chang C, Olson D, Ward KR, Mulholland MW, Cohen MS. The surgery innovation and entrepreneurship development program (SIEDP): an experiential learning program for surgery faculty to ideate and implement innovations in health care. *J Surg Educ.* 2018;75(4):935-941. PMID: 28989009.
6. https://medicine.umich.edu/dept/surgery/news/archive/201810/surgical-innovation-prize-development-accelerator-course.
7. https://medicine.umich.edu/dept/surgery/about-us/faculty-resident-life/our-initiatives/innovation-strategies.
8. https://medicine.umich.edu/dept/surgery/innovation/surgical-innovation-development-accelerator-course/sidac-msia-impact.
9. Cohen MS, Kao L, eds. *Success in Academic Surgery: Innovation and Entrepreneurship.* New York: Springer Nature; 2019:217-234:chap 15.

10. https://innovation.medicine.umich.edu/innovation-and-entrepreneurship/.
11. https://medicine.umich.edu/medschool/education/md-program/curriculum/impact-curriculum/paths-excellence/innovation-entrepreneurship.
12. https://innovateblue.umich.edu/event/mi-pitch-club-the-path-of-excellence-in-innovation-entrepreneurship/.
13. https://cfe.umich.edu/certificate/#approvedcourses.

9

Outreach, Global Health, and Working Beyond Boundaries

Megan Johnson
Mark G. Shrime
Krishnan Raghavendran

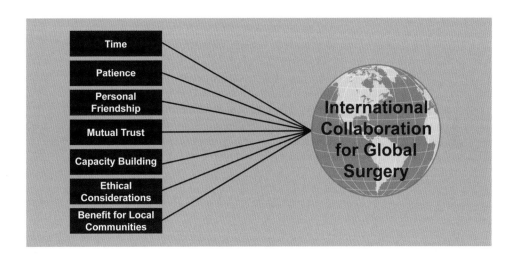

GLOBAL BURDEN OF DISEASE

Quantifying the magnitude of morbidity and mortality worldwide is difficult, with complicating factors at all levels of care.[1] The most common metric used to quantify the loss of healthy life due to disease is the disability-adjusted life year (DALY),[2] which is the sum of years of life lost to premature mortality and years of life spent living with morbidity and disability.

The Global Burden of Disease Study (GBD) is a worldwide comprehensive study that examines trends from 1990 to present with annual updates beginning in 2015. In many low-income and middle-income countries, country-specific health data remain scarce, leading to extrapolation and modeling based on demographics, surveillance systems, household surveys, verbal autopsies, and facility-level data inquiries.[3-7] Caveats aside, the GBD project has documented that cardiovascular diseases are the leading cause of death in almost every region of the world,[8] accounting for approximately one-third of all deaths globally.[9] Cardiovascular mortality has increased by 12.5% over the past decade.[10]

Noncommunicable diseases in general have shifted to the forefront of the global burden of disease as part of what has been called the "demographic transition": aging of the global population, improved childhood mortality, and declines in death due to the infectious causes which had previously been at the forefront.[11] Between 2005 and 2015, cancer cases increased by 33% and are expected to increase in the future.[12] However, while deaths from noncommunicable disease now account for more than one-half of global health loss,[13] infectious diseases such as tuberculosis still kill more than 1 million people every year.[11,14] The combination of HIV, tuberculosis, and malaria accounts for approximately 10% of the world's overall disease burden.

The global burden of disease is not limited to DALYs and mortality rates. The economic burden of diseases is tremendous and is a problem for global economies. The cost of diabetes worldwide has been estimated at $1.31 trillion, or 1.8% of the global gross domestic product in 2015[15] and chronic hepatitis C expenses exceed $10 billion annually in the United States alone.[16]

GLOBAL BURDEN OF SURGICAL DISEASE

The global burden of surgical disease is substantial but difficult to quantify, particularly in the developing world. Diseases that require surgical and anesthesia care constitute a considerable proportion of the global burden of disease. In 2006, Debas and colleagues estimated the fraction of disease treatable by surgical intervention as 11% of overall disease burden.[17] More recently, Shrime and colleagues, based on survey results, estimated that the burden of disease requiring surgical intervention approximates 30%.[18] Other estimates put the global burden of surgical disease at 30% to 35%[18,19] of the world's overall disease burden, on par with the disease burden attributable to cardiovascular conditions. Close to 17 million deaths are caused by surgical diseases every year,[20] and surgical conditions are estimated to result in losses of 1.25% of the potential GDP each year.[21] An estimated 12.3 trillion dollars are lost in the GDP of low- and middle-income countries due to surgical conditions.

At least 4.8 billion people do not have access to surgery,[22] and despite high surgical rates worldwide, cases are not spread evenly throughout the world. Middle-expenditure and high-expenditure countries, accounting for 30.2% of the world's population, provided 73.6% of surgeries worldwide in 2004, whereas poor-expenditure countries accounting for 34.8% of the global population yet undertook only 3.5% of all surgical procedures.[23] Greater than 95% of the population of South Asia, central, eastern, and western sub-Saharan Africa do not have access to surgical care, compared to overwhelming access in most regions of the developed world.[22] With increasing efforts from institutions such as the Lancet Commission on Global Surgery, launched in 2014, and the World Health Assembly, attention to the global burden of surgical disease has increased in recent years.

The ability to provide surgical care requires an intricate web of factors. Not only are the staff and facilities to perform surgery essential, but demand-side barriers, such as the ability of the population to reach the facility in a timely manner and to receive surgery without catastrophic expenditure, must also be considered.[22] In resource-constrained countries, surgical services are concentrated almost wholly in cities and reserved for those who can pay for them.[24] Almost 3.7 billion people, or half of the global population, are at risk of catastrophic expenditure if surgery becomes necessary and 81.3 million people experience financial catastrophe each year.[25]

The wide scope of surgical needs complicates measurement of the prevalence and the effect of surgical conditions.[26] In 2015, the Lancet Commission on Global Surgery found that the consequences of untreated surgical conditions in low- and middle-income countries are large and for many years have gone unrecognized.[20] One hundred forty-three million additional surgical procedures are needed each year to save lives and prevent disability.[20] Recent efforts to define necessary steps toward global surgery have been taken.[20,27,28]

Six core indicators to measure surgical access were outlined by the Lancet Commission on Global Surgery which help set standards for surgical care: geographical accessibility, density of surgical providers, number of procedures performed, perioperative mortality, risk of impoverishing expenditure, and risk of catastrophic expenditure.[20] Furthermore, in 2016, researchers proposed three Bellwether procedures, finding that hospitals with the ability to perform caesarean delivery, laparotomy, and treatment of open fracture were more likely to be able to deliver emergency and essential surgical care.[27] The Bellwether procedures provide a benchmark to first-level hospitals, anticipating ability to provide essential surgical care.

GLOBAL BURDEN OF TRAUMA

In the year 2013 it was estimated that 973 million people sustained injuries that warranted health care and that injury accounted for 4.8 million deaths.[29] It is estimated that about 16,000 people die from injuries every day. Eighty-five percent of all traumatic injuries occur in developing countries, and worldwide trauma is the leading cause of mortality in the 5 to 40 age group. Even in high-income countries, traumatic unintentional injuries, self-inflicted injuries, and injuries related to interpersonal violence account for the majority of deaths in the 15 to 45 age group.[29] The additional burden of the sequelae from trauma with significant morbidities accounts for a very large part of the disability spectrum.

The majority of traumatic deaths are due to road traffic accidents. Traffic accidents are estimated to account for 30% of deaths, globally.[29] This number is higher in the low- and middle-income countries with 37% in India as per National Crime Record Bureau report in 2014. A vehicular accident is reported every 2 minutes and a death every 5 minutes on Indian roads.[30] In India, the mortality rate for severe injuries (injury severity score of >16) is six times that of developed countries.[30]

There has been an increase in the incidence of intentional injuries that include self-inflicted and interpersonal violence. Data reported from the United Nations Office on Drugs and Crime suggest while the incidence of homicide is decreasing in Asia and Europe, it is increasing in South America and Eastern and Southern Africa.[31] Self-harm is the second leading cause of death from injuries, and global trends suggest an uptick, particularly observed during the recent economic global downturn.

Disability remains the major sequelae of trauma. Disability can be categorized as short and long term. Most epidemiologists have adopted disability-adjusted life years (DALY) as a global reflection of the burden of disease at a population level and as a means of comparative assessment of different diseases. DALY is obtained by adding the years of lost life (YLL) reflecting fatalities and years lived with disability (YLD) for nonfatal injuries. Injury is responsible for 10% of the global disease burden (measured by DALY). YLL accounted for 85% of injury DALY.[29] The major contributors to injury DALY are road traffic accidents (29%) and self-harm (14%).

There are major economic effects of trauma. In the United States, trauma accounts for a substantial burden. Estimates from the year 2005 suggest that mortality from unintentional injuries resulted in $1.3 billion in medical costs. The economic burden of disability for the same year was much higher at $82 billion. Economic effects in developing countries are dramatic; India forfeits 3% of annual GDP to accidents. Major disability imparts tremendous societal and economic burdens.

There are several potential approaches to these problems. Most important are the public health programs aimed at educational and injury prevention. While a multidisciplinary injury prevention program has been shown to be most effective, especially in the developed world, lack of good data precludes its application in the low- and middle-income countries. It is important to realize that transfer of these preventive measures from one area to another must take into consideration the local environment, culture, and social structure of the population. Prioritized research with the goal of improving delivery of care to surgical patients in the developing world is also required.

BUILDING INTERNATIONAL COLLABORATIVES

Unique Strategies for Individual Countries

For international institutions interested in developing surgical care in low- and middle-income countries, understanding the needs of the community from an epidemiological perspective, implementing proven pathways of improving access to surgical care, and measuring progress over time through research are of utmost importance. For international institutions in high-income countries and for healthcare systems in low resource environments, symbiotic collaborations form the foundation of success.

Developing relationships is the first step in this process. Successful initiatives within other fields particularly in the management of HIV, malaria, and tuberculosis were founded on this principle. It is equally important to understand the local environment and the prevailing culture at the foreign institutions. Building a collaborative relationship takes time and varies with the host country involved. Success usually involves personal friendships and mutual trust. Such collaborations may take many years to develop and must focus on the needs of the local environment in the developing world to be successful. To ensure continued development and quality improvement, research is a critical component of sustainability.[32]

Capacity Building

An essential prerequisite for successful collaborations across the developing world is capacity building by academic institutions. Capacity building is defined as a conceptual approach to development that focuses on understanding the various obstacles that prevent realization of specific goals while enhancing the capabilities to achieve sustainable results. Capacity building has been defined across multiple

Table 9.1 Seven Steps to Create Capacity Building in LMIC[33]

Good Practice Document
1. Network, collaborate, communicate, and share experiences
2. Understand the local context and accurately evaluate existing research capacity
3. Ensure local ownership and secure active support
4. Build in monitoring, evaluation, and learning from the start
5. Establish robust research governance and support structures, and promote effective leadership
6. Embed strong support, supervision, and mentorship structures
7. Think long-term, be flexible, and plan for continuity

strata including individual, organizational, institutional, and national settings. The concept outlined here describes capacity building with reference to academic institutions and research in surgical disciplines. In an attempt to define capacity building for research in the low- and middle-income countries, a group of organizations including the National Institutes of Health, the Fogarty Foundation, and the Swedish Cooperative Agency published a document that outlines simple steps toward achieving the goal of fostering research in the developing world.[33] Details are provided in *Table 9.1*.

Building research capacity, particularly in the developing world, involves certain key elements. Prominent aspects include (1) mentoring of clinicians and scientists; (2) accessibility to resources including scientific journals, databases, and services of a health service librarian; (3) building a research culture in which people actively discuss and think about research, seeing it as part of their daily professional lives; and (4) engagement of external collaborators in research initiatives. Confidence building and encouragement are critical elements for long-term success (*Figure 9.1*).

An Example

The University of Michigan–All India Institutes of Medical Sciences (UM–AIIMS) collaborative that began in 2010 has adopted these core principles.[34] At the outset, there was a signing of a memorandum of understanding between the trauma burn center at UM and AIIMS. The apex trauma institute within AIIMS is committed to the establishment of all components of a trauma system, involving not only policymakers but also healthcare professionals (general surgeons, orthopedic surgeons, neurosurgeons, anesthesiologists, emergency physicians, and nurses) in India. University of Michigan surgical leaders were involved in bilateral discussions and visits pertaining to the development of a curriculum for development of trauma and surgical critical care programs in India while also providing technical background relevant to contemporary research. A traveling program, whereby faculty from AIIMS visit the UM trauma burn and critical care program, was established. This program included a 2-month visit by the chief of surgery at AIIMS. At the

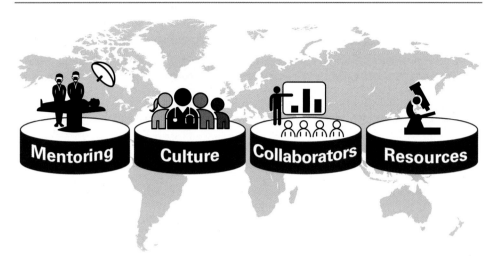

Figure 9.1 Building research capacity.

conclusion of this visit, faculty members were able to write grant proposals that led to successful awards from the Indian Council of Medical Research (ICMR) and the Department of Bio-technology in India.

A week-long, intensive course in research methods was undertaken as part of the UM–AIIMS collaboration. The course was designed to build bidirectional opportunities for research between the two institutions and countries. The course addressed a stated need at AIIMS for a formal, structured experience that would assist junior faculty in developing best practices for translational and clinical research. The goals of the course were achieved by a combination of didactic and small group sessions applied to both clinical outcomes and translational research. Fifty Indian junior faculty members participated. They were asked to develop and refine 5-page grant projects using group mentoring and feedback sessions. The sessions also focused on methods to develop and justify feasible scientific questions pertaining to human subject research. Ten successful concept ideas were initiated across multiple disciplines and then developed into full proposals with mentorship from both the institutions.

As a result of these exchanges, the collaborative was able to obtain joint funding from the NIH through the US–India Collaborative Award examining the use of ultrasound to measure optic nerve sheath diameter as a surrogate marker of intracranial pressure elevation in traumatic brain injury (TBI). A reciprocal award was issued by ICMR to AIIMS. Multiple abstracts, oral presentations, and manuscripts reflected important metrics of success. The awards from NIH/ICMR further strengthened the research coordination center at AIIMS by enabling employment of research staff. A joint proposal involving clinical trial of very early decompressive craniectomy in patients with severe TBI in India was submitted to the NIH. A summary of important events with the respective timeline is provided in *Table 9.2.*

An important benefit of such an initiative pertains to surgical education. Surgical residents and medical students from the University of Michigan may spend a month at the apex trauma center and AIIMS working with local surgeons who practice in a resource-limited environment. These learners understand firsthand the magnitude of health burden in a developing country. The feedback provided by these individuals has been very positive.

Table 9.2 Timeline of Major Events of the University of Michigan and AIIMS Collaborative[34]

Event	Timeline
Signing of MOU between AIIMS and trauma-burn service	2010
Visiting faculty from AIIMS to UM (6-8 wk)	2011 to present
UM faculty and Presidential visit	November 2013
Research methods course co-organized by AIIMS and UMHS, New Delhi	November 2014
Mentoring program and development of research projects	2014 to present
Joint proposal, manuscripts, oral presentations, and funding through US–India collaborative (NIH/DBT–India)	2014 to present
Submission of joint proposal for a clinical trial involving DC to the NIH and inclusion of global health research in a T32 application to NHLBI	2016

THE CENTER FOR GLOBAL SURGERY EVALUATION

Because of the immense burden of surgical disease and the deficit in provision of surgical care for those who need it, a concerted effort is underway in the global community to meet the unmet need. In 2015, the World Health Assembly adopted resolution 68.15, aimed at strengthening emergency and essential surgical care and anesthesia, with a recognition that doing so was necessary to achieve the goal of universal health coverage. Since then, the world has seen a groundswell of efforts primarily focused on the creation of national surgical, obstetric, and anesthetic plans (NSOAPs). Aimed at incorporating surgery within a country's overall health plan, these NSOAPs are built on six pillars: workforce, infrastructure, financing, information management, service delivery, and governance.

Simultaneously, a large and growing charitable sector has stepped in to alleviate the burden of surgical disease. At last count, in 2016, 403 surgically oriented nongovernmental organizations were operating in all 139 low- and middle-income countries.[35] The market for these organizations is massive: a survey of the financial records of 160 of them found that their total aggregated expenses over 5 years exceeded $3 billion.[36]

A push to *do* something to fix the problem of global surgery has not, however, been accompanied by a commensurate push to evaluate what the international community has decided to do. The $3 billion investment has largely gone unexamined. The work of many implementers across academia, industry, ministries, and the charitable sector is often predicated on an assumption that doing *something* is better than doing nothing at all. This stance is fundamentally problematic: good ideas often fail in the implementation.

To combat the paucity of data in the global surgery space, the Center for Global Surgery Evaluation was established.[37] The goal of the center is to drive impact evaluation at all levels of global surgical intervention. In line with

WHA68.15 (Sixty-eighth World Health Assembly), it works to include impact evaluation at every level of national surgical planning, within the mandates of charitable organizations, and in collaboration with implementers and academia. Its goal is to assure that the impetus to *do* is elevated to a mandate to *do well* within the field of global surgery.

ROLE OF ACADEMIC INSTITUTIONS

The number of global health programs supported by universities in the Unites States has increased steadily. In 2000, only three institutions had formal programs in global health. By 2012, 35 institutions had developed similar offerings. However, to date few programs in the United States have included global health training with respect to surgical disciplines, although the surgical expertise represented within American academic institutions has much to contribute.

The goals of surgical education, patient care, and research can be seamlessly integrated in a model of "convergence science." Education and training provided to surgical trainees through collaboration with international partners can be integrated into a meaningful academic curriculum. This form of education, and the opportunity to study and train abroad, will both attract talented residents and also prepare them for the future as citizens of the world. With this effort, American institutions have the potential to improve the health of the underprivileged by sharing best practices and care models.

Recently, a new concept of academic global health has been instituted by Wernli and associates.[38] These authors argue for an integration of research and implementation science. They have defined academic global health as a "system based, ecological and trans-disciplinary approach to research, education, and practice which seeks to provide innovative, integrated, and sustainable solutions to address complex health problems across national boundaries and improve health for all." They have also defined the scope of research outlined in *Figure 9.2.*

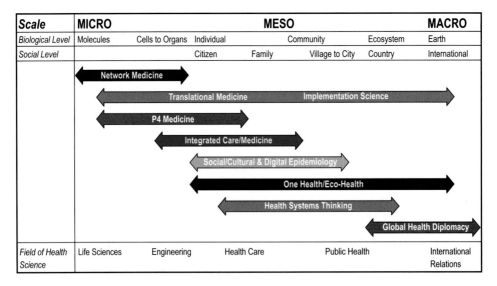

Figure 9.2 Scope of interdisciplinary research in global health.

Research institutions have critical roles in setting the agenda for global science. Transnational projects provide a venue for furthering science and serve as scientific springboards for faculty initiatives. These goals are best addressed by the adoption of quality, high-throughput technologies that have the potential to translate science into practices that benefit local populations.

ETHICAL CONSIDERATIONS

Ethical Principles

With increased awareness and interest among the medical profession in global health, an area of intense scrutiny relates to the consideration of ethics in the conduct of clinical rotations, clinical trials, and research in general. A wide variety of authors have commented on this evolving subject including sentinel work performed by the World Health Organization in addressing the specific ethical issues related to global health. A number of frameworks have been provided that encompass the guiding principles of effectiveness, proportionality, necessity, least infringement, and public justification.[39] Stapleton et al. argue that ethics involves the application of moral values to health issues characterized at a global level.[40] Regardless of the definition, the nature and cultural diversity of the population at large make the consideration of ethical issues in global health particularly complex.

Research and Ethics in Global Health

An approach that has been well described in research in the global context is the concept of community-based participatory research (CBPR). The basic principles of CBPR have been very well articulated by Israel et al. It adopts nine principles all targeted to the final goal of benefitting the local community involved with research.[41] It also provides an opportunity for the community to enumerate the most relevant problems or questions that affect their lives. Though the process can be time-consuming, in the longer term specific relationships are established that lead to stability of the research environment. In addition, CBPR challenges the notion that the researchers are more knowledgeable than the local community. As an example, a project involving mapmaking by the local community can help identify areas of disparities within that population.[41] Photovoice is another tool where the community members are given video cameras and asked to record voices that represent the community and help promote a critical awareness of a particular problem or a disease process.[41] These basic principles of transparency in the project and funding along with shared knowledge go a long way in establishing international collaborations in the developing world.

Academic Publication Across Global Communities

While publications and sharing knowledge in conferences are considered important elements of academic achievement, it is important to remember that the community at large needs to be informed. The economic and telecommunication disparities between the West and low- and middle-income countries are substantial. Therefore, it is important to disseminate the information obtained at the conclusion of the research activity with the local community in a language and format that is well understood. These could include conduct of community forums, discussion with local elders, and dissemination through visual media. A channel for feedback is also a necessary tool in fostering this relationship. A major issue that has led to conflicts in the past has been the exclusion of the local researchers from authorship. These practices could be construed as imperialistic and do not promote an equal partnership, a process so integral to research across the global community.

Ethical Dilemmas in International Collaborations

Broad international collaborations between researchers in areas across the world have the potential to inform the local community involved with capacity building. These areas of converging science also have unique issues related to cultural and economic differences in addition to the so-called "privilege dynamics." Anderson et al. have published on their efforts of a collaboration between the ministry of health in Ghana and the University of Michigan.[42] The "Elmina Declaration" describes a charter of collaboration in addition to the provision of moral and ethical framework. The major principles adopted here include sharing data and technology, improving infrastructure for skills training and clinical care, and translating research to policy and national initiatives.

In summary, a focus on the local community, transparency, and mutual trust combined with appropriate bilateral communication strategies and introduction of capacity building and sustainability are key to a long-lasting friendship and collaboration across the globe.

SUMMARY

The global burden of surgical diseases is substantial and has widespread effect on the population at large. Surgical departments within American academic institutions can play key roles in establishing programs in global health that have the potential not only to change the landscape of research but also to provide an opportunity for faculty and residents to embark on new frontiers. International collaboration across the developing world takes time, patience, personal friendship, and mutual trust. Capacity building for research activities in the low- and middle-income countries is a necessary first step in establishing long-term relationships leading to clinical trials and meaningful translational research in the future. Ethical considerations across international partnerships are unique, and a considerable emphasis has to be placed on mutual trust and the benefit of the local communities.

REFERENCES

1. Byass P. The imperfect world of global health estimates. *PLoS Med.* 2010;7(11):e1001006.
2. Salomon JA, Haagsma JA, Davis A, et al. Disability weights for the global burden of disease 2013 study. *Lancet Glob Health.* 2015;3(11):e712-723.
3. Byass P, de Courten M, Graham WJ, et al. Reflections on the global burden of disease 2010 estimates. *PLoS Med.* 2013;10(7):e1001477.
4. Hill K, Lopez AD, Shibuya K, Jha P; Monitoring of Vital Events. Interim measures for meeting needs for health sector data: births, deaths, and causes of death. *Lancet.* 2007;370(9600):1726-1735.

5. Mathers CD, Fat DM, Inoue M, Rao C, Lopez AD. Counting the dead and what they died from: an assessment of the global status of cause of death data. *Bull World Health Organ.* 2005;83(3):171-177.

6. Setel PW, Macfarlane SB, Szreter S, et al. A scandal of invisibility: making everyone count by counting everyone. *Lancet.* 2007;370(9598):1569-1577.

7. Tichenor M, Sridhar D. Metric partnerships: global burden of disease estimates within the World Bank, the World Health Organisation and the Institute for Health Metrics and Evaluation. *Wellcome Open Res.* 2019;4:35.

8. Benziger CP, Roth GA, Moran AE. The global burden of disease study and the preventable burden of NCD. *Glob Heart.* 2016;11(4):393-397.

9. Joseph P, Leong D, McKee M, et al. Reducing the global burden of cardiovascular disease, Part 1: the epidemiology and risk factors. *Circ Res.* 2017;121(6):677-694.

10. GBD 2015 Mortality and Causes of Death Collaborators. Global, regional, and national life expectancy, all-cause mortality, and cause-specific mortality for 249 causes of death, 1980-2015: a systematic analysis for the Global Burden of Disease Study 2015. *Lancet.* 2016;388(10053):1459-1544.

11. GBD 2013 Mortality and Causes of Death Collaborators. Global, regional, and national age-sex specific all-cause and cause-specific mortality for 240 causes of death, 1990-2013: a systematic analysis for the Global Burden of Disease Study 2013. *Lancet.* 2015;385(9963): 117-171.

12. Global Burden of Disease Cancer Collaboration; Fitzmaurice C, Allen C, Barber RM, et al. Global, regional, and national cancer incidence, mortality, years of life lost, years lived with disability, and disability-adjusted life-years for 32 cancer groups, 1990 to 2015: a systematic analysis for the global burden of disease study. *JAMA Oncol.* 2017;3(4):524-548.

13. Murray CJ, Vos T, Lozano R, et al. Disability-adjusted life years (DALYs) for 291 diseases and injuries in 21 regions, 1990-2010: a systematic analysis for the Global Burden of Disease Study 2010. *Lancet.* 2012;380(9859):2197-2223.

14. GBD Tuberculosis Collaborators. The global burden of tuberculosis: results from the Global Burden of Disease Study 2015. *Lancet Infect Dis.* 2018;18(3):261-284.

15. Bommer C, Heesemann E, Sagalova V, et al. The global economic burden of diabetes in adults aged 20-79 years: a cost-of-illness study. *Lancet Diabetes Endocrinol.* 2017;5(6):423-430.

16. Stepanova M, Younossi ZM. Economic burden of hepatitis C infection. *Clin Liver Dis.* 2017;21(3):579-594.

17. Debas HT, Gosselin R, McCord C, Thind A. Surgery. In: Jamison DT, Breman JG, Measham AR, et al, eds. *Disease Control Priorities in Developing Countries.* Washington, DC: World Bank Publications; 2006.

18. Shrime MG, Bickler SW, Alkire BC, Mock C. Global burden of surgical disease: an estimation from the provider perspective. *Lancet Glob Health.* 2015;3(suppl 2):S8-S9.

19. Fehlberg T, Rose J, Guest GD, Watters D. The surgical burden of disease and perioperative mortality in patients admitted to hospitals in Victoria, Australia: a population-level observational study. *BMJ Open.* 2019;9(5):e028671.

20. Meara JG, Leather AJ, Hagander L, et al. Global Surgery 2030: evidence and solutions for achieving health, welfare, and economic development. *Lancet.* 2015;386(9993):569-624.

21. Alkire BC, Shrime MG, Dare AJ, Vincent JR, Meara JG. Global economic consequences of selected surgical diseases: a modelling study. *Lancet Glob Health.* 2015;3(suppl 2):S21-S27.

22. Alkire BC, Raykar NP, Shrime MG, et al. Global access to surgical care: a modelling study. *Lancet Glob Health.* 2015;3(6):e316-e323.

23. Weiser TG, Regenbogen SE, Thompson KD, et al. An estimation of the global volume of surgery: a modelling strategy based on available data. *Lancet.* 2008;372(9633):139-144.

24. Farmer PE, Kim JY. Surgery and global health: a view from beyond the OR. *World J Surg.* 2008;32(4):533-536.

25. Shrime MG, Dare AJ, Alkire BC, O'Neill K, Meara JG. Catastrophic expenditure to pay for surgery worldwide: a modelling study. *Lancet Glob Health.* 2015;3(suppl 2):S38-S44.

26. Dare AJ, Grimes CE, Gillies R, et al. Global surgery: defining an emerging global health field. *Lancet.* 2014;384(9961):2245-2247.

27. O'Neill KM, Greenberg SL, Cherian M, et al. Bellwether procedures for monitoring and planning essential surgical care in low- and middle-income countries: caesarean delivery, laparotomy, and treatment of open fractures. *World J Surg.* 2016;40(11):2611-2619.

28. Shrime MG, Daniels KM, Meara JG. Half a billion surgical cases: aligning surgical delivery with best-performing health systems. *Surgery.* 2015;158(1):27-32.

29. Haagsma JA, Graetz N, Bolliger I, et al. The global burden of injury: incidence, mortality, disability-adjusted life years and time trends from the Global Burden of Disease study 2013. *Inj Prev.* 2016;22(1):3-18.

30. Gururaj G. Road traffic deaths, injuries and disabilities in India: current scenario. *Natl Med J India.* 2008;21(1):14-20.

31. UNODC Global Study on Homicide. 2013. United Nations publication, Sales No. 14.IV.11.

32. Ranganathan K, Habbouche J, Sandhu G, Raghavendran K. Cultivating global surgery initiatives abroad and at home. *J Grad Med Educ.* 2018;10(3):258-260.

33. Seven principles for strengthening research capacity in low- and middle income countries: simple ideas in a complex world (2014) by ESSENCE on Health Research is licensed by the Wellcome Trust of the United Kingdom under a Creative Commons Attribution-NonCommercial-ShareAlike 3.0 Unported License. Based on work at: http://www.who.int/tdr/publications/seven-principles/en/2014:1-36.

34. Raghavendran K, Misra MC, Mulholland MW. The role of academic institutions in global health: building partnerships with low- and middle-income countries. *JAMA Surg.* 2017;152(2):123-124.

35. Ng-Kamstra JS, Riesel JN, Arya S, et al. Surgical non-governmental organizations: global surgery's unknown nonprofit sector. *World J Surg.* 2016;40(8):1823-1841.

36. Gutnik L, Yamey G, Riviello R, Meara JG, Dare AJ, Shrime MG. Financial contributions to global surgery: an analysis of 160 international charitable organizations. *Springerplus.* 2016;5(1):1558.

37. The center for global surgery evaluation. Available at http://www.globalsurgeryevaluation.com.

38. Wernli D, Tanner M, Kickbusch I, Escher G, Paccaud F, Flahault A. Moving global health forward in academic institutions. *J Glob Health.* 2016;6(1):010409.

39. Kekulawala M, Johnson TRB. Ethical issues in global health engagement. *Semin Fetal Neonatal Med.* 2018;23(1):59-63.

40. Stapleton G, Schroder-Back P, Laaser U, Meershoek A, Popa D. Global health ethics: an introduction to prominent theories and relevant topics. *Glob Health Action.* 2014;7:23569.

41. Israel BA, Eng E, Schulz A, Parker EA. *Introduction to methods for CBPR for health.* In: *Methods for Community-Based Participatory Research Health.* Hoboken, NJ: John Wiley & Sons; 2012:337.

42. Anderson F, Donkor P, de Vries R, et al. Creating a charter of collaboration for international university partnerships: the Elmina declaration for human resources for health. *Acad Med.* 2014;89(8):1125-1132.

10

Research Development

Amir A. Ghaferi
Peter K. Henke
Marina Pasca di Magliano

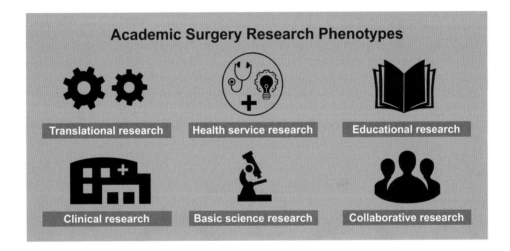

Academic Surgery Research Phenotypes

Translational research Health service research Educational research

Clinical research Basic science research Collaborative research

ACADEMIC PHENOTYPES

There are numerous academic surgery phenotypes. The stereotype of the academic surgeon is a busy clinical surgeon who has an NIH-funded basic science laboratory that is studying the pathophysiology of a specific condition in his or her clinical specialty. While this may have been true in the past, there are now a variety of academic pathways that are embraced by academic surgical departments. Some of the most common include basic science research, translational research, health service research, clinical research, education research, and collaborative or team science. There may be many others and this list is not meant to be exhaustive.

Basic science–focused surgeons perform laboratory experiments to answer biologic questions related to the molecular and cellular mechanisms underlying disease. Translational research relates to work aiming to link laboratory findings directly to clinical care. This research has a clearer impact on the day-to-day practice of surgery and its associated diseases. Health services research, sometimes referred to as outcomes research, seeks to understand and often improve the result of healthcare interventions or policies. Clinical research, which may include clinical trials, examines the direct clinical effects of treatments by using human subjects both retrospectively and prospectively. Educational research is a rapidly expanding field in surgery and seeks to understand and improve training paradigms at all stages of a surgical career (i.e., medical school, residency, independent practice). Another area of significant growth and value is collaborative or team science, whereby surgeons contribute important clinical or preclinical insights into disease processes that enable nonclinical basic scientists, health services researchers, or education researchers to maximize the novelty, relevance, and impact of their work.

ESTABLISHING RESEARCH GOALS

Short-term Research Goals

Surgeons are accustomed to quick results with operations or interventions that yield dramatic and immediate benefits. They are accustomed to seeing a problem, identifying a solution, and implementing that solution with measurable and often immediate impact. This logic can be applied to research as well. Unfortunately, surgeons also strive for perfection. As such, some surgeon-scientists get so bogged down in trying to hit a home-run that they forget base hits are also important. Investigators may work diligently for years on projects that have significant scientific potential. However, during that intense period, some fail to publish on that work for fear of piecemeal publication. This is a recipe for failure as tenure clocks keep ticking.

While academic surgery is a marathon, it requires an understanding that short-term "wins" or progress is important and needs to be part of a larger, long-term strategy (*Figure 10.1*). For example, even while one is working on experiments

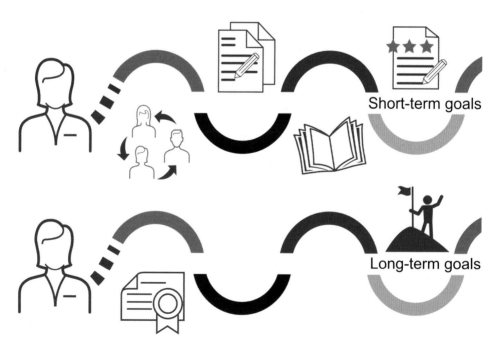

Short-term goals

Long-term goals

Figure 10.1 Short-term (top) and long-term (bottom) research goals.

designed to yield a high-impact publication, attention should be given to maintaining and honing the writing and publishing skills needed to be a successful academic surgeon. This is called "paying the academic bills." One can also visualize an academic career as two parallel paths that may or may not come into contact or overlap. The first path consists of short-term goals and productivity. This is the "churn" that should yield results within months. Examples of productivity include submitting abstracts for meetings, writing clinical papers about clinical areas of expertise, writing book chapters, or preparing narrative reviews about a clinical or research topic. These endeavors help growing academic surgeons overcome "bibliopenia" and provide opportunities to establish their area of clinical and academic expertise. This path cannot be underestimated in its importance for academic success. The second path is about the "moon shot." This is the larger vision for a better world, surgical discipline, etc. One may or may not even be able to achieve this, but one will chip away at it with multiple research projects, grants, collaborations, and more. It is important to avoid being discouraged as there will be road bumps with that path. One can fall back on the first path to maintain a positive spirit needed to keep an academic career alive and healthy.

Secondary benefits of maintaining a healthy set of short-term research or academic goals are the opportunities for mentorship that come along. Every medical school has numerous eager, talented, and inspiring students who are looking to apply the scientific method. In fact, broadening one's horizons beyond the medical school opens even more opportunity to a diverse set of students from undergraduates to nonmedical graduate students to postdoctoral fellows. Some of the most enlightening projects have been a result of working with students who are passionate about a topic and bring a unique perspective to the field. It is important to begin flexing mentorship muscles as this may come naturally to some but require intentional effort and improvement for others.[1]

Long-term Research Goals

During one's surgical career, an overarching academic focus will be primarily in one of three areas: basic-translational, health services, or educational research. What is sometimes called the "moonshot work" will be a multiyear focus and typically a subject that requires long-range experiments or analyses that should result in a cogent and broad research theme. For example, this may be multiyear experiments related to a basic pathobiological mechanism of a disease process that is relevant to humans, a multiyear clinical trial program, extensive database interfacing and development, or developing an educational platform for validation. These projects are usually the subject of one or more extramural grant(s). This work should generally answer a big clinical question, with logical hard endpoints that are achievable and that will generate sustained interest over at least 5 or more years.

The broad, long-range narrative of a research career is generally one of two paradigms. Many choose to coordinate their clinical specialty with their research focus. For example, a surgical oncologist investigating the role of T-cell subtypes in liver cancer or investigating health disparities for colon cancer outcomes is typical. Alternatively, one may have their major research focus in an area that does not mirror their surgical practice. The narrower focus in the same topic allows one to develop a great depth of knowledge and relevant supportive publications. However, one of the joys of academia is the ability and freedom to answer different questions that may come to the forefront in one's clinical practice, often outside of the main research focus. This strategy allows one to bring in people from various backgrounds and other expertise to disseminate that knowledge to a wider audience than would otherwise be possible. In the authors' opinion, productivity and impact in the research arena is more important than whether the science dovetails specifically with the clinical specialty.

Collaborators are critical for one's main research focus, and diversity of relevant expertise is critical. For example, basic science–focused surgeons may be primarily mentored by a senior surgeon with an independent lab, yet it is beneficial for that same junior faculty to have mentors in the basic sciences disciplines, such as immunology, cell biology, oncology, etc., depending on the project specifics. This provides for a diverse cognitive input in terms of experimental planning, experiences and knowledge related to the disease process, and modeling of the disease process itself. Similarly, bringing in a behavioral scientist, economist, and education specialist with regard to non-basic-translational work is highly beneficial for those involved in this area. This diversity not only increases the junior faculty's collaborative mentors and colleagues but also exposes them to different areas that may be fruitful long term. Nonsurgeon and nonclinician experts will often bring a markedly different viewpoint and can elevate innovation and novelty of the research approach. These collaborations take time, effort, and open-mindedness to develop but are well worth the investment. These collaborator networks are often dependent on the primary mentor's connections, underscoring an often overlooked asset of a good mentor.

Mentors change over one's career. The junior faculty will likely engage with a relatively diverse group of mentors over time both within and outside of the institution. Similarly, an early stage mentor may be different from a midcareer mentor depending on the project. Clinical practice mentors are often not the same person as the academic mentor. Having this open mind framework allows both the mentor and mentee to flourish. Picking a good mentor and being a good mentee is a topic unto itself, but suffice it to say, this is a critical relationship for one's career success.[2,3]

Extramural support is expected for one's "moonshot" research enterprise. The types of grants that are the highest currency in academic medical centers are typically extramural, peer-reviewed grants, and quite competitive. K-awards are a usual path for junior faculty to directly gain mentored experience, and receipt of a K-award enhances one's credentials to then compete for an R01 level grant. Indeed, having a K-award directly increases the chances of transitioning to R level grants.[4] Veterans Administration (VA) funding, in the form of a Merit Review grant, has a similar level of competitiveness as NIH funding. This usually requires that one has at least some lab space, human samples, or experiments performed in the VA system, often on site. Department of Defense (DOD) funding is more of a contractual nature, based on a topic area, but can provide significant funding as well as indirect funding support to the institution. Persistence is critical, and indeed, early career investigators who came close to a fundable score succeed as well as those having an early grant win.[5]

It is often hard to progress directly from postdoctoral training to being competitive for an R-award, unless perhaps, as a Co-Principal investigator. This route may be appropriate with a senior mentor who will ultimately transfer their project to the junior mentee over time. Team science is now a more viable route for scholarly activity and academic promotion. An excellent example of team science is large genome-wide analysis, requiring many partners to complete the analysis.[6]

Program project grants (PPG) from the NIH are generally reserved for those who are heading up a large group of independent scientists and may be more appropriate for later in one's career. This mechanism provides funding for common service cores, i.e., animal core, antibody core, etc. Here again, the opportunity to harness diversity of experience and thought is critical. Although perceived barriers and attitudes often exist between surgical and medical fields, this bias doesn't benefit patients long term.

T32 grants are another way to involve multiple investigators and build a pipeline of student and postdoctoral researchers. This grant mechanism provides salary support and some modest amount for supplies for 2 years, including predoctoral, postdoctoral, MD, or PhD. The Principal Investigators (PIs) of this grant type need to have a track record of independent funding and of successful mentees. T32 training grants provide an opportunity to diversify trainees via selection processes to the benefit of both the applicant and the lab in which they train.

The NIH has put efforts into deliberately encouraging underrepresented minorities (URMs) to apply for research funding.[7] Specifically, the Research Supplements to Promote Diversity in Health-Related Research program has been implemented and evaluated.[8] The most successful approach is building a pipeline of URMs.[9] This is also enhanced through the National Research Training Network. For example, focused efforts to enhance grant writing have been done at faculty and postdoctorate levels.[10] Successful strategies to recruit and retain URM faculty include competitive salaries and support, a flexible working environment, and leadership positions.[11] Similarly, recruiting URM students is associated with URM faculty recruitment, although in a delayed fashion.[12] Various new strategies to eliminate the learning gap between URM and non-URM students may also increase the pipeline of students and ultimately faculty.[13]

RUNNING AN EFFECTIVE RESEARCH "LAB"

Establishing Infrastructure

Promoting outstanding laboratory research in a Department of Surgery requires intentional effort and careful allocation of resources. Laboratory research is a highly competitive field, where the attrition rate is very high even for PhD scientists or physician/scientists in less demanding disciplines than Surgery. Yet, the rewards of promoting a basic research program within surgery are high. Surgeons have first-hand experience of the patient condition, thus bring unique insights in disease-focused research. For a bench research enterprise to succeed within a Department of Surgery, an ideal setup is to facilitate collaborative groups that extend beyond the Department, and include a diversity of backgrounds and expertise within the department itself. Furthermore, a well-developed individualized mentoring plan is of the essence. Although women compose half of medical and graduate students, they are underrepresented on faculty, and even more so in leadership positions.[14] Similarly, the proportion of underrepresented minority on faculty is extremely low.[15] Thus, for those surgeon-scientists that have a basic research program, and in particular women and URMs, creating a supportive environment and setting the stage for success is paramount. Specific practical approaches to foster thriving research and successfully start an independent laboratory are discussed below.

Starting a Lab: Different Models

Most tenure-track Assistant Professors who establish a research laboratory start with their own independent space and equipment. This is also true for tenure-track PhD scientists in clinical departments and physician-scientists in less demanding specialties. A second model, which the Department of Surgery at the University of Michigan uses for surgeon-scientists, is embedding the new faculty in an established laboratory that provides support and mentorship. The host laboratory can be within the Department of Surgery or in a separate department.

Advantages and Disadvantages of Starting With Independent Laboratory Space

Having an independent lab space is how most tenure-track assistant professors start. This arrangement requires a substantial investment in equipment, and significant startup funds. Additionally, hiring the right people is challenging. However, having an independent lab space allows the PI to foster their own lab culture, have access to more space (even the smallest laboratory unit or bay in a shared space model will accommodate at least four researchers), and develop an independent program. It is difficult, or impossible, to provide an equipment list that is useful for all, as needs are dependent on each investigator's unique research program. Furthermore, equipment changes as technology evolves and some machinery becomes obsolete while others become common. Obtaining equipment lists from peers who have recently gone through the job market, as well as noting all the equipment used during postdoctoral or academic-development training is important. It is important to determine what shared resources are available and how accessible (in terms of both cost and wait-time) to each investigator. Likely the biggest challenge of this model is to hire, train, and retain lab personnel when the PI is away from the lab due to clinical obligations.

Advantages and Disadvantages of Being Embedded in a Larger Lab

At the University of Michigan, most Assistant Professors in Surgery are initially embedded in a larger, established lab. This arrangement has several advantages, including a shorter ramp-up time (as the lab is functional from day 1), lower cost, and easier supervision of lab personnel. It might also obviate the need to hire a lab manager, thus saving resources which may be used for other purposes.

It is of the essence that the host PI be highly committed to the junior faculty, and a clear conversation needs to be maintained to make sure that the junior faculty has a well-delineated independent research direction that should be related, but not overlapping. Choosing a host lab is fundamental, as this choice is harder to change later. In addition, changing laboratories would inevitably lead to slower research progress, thus having a negative impact on the promotion timeline. This model has generally been very successful at the University of Michigan, with host laboratories being either within Surgery or in other departments, and led by surgeon-scientists or by PhD scientists.

Taking Diversity Into Account

Basic sciences, here referring to any type of laboratory-based research, or wet-lab research, has historically retained very few women. While graduate students and postdocs are about half female, the proportion decreases on tenure-track faculty and then continues to decrease going up the ranks.[16,17] This decline cannot be explained by a lack of people training to become scientists. The problem is compounded for clinician scientists, including surgeon-scientists, who carry a burden of higher clinical duties than many other specialties.

It goes without saying that men can be exceptional mentors for junior women. However, it is important to consider the lack of a peer group as a factor that might discourage junior women surgeons from following a basic research path. Furthermore, the lack of a peer group can be an obstacle to career advancement, as is the reduced opportunity to network informally at conferences and similar settings. Institutional efforts to increase faculty diversity often begin with initiatives (committees, mentoring efforts, visibility for women, and URM faculty) that paradoxically increase the burden of institutional service for the same group of people. A simple example is committee representations: if women faculty are the minority, and committee membership is balanced, then women will serve on more committees than men on faculty. A possible solution that would benefit all faculty, men and women, that take on a disproportionate amount of service would be to reward service both in the short term (e.g., with discretionary funds to the lab to account for the diminished amount of time to write grants) and in the long term (e.g., taking service into account for promotion).

How to Manage and Obtain Appropriate Resources

Space is a fundamental resource and scarce at most academic medical schools. In addition to laboratory space, and depending on the type of research, cell culture space and/or animal housing space may be equally important. At most Institutions, space is a limiting factor and it is important to have a clearly outlined space allocation. As mentioned above, an equipment list is essential, and a combination of sharing and acquiring new equipment is an efficient way to start the laboratory. Importantly, most equipment needs to be in place to be able to successfully apply for external funding. Only limited equipment can be budgeted for grants—and it is a part of the budget often cut in study section. Thus, proposing to use equipment that is not in place is likely to result in a lower grant score due to lack of feasibility. It is therefore important to negotiate realistic startup packages that account for the cost of acquiring suitable equipment.

Internal pilot funding mechanisms provide an opportunity to receive feedback as well as funds to generate preliminary data. Career-development mechanisms, some restricted to physician-scientists or surgeon-scientists, contribute to establishing a funding history. A timeline to the first K08 application should be developed early. Since K08 grants do not usually provide sufficient research funds for supplies, it is important to obtain additional grant funding or departmental support to successfully run the laboratory.

Managing Teams

Managing people in the lab is one of the most important, challenging, and potentially rewarding aspects of running a research laboratory. People are inherently different, and their team interactions are complex. The challenges are compounded if clinical duties limit lab time to a few days each week. Mentoring and managing styles vary, and trainees have different needs. To compound the challenge, most new investigators have little training in people management.

Most new PIs spend time at the bench, to do experiments as well as to train trainees. Training laboratory personnel so that they can reliably perform most/all lab work is essential to the success of the laboratory, and probably a necessity for surgeon-scientists: most biomedical projects rely on living organisms (cells, mice) that cannot be left unattended several days each week. Time is well-spent ensuring that laboratory personnel are adequately trained, and discussing experimental planning, data analysis, and interpretation. Writing grants and manuscripts will take the majority of the time not spent with other obligations.

It follows then that hiring appropriate lab personnel is critical for a laboratory's success. The initial hire is often a career technician who can supervise lab operations as well as be at the bench. While such individuals exist, they are rare. However, many recent graduates with a desire to apply to medical school or graduate school seek to obtain research experience. A recent graduate will be relatively inexperienced, yet might be ideal for new PIs as long as they have enough time to dedicate to training or are embedded in a lab situation which allows training by other laboratory members. Those individuals are usually highly driven and hardworking; the disadvantage, of course, being that their time in the lab is usually limited to 1 or 2 years (a 1-year arrangement is likely to be undesirable, as several months of training is usually needed at the start). Similarly, postdocs—particularly if interested in an academic career—are very motivated. However, postdocs who do want to start their own laboratory will need to develop an independent research direction, something a small lab might lack the resources to allow. If postdocs are hired, it is important to pay attention to their career development and it might be beneficial to identify a PhD co-mentor who will help guide their career as well as their academic job search later (which is quite different for PhD scientists vs. MDs). Surgery residents or residents in other specialties who are engaging in their research time may be ideal, as they tend to gravitate toward surgeon-run laboratories, are hardworking and driven, and do not have the same pressing need to develop a separate research direction. Both postdocs and surgery residents will have the same drive to publish as starting PIs, thus aligning their career goals. In addition, both postdocs and residents need to build a funding history, so they will be motivated to apply for fellowships—potentially relieving the financial burden and freeing resources to hire new laboratory members.

Graduate students are the driving force in many academic laboratories. They need significant supervision and entail a number of administrative commitments, and they might be a difficult fit for surgeon-scientists. Undergraduate students are available through many different mechanisms, some that require the PI to pay salary while others that don't (usually based on the students acquiring credit).

Cadence of Research Meetings

The PI needs to meet with laboratory personnel through a variety of modalities to keep projects moving forward efficiently. Even though there are variations, typically meetings follow some combination of 1:1 meetings, lab meetings, and ideally joint meetings that bring together multiple laboratories sharing common interests. Managing people is a fundamental skill, although it is rarely taught. One-on-one meetings are essential, as they allow the PI to set an experimental plan, analyze and interpret data, and adjust the experimental plan as needed. These meetings are important to ensure that work in the lab is directed to the end goal (publication) and that not too much time and energy is spent on dead-end projects, and that there are not unnecessary delays. A weekly meeting with each lab member is ideal, possibly at a set, constant time. It is important to set expectations for the meeting: trainees/lab personnel should talk about the goals of their experiments, show data, and be involved in developing a plan for future experiments. In addition, it is important to discuss literature and ensure people in the lab are reading widely. This is a setting to discuss training goals, provide mentorship, but also address any issue of work performance.

In laboratory science, technical difficulties are common. It is important to be mindful of the time spent troubleshooting (finding experts who can train lab personnel can save time; it is worth using resources for that, even if it means covering travel for a trainee to a collaborator's lab). It is equally important to design experiments so that a "go/no go" decision for each project is made early. Reasons for a "no go" decision might be: lack of a clear phenotype/effect; technical difficulties that do not seem to be solvable in a reasonable time; and excessive competition on the topic by bigger players in the field.

Lab meetings should also occur weekly (they could initially be combined with the host lab). Different modalities can be used or alternated. A presentation by a single lab member gives everybody on the team the opportunity to keep up-to-date with other people's work and identify areas of common interest. It is important to discuss technical or conceptual difficulties so that they might be addressed as a group. A roundtable format can also be used for updates by all laboratory members. Journal clubs can be interspersed, especially when an article of interest to the whole laboratory is published. Lab meeting is the best setting to discuss general lab management issues, including lab finances, ordering policy, and lab chores. Following lab meeting with a 1:1 meeting with the person who presented their data is a great opportunity to provide feedback on the presentation itself. Lab meetings should promote active participation by lab members, some of whom might need encouragement to speak up.

A key aspect of lab management is to ensure that personnel keep accurate and timely records of their work. Discussing lab notebook keeping and the integration and appropriate storage of electronic data is essential to run an effective research operation, avoiding the need to duplicate troubleshooting and setting new techniques. Equally important is the legal aspect of lab book keeping, which comes into play for patent applications but also if any doubt is raised as to the rigor of published research.

Keeping people on task is essential, even more so when the lab is small. People vary widely in their commitment, work ethic, and career goals. It is important to set clear expectations, provide constant feedback, and identify performance issues early. Conversely, for high-performing postdocs or staff, it might be valuable to provide them with additional manpower (often in the form of an undergraduate student or junior technician). That will allow them to practice their own mentorship skills, as well as devote their time to the more important experiments while delegating routine tasks. Postdocs are often attracted to established laboratories rather than small newly formed labs. Teaming up with senior faculty members and even co-mentoring postdocs can benefit both the postdoc and the faculty member. The postdoc gets the benefit of a mentor that is better known on the national scale—important for the later job search—while also benefiting from the frequent interactions that are only possible with new faculty members. Furthermore, having two mentors makes it easier for the postdoc to identify their own, independent research direction.

It should be emphasized that postdoctoral fellows are training with the goal to pursue an academic career (or alternative careers such as teaching, industry, and so on) and are not long-term employees. In fact, most institutions cap the postdoctoral time to 5 years. The transition to independence, especially within academia, is highly competitive, with several applicants for each job opening. While career development for postdocs is not the topic of this chapter, it is important to be aware of this responsibility, and to be willing to support the postdoc's career—or alternatively staff the lab with technicians or senior scientists whose goal is not to become independent.

Surgeon-scientists are unlikely, at least initially, to have the time to devote to training a graduate student, in addition to the additional time commitment to devote to joining a graduate program. In contrast, PhD scientists who join the faculty in a clinical department, including Surgery, should become involved with a graduate program as soon as possible after starting their faculty job. This can be achieved by joining a program that has no departmental affiliation, or by obtaining a joint appointment in a basic science department.

Engaging Collaborators

Engaging collaborators is essential for success. Ideally, a new PI will find a community of people sharing a common research interest, who hold regular joint meetings and share resources, reagents, and expertise. Potential collaborators should be sought during the interview process. It is also often productive to design research projects that take advantage of unique resources at a specific institution. For example, when I started my academic career, I took advantage of a colleague's expertise in Notch signaling and merged it with my focus on pancreatic cancer. This resulted in a great collaboration (my colleague was interested in hematopoietic malignancies, thus there was no potential for competition), my very first career development grant, and a joint publication down the line. Currently, one of the junior faculty I mentor, a surgeon-scientist, is taking advantage of genetically engineered mouse models generated in my laboratory to explore the epigenetic regulation of cancer, his area of interest and a clearly distinct topic from my laboratory's research.

Regular meetings, setting expectations, and breaking tasks into smaller units all contribute to trainees' success, which in turn is linked to the faculty member's success. Maximizing collaboration within the laboratory, or with members of collaborators' laboratories, allows trainees to overcome initial technical challenges. A useful practice is to keep a shared folder for articles that are fundamental knowledge for all in the laboratory. Encouraging trainees to read widely is necessary—a trainee-organized journal club during lab meeting or even separately is a great addition to other research meetings. Co-mentors, members of a mentoring committee, or thesis committee can similarly contribute to ensuring that projects advance steadily. It is also important to promote trainees' presentation skills, written and oral, so that they might contribute to writing manuscripts describing their work. Great insights in managing teams and promoting productivity in the lab are provided in "*At the Helm, Leading your Laboratory*, Kathy Barker, Cold Spring Harbor Laboratory Press." The companion volume *At the Bench* is a useful guide for laboratory staff.

Most journals provide clear authorship standards. Authorship requires an intellectual contribution to the work, whether experimental, data analysis, or writing/editing of the manuscript. In most biomedical sciences fields, the first author has done most of the experiments, and often written the initial draft of the manuscript; the last authors have provided the conceptual framework for the project as well as resources, laboratory space, and so on. The last author is ultimately responsible for the content of the publication and is usually in charge of a significant proportion of writing and editing.

Most articles have several authors; trainees and people responsible for the experimental work go in order of contribution (a rule of thumb is to see how many figures/panels each person contributed) from the first. Somewhat confusingly, collaborators and senior co-authors, who provided essential intellectual contributions or shared key resources, are listed from the end. In other words, the second author will have done fewer experiments than the first author; the second-to-last author will have provided a meaningful contribution but less than the last author. Sharing of first authorship and least authorship, and variations such as first authors serving as co-corresponding authors are increasingly common, as science becomes more of a team effort. Different approaches can be used to discuss authorship. It is important to be clear from the beginning that a project is to be considered a collaboration, while possibly leaving details regarding the order of authors to a later time, when the contribution of each person to the project is clear. Authorship might have to be re-discussed if a party fails to do their assigned work, or, conversely, takes on a larger share of the work.

ENSURING EQUITABLE INTERVIEWS AND AVOIDING BIAS

While diversity is problematic at the faculty and medical school leadership level, it is much less so among trainees and laboratory staff. That said, opportunities for trainees are not equal, as bias in hiring occurs.[18] Strategies that are useful to hire diverse faculty can be used when hiring for a laboratory, such as asking similar questions of each candidate, and critical reading of recommendation letters(*Figure 10.2*).

As Admissions Chair for the Cancer Biology Graduate Program at the University of Michigan and one of 14 Admissions Chairs for the different programs under the Program in Biomedical Sciences (PIBS) umbrella, the author has followed closely and implemented strategies to ensure a diverse graduate class. Of note, incoming graduate students are at least 50% female. Our effort, as Admission Chairs has been focused on recruiting URM students. Strategies that have been successful include *outreach, programmatic review of applications* and *intentional interview strategies.* For outreach, we ensure faculty and student participation at minority scientific conferences and promote both on-campus and off-campus initiatives such as "Developing Future Biologists" as well as a number of summer programs aimed at bringing in URM trainees heading to graduate or medical school.[19,20]

For the programmatic review, every candidate application is carefully reviewed, GREs are not provided (recent studies have demonstrated Graduate Record Examination is a better representation of the student's family income than the student's potential to do well in graduate school), and factors such as past research experience are considered in relation to the opportunities each student had. During the interview process, applicants get to meet trainees on campus who represent diversity. Similarly, although more challenging, the program strives to have each trainee meet diverse faculty. Parallel approaches can be used when interviewing for one's own laboratory, including having applicants meet members of collaborators' groups. Different training history and cognitive differences are as important as other parameters of diversity when recruiting laboratory members.

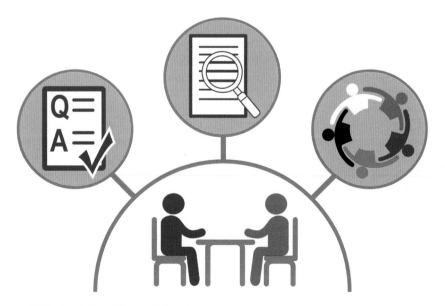

Figure 10.2 Avoiding bias in interviews.

FUNDING SOURCES THAT REWARD DIVERSITY

Academic laboratories are based on external funding, most of which is obtained through the NIH. Physician-scientists often apply initially to K08 mentored awards (mechanisms open to both MD and PhD scientists include the K22 award and the "transition to independence" K99/R00 award that includes a mentored phase and an independent phase and needs to be secured during postdoctoral training). Later, R01 funding is usually the main financial support for a lab. Unfortunately, NIH funding is unevenly distributed, with most funding going to a relatively small number of laboratories and with evidence of gender and racial discrimination in the allocation of funding.[21-25] The percentage of women holding an R01 award is about 30%, consistent with the percentage of women on faculty. However, the percentage of women PIs decreases steadily for two or more R01 grants, with the grantees holding 4 R01 awards being only 13% female. Diversity focused initiatives can increase the funding available to the laboratory as well as promote trainees' career.

R01 grants funded by the NIH can be the basis to apply for a "minority supplement" (research supplement to promote diversity). Preconditions apply: the end date of the parent R01 must be multiple years in the future; an eligible candidate must be working in the laboratory; and the salary of the applicant may not be paid from the parent grant at the time of application. The application process requires writing a research project that is related to, but not overlapping, the parent R01. Two separate supplements can be requested for a single R01. The supplements are administratively reviewed, not peer reviewed, and require an annual progress report that is separate from that of the parent R01.

In addition, postdocs and graduate students that are classified as "underrepresented minority" can apply to individual F30, F31, and F32 grants as a diversity applicant, which usually allows a slightly higher payline than the regular mechanism. These grants are reviewed by standing study sections, together with non-diversity counterparts. For the candidate, the F mechanism is more beneficial as it helps establish a funding history. Diversity supplements and F grants can be held concurrently, as supplements can be rebudgeted to cover supply costs; however, rebudgeting requires permission from the NIH and is not guaranteed. It is important to note that both diversity supplements and F-series grants require the applicant to be a permanent resident of the United States or a citizen, and visa holders are not eligible.

Institutional training grants (T32) are an excellent option for trainee funding. These offer both predoctoral and postdoctoral slots, allow the trainees to be integrated in the program's activities, and generally cover salary and, if applicable, tuition. In addition, they often provide travel funding to allow trainees to attend conferences. While not specifically designed for URM trainees, these opportunities are open to all who meet residency/citizenship requirements.

For cancer researchers, the American Cancer Society has mechanisms that parallel both the K08 award, for junior faculty, and support postdoctoral training. Citizenship requirements exist for both. For trainees (both graduate students and postdocs) who are visa holders, NIH grants are not an option. Some postdoctoral opportunities exist through foundations, which are field-specific and highly competitive. Internal funding mechanisms are also sometimes available, often paired with T32 training grants.

BALANCING RESEARCH AND SERVICE

Typically, one's academic surgical career is composed of three main areas: teaching, research, and service. Certainly, the two most intuitive and "fun" are research and teaching. Education is inherent to the job as a minimum expectation of being an academic surgeon by teaching medical students, residents, and fellows. Teaching takes investment of time, but also brings the joy of seeing junior residents progress to chief level with competence and confidence, or when inspiring a medical student to pursue scientific investigation. Similarly, directly mentoring PhD students and nonphysician postdoctorates and fellows is a bedrock part of running a research enterprise.

Service activities encompass multiple venues. Manuscript reviews are a useful and important activity. All manuscripts are peer-reviewed and performing that same service for others is important. Peer review of manuscripts educates one on how excellent and lesser papers are written and presented, how the papers are structured, and the organization of the critiques. One needs to be fair and constructive but to also realize that some manuscripts are not acceptable for the journal to which they have been submitted. The journal impact factor may drive the level and depth of the review itself. For example, reviews for a journal that has an impact factor of 1.5 compared with one that has an impact factor of 15, likely have differing levels of scrutiny reflecting different degrees of selectivity.

Grant reviews are another service activity that is both important for one's academic career as well as providing a service to those who submit grants. Grant reviews require a lot of work and thus the reviewers need to be respectful and put in the work to review in a conscientious, unbiased, and fair fashion for the sponsoring agency. This often takes the form of an NIH, DOD, or VA study section. Care must be taken to be aware of unconscious bias that may unfairly penalize an applicant. The issue of reviewer bias in the NIH has been controversial, with some suggesting that black applicants were less likely to get fundable scores than white applicants, while other data suggest that this may not be the case.[24,26] Similarly, data suggest women applicants may be at a greater disadvantage than men in grant resubmission.

Other service obligations are institutional. Institutional Review Board (IRB) and animal committee review participation are examples. It is recommended these two committee activities be sought at the late Associate or Full Professor level, due to experience needed and the time commitment involved. Often, shorter committee obligations can be done and are useful for promotion and good citizenship. These are often dictated by departmental leadership.

National and international societal committee participation is a currency that is important for promotion and can be a great networking activity. This service is generally both specialty and subspecialty specific. These committees are other ways to meet colleagues and interact with others of diverse scientific interest. These experiences allow one to see how meetings are conducted and how certain committees accomplish much while others do not. These experiences provide important career lessons on leadership style.

The promotions process varies by institution but is generally rigorous and standardized. The Promotions Committee evaluates the three missions of research, education, and service for the individual faculty. Some faculty may be assigned to the primary clinical track where the expectation of the surgeon is to build and drive a clinical program and teach residents without the requirement of the extramural grant funding or publications. Conversely, a tenure research track faculty has grants obtained and papers published, as well as consideration of mentee's success as their academic currency, and less of a focus on a high-volume clinical practice. Determining the promotion requirements and standards early is important, and the Section and Departmental leadership can often guide this process.

REFERENCES

1. Chopra V, Edelson DP, Saint S. A piece of my mind. Mentorship malpractice. *J Am Med Assoc.* 2016;315(14):1453-1454.

2. Ortega G, Smith C, Pichardo MS, Ramirez A, Soto-Greene M, Sánchez JP. Preparing for an academic career: the significance of mentoring. *MedEdPORTAL.* 2018;14:10690.

3. Valsangkar NP, Zimmers TA, Kim BJ, et al. Determining the drivers of academic success in surgery: an analysis of 3,850 faculty. *PLoS One.* 2015;10(7):e0131678.

4. Nikaj S, Lund PK. The impact of individual mentored career development (K) awards on the research trajectories of early-career scientists. *Acad Med.* 2019;94(5):708-714.

5. Wang Y, Jones BF, Wang D. Early-career setback and future career impact. 2019. Available at https://ssrn.com/abstract=3353841 or http://dx.doi.org/10.2139/ssrn.3353841.

6. Klarin D, Damrauer SM, Cho K, et al. Genetics of blood lipids among ~300,000 multi-ethnic participants of the Million Veteran Program. *Nat Genet.* 2018;50(11):1514-1523.

7. Guerrero LR, Ho J, Christie C, et al. Using collaborative approaches with a multi-method, multi-site, multi-target intervention: evaluating the National Research Mentoring Network. *BMC Proc.* 2017;11(suppl 12):14.

8. Duncan GA, Lockett A, Villegas LR, et al. National Heart, Lung, and Blood Institute workshop summary: enhancing opportunities for training and retention of a diverse biomedical workforce. *Ann Am Thorac Soc.* 2016;13(4):562-567.

9. Sánchez JP, Castillo-Page L, Spencer DJ, et al. Commentary: the building the next generation of academic physicians initiative: engaging medical students and residents. *Acad Med.* 2011;86(8):928-931.

10. Jones HP, McGee R, Weber-Main AM, et al. Enhancing research careers: an example of a US national diversity-focused, grant-writing training and coaching experiment. *BMC Proc.* 2017;11(suppl 12):16.

11. Peek ME, Kim KE, Johnson JK, Vela MB. "URM candidates are encouraged to apply": a national study to identify effective strategies to enhance racial and ethnic faculty diversity in academic departments of medicine. *Acad Med.* 2013;88(3):405-412.

12. Page KR, Castillo-Page L, Wright SM. Faculty diversity programs in U.S. medical schools and characteristics associated with higher faculty diversity. *Acad Med.* 2011;86(10):1221-1228.

13. Ballen CJ, Wieman C, Salehi S, Searle JB, Zamudio KR. Enhancing diversity in undergraduate science: self-efficacy drives performance gains with active learning. *CBE Life Sci Educ.* 2017;16(4):ar56.

14. Plank-Bazinet JL, Heggeness ML, Lund PK, Clayton JA. Women's careers in biomedical sciences: implications for the economy, scientific discovery, and women's health. *J Womens Health.* 2017;26(5):525-529.

15. Meyers LC, Brown AM, Moneta-Koehler L, Chalkley R. Survey of checkpoints along the pathway to diverse biomedical research faculty. *PLoS One.* 2018;13(1):e0190606.

16. Carr PL, Raj A, Kaplan SE, Terrin N, Breeze JL, Freund KM. Gender differences in academic medicine: retention, rank, and leadership comparisons from the National Faculty Survey. *Acad Med.* 2018;93(11):1694-1699.

17. López CM, Margherio C, Abraham-Hilaire LM, Feghali-Bostwick C. Gender disparities in faculty rank: factors that affect advancement of women scientists at academic medical centers. *Soc Sci.* 2018;7(4):62.

18. Sheltzer JM, Smith JC. Elite male faculty in the life sciences employ fewer women. *Proc Natl Acad Sci USA.* 2014;111(28):10107-10112.

19. Developing Future Biologists University of Michigan 2019. Available at https://www.developingfuturebiologists.com/. Accessed July 18, 2019.

20. Postbac Research Education Program (PREP) University of Michigan Medical School: Regents of the University of Michigan; 2019. Available at https://medicine.umich.edu/medschool/education/non-degree-programs/postbac-research-education-program-prep. Accessed July 18, 2019.

21. Wahls WP. The NIH must reduce disparities in funding to maximize its return on investments from taxpayers. *Elife.* 2018;7:p.e34965.

22. Pohlhaus JR, Jiang H, Wagner RM, Schaffer WT, Pinn VW. Sex differences in application, success, and funding rates for NIH extramural programs. *Acad Med.* 2011;86(6):759-767.

23. Magua W, Zhu X, Bhattacharya A, et al. Are female applicants disadvantaged in National Institutes of Health peer review? Combining algorithmic text mining and qualitative methods to detect evaluative differences in R01 reviewers' critiques. *J Womens Health.* 2017;26(5):560-570.

24. Ginther DK, Schaffer WT, Schnell J, et al. Race, ethnicity, and NIH research awards. *Science.* 2011;333(6045):1015-1019.

25. Tabak LA, Collins FS. Sociology. Weaving a richer tapestry in biomedical science. *Science.* 2011;333(6045):940-941.

26. Forscher PS, Cox WTL, Brauer M, Devine PG. Little race or gender bias in an experiment of initial review of NIH R01 grant proposals. *Nat Hum Behav.* 2019;3(3):257-264.

Part 2

ATTRACTING TALENTED MEDICAL STUDENTS

11

Outreach Before Medical School

Jason Hall
Miles B. Cahill
Jennifer F. Tseng

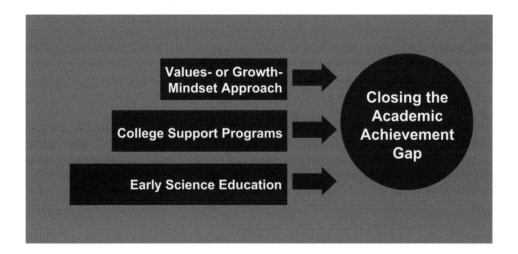

INTRODUCTION

The pervasive oppression of underrepresented minority groups in the United States through inferior education, housing, health care, employment opportunities, and uneven application of criminal injustice has been well established.[1-6] In the medical literature, disparities in healthcare outcomes have also been widely documented in minority communities in the United States. These differences are often attributed to genetics,[7] socioeconomic factors,[5] and provider implicit bias.[6] The larger societal conditions in which communities of color navigate are discussed less often. In spite of these circumstances, black and African-American applications to medical school have increased by nearly 1500 between 2002 and 2015.[8] Unfortunately, the number of acceptances only increased by 215.[8] Although African-Americans represent approximately 13% of the population, they only compose 4% of the physician workforce.[9] Some data suggest that white patients who are able to choose their own doctor are more likely to choose a race concordant provider. Satisfaction was rated higher across all racial groups when the patient and physician were of the same race.[10] Therefore, increasing the numbers of underrepresented minorities entering medical fields is a major priority for an increasingly diverse society.

There are significant challenges to meeting this objective. It is well documented that large segments of the population have been historically underrepresented in medicine and in science and engineering fields. As the National Science Foundation report summarizes,

> The representation of certain groups of people in science and engineering (S&E) education and employment differs from their representation in the U.S. population. Women, persons with disabilities, and three racial and ethnic groups—blacks, Hispanics, and American Indians or Alaska Natives—are underrepresented in S&E. While women have reached parity with men among S&E degree recipients overall, they constitute disproportionally smaller percentages of employed scientists and engineers than they do of the U.S. population. Blacks, Hispanics, and American Indians or Alaska Natives have gradually increased their share of S&E degrees, but they remain underrepresented in educational attainment and the S&E workforce.[11]

Byars-Winston et al. report 2014 National Center for Education Statistics data that show that while a majority of underrepresented students enter college with plans to major in a STEM discipline, only about 17% earn bachelor's degrees in those areas.[12] They conclude "underrepresentation, instead, appears to be a problem of translating the abilities and interests of students from racial/ethnic groups historically underrepresented in the sciences into persistence."[2] This disparity is a particularly concerning issue in medicine, as there is good evidence that this may affect patients' health.[13]

Efforts to increase minority enrollment in medical school that focuses exclusively on undergraduate students are less likely to affect the kind of changes that will be necessary to change the medical workforce significantly. This chapter will argue that increasing medical school enrollment will only be achieved through significant societal change that works to eliminate a racially based academic achievement gap in early education. Thus, the content of this chapter focuses upon improving medical school admission for underrepresented minorities argues for broader societal change.

THE ACADEMIC ACHIEVEMENT GAP

In 2018 to 2019, women made up 51.6% of matriculants to US medical schools.[14] However, several racial and ethnic groups have not experienced similar gains in representation. African-Americans, Native Americans, and Hispanic students continue to be underrepresented in US medical schools.[15] Morgan et al. cite several studies that show that students from groups underrepresented in medicine (URM) and from underprepared populations abandon premedical preparation at rates much higher than majority and privileged students. There is also evidence that some groups face challenges in the medical school admissions process.[16]

While most agree that medical students should be admitted based on "merit," there is some disagreement as to what this term means. In the United States, the predominant way of quantifying merit is the Medical College Admissions Test (MCAT) and undergraduate grade point average (GPA). These metrics do quantify academic achievement but do not measure fitness for a medical career. Although subjective, there is some suggestion that exclusive admission of students in the top end of this distribution can result in admission of students poorly suited for a medical career.[17,18] Students in underrepresented groups are often characterized as not having the essential skills to succeed in medical school as quantified by the aforementioned metrics.[19] For example, it is often pointed out that black and African-American applicants have significantly lower MCAT scores than other ethnic groups.[20] This type of summary assessment of the data misses significant nuances. When carefully examined, the mean MCAT score for all students is 506 ± SD 9.3. The African-American mean is 497 ± SD 9.1 and white 507 ± SD 8.2. The standard deviations suggest significant heterogeneity within each racial group.

Although there is discussion regarding high-stakes testing such as the MCAT, data suggest that the academic achievement gap between white and underrepresented minority groups begins in childhood.[1,21] The National Assessment of Educational Progress measures performance of students on mathematics and reading tests at the 4th, 8th, and 12th grade levels. This assessment found a significant but stable gap between black and Hispanic scores compared with those of white students in years 2013 to 2015. A socioeconomic component was also notable as children who received free or reduced-cost lunches performed worse than children who did not receive support for lunch.[22] Over the past 20 years, average scores have improved for all groups. However, the gap between the average scores of underrepresented groups and those of white students has not changed significantly over this period of time.[23,24]

As students consider preparation for advanced studies in science, further gaps emerge as white and Asian students tend to enroll in "rigorous" curricula (4 credits in math [1 credit precalculus or higher], 3 credits in science [with biology, chemistry, physics, all being represented], 3 credits in English, 3 credits in social studies, and 3 credits in foreign language) more often than other racial groups.[21] At the lowest rung of entry into the workforce, African-Americans graduate high school at much lower rates than their white peers.[25] Thus, it is no surprise that underrepresented minority groups abandon premedical preparation at much higher rates than other groups.[16]

There are a number of explanatory models for these performance differences. While discrimination has been invoked, it is unlikely to be the only explanatory factor.[26-28] One group of authors found that students from underrepresented groups are less likely to have higher social capital, leading to underachievement. This effect could be accentuated by ethnic and religious self-segregation.[29] "Stereotype threat" has also been proposed as a mechanism. This phenomenon suggests that actual poor performance is mediated by a societal expectation of poor performance.[30,31] Beyond ethnicity, Grace finds that subjective social status leads premedical students who perceive themselves to have lower social status to have more doubts about their fitness for medical school.[32,33]

MCAT REDESIGN AND DIVERSITY

Racial and Ethnic Diversity

The Association of American Medical Colleges spent many years reformulating the MCAT and adjusting guidelines for medical school requirements. When the current 2015 reformulation was unveiled, it quickly became clear that a typical undergraduate student needs to take at least 15 courses to prepare for application. Kaplan et al.[34]

posit that one of the motivations for the redesigned MCAT was to respond to the fact that "disparities in health outcomes among races and ethnic groups persist." Requiring undergraduate training in behavioral and social sciences to set a foundation for understanding nonbiological factors that can affect health is a laudable goal. However, the requirement of eight semesters of laboratory science plus biochemistry makes it challenging for an underprepared student to transition to college and complete the requirements on time. Even if a college offers a preparatory course in advance of the standard introductory science courses, the result is students must double up on laboratory sciences, typically early in their careers. For some students, this heavy load can be too much to manage.

Improving the Pipeline

Because of poor representation at lower levels of academic achievement, it is no surprise that underrepresented minorities on average are less "prepared" for the rigorous academic competition that is commonplace among undergraduates seeking admission to medical school. The pace and sheer volume of information that students are expected to master in order to be competitive on the MCAT examination are significant. For example, a typical undergraduate student needs 15 courses to prepare for the MCAT. In addition to the original requirements of a semester of calculus (or college mathematics), two semesters of general chemistry, two semesters of organic chemistry, two semesters of physics, and two semesters of English, the new examination expects a semester each of statistics, introductory psychology, introductory sociology, and biochemistry. For many colleges with a four course per semester load, this is nearly half of available course choices, on average two courses per semester. If a premedical student plans to attend medical school directly from college, the strain is even greater, as the student would need to finish these courses in 3 years. This level of academic performance is unlikely to be met if students do not have a history of significant class loads with challenging courses before starting college.

Barr, Matsui, Wanat, and Gonzalez found that chemistry courses in particular discourage many premedical students from continuing their studies, even at highly selective universities like University of California at Berkeley and Stanford University. This is especially true for groups underrepresented in medicine (URM).[35] This study's conclusion is consistent with literature that has found this barrier is present at both universities and liberal arts colleges[36] and for URM students who have had high-school enrichment programs in STEM.[37] Barr et al. conclude, "It appears that the time is right to undertake a fundamental reassessment of the historical role chemistry courses have played in the premedical curriculum at colleges and universities throughout the country."[35]

PREUNDERGRADUATE PROGRAMS

There have been a number of proposals to improve competitiveness. One example of a program aimed at an elementary school cohort is Project Excite sponsored by Northwestern University's Center for Talent Development.[21] The objective of this program was to better prepare minority students from the third to the eight grade for advanced math and science courses in high school. Importantly, this program included 445 required and 180 optional hours of Saturday, summer and after-school activities. The authors compared the performance of Project Excite participants with that of students from their local school districts on the Illinois Standards Achievement Tests and a number of other standardized examinations. Students who participated in Project Excite performed better than their black, Latino, and low-income peers. Their scores approached those of white, Asian, and non–low-income students. Because of this, participants in the program were more likely to be placed in above grade-level math courses.[21]

There are other examples of university-sponsored programs designed to increase the interests of underrepresented precollege students in medical careers. Boston University School of Medicine created a partnership with Boston Area Health Education Center (BAHEC), a division of the Boston Public Health Commission. BAHEC is "a youth pathway to health careers program." BAHEC sponsors a summer program as well as after-school programs during the school year. In the summer session, BUMC offers four electives—a course which provides exposure to basic scientific research, one that provides experience with public health issues, a clinical course that focuses on physical examination skills, and another clinically related course which focuses on different careers in health sciences. During the academic year, BUMC offers an introduction to clinical medicine course, an introduction to dental medicine course, and a course in global health taught by BU undergraduate students. During the clinically related courses, students experience hands-on activities such as suturing, physical examination, mock dental procedures, brain dissection, and EKG analysis. Students are selected by BAHEC, and approximately 15 enroll in each of the various electives. Initial feedback from participants has been outstanding.

COMPREHENSIVE SUPPORT

Morgan et al. make several suggestions for improving undergraduate outcomes for underprepared students, with an emphasis on the first year of college. Successful programs include forming living and learning communities and pathway programs set up in partnership with medical schools.[16] A program at the University of Michigan (Health Sciences Scholars Program) helps students academically but also gives them a sense of ownership and belonging in STEM and medical fields. Toven-Lindsey et al. describe a similar program at University of California, Los Angeles, which has been successful in helping students from underrepresented groups persist and succeed in STEM disciplines, including gateway courses.[38]

The University of Massachusetts Medical School has offered a number of programs to support underrepresented groups, providing a continuity of programs from high school through postcollege years. According to Dr Deborah-Harmon Hines, PhD, Professor Emeritus at the medical school, success is based on "high expectations of students," having the programs "highly structured," with staff participating in the program for long periods of time. Also critical to success is "strenuous tracking and follow-up," with tracking of over 80% of participants and providing "specific recommendations: for each participant" (*Figure 11.1*). Goonewardene et al. make a number of similar suggestions for supporting underrepresented students in STEM at small universities, citing an example at Lock Haven University, noting that a "comprehensive program fostering engagement through individualized attention, a robust learning community, meaningful research opportunities, and peer and alumni support is essential."[39]

Authors from Cornell University reported similar results through the Biology Scholars Program (BSP). BSP is structured as a diversity support program to enhance underrepresented racial minority (URM) student performance. Although BSP matriculants are less academically prepared when they enter college, by graduation they appear to have closed the achievement gap. These students finish college with GPAs similar to those of majority students.[40]

High expectations   Structured programs   Follow-up

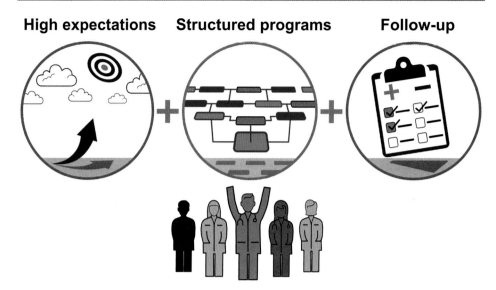

Figure 11.1 Elements of student support.

Support for at-risk students has been implemented at 4-year colleges as well. At the College of the Holy Cross, a cohort of students each year who have a demonstrated interest in STEM but have some factor that puts them at risk (e.g., identification as an underrepresented minority, first-generation college student, Pell Grant eligibility) are identified. They are invited to participate in the First-Year Research Advancement Program (FRAP). According to Associate Professor of Biology Julia Paxson, PhD, DVM, "FRAP students are paid to work in teams of two with a research student mentor in a faculty lab for 8 hours a week throughout the academic year. As part of the program, participants attend a weekly cohort meeting consisting of lively discussions on a variety of topics related to science, careers, study strategies, and adapting to life at college. We bring in experts from around campus including the Center for Career Development, Academic Services and Learning Resources, the Counseling Center, and the Office of Multicultural Education, as well as the internal earned expertise of our senior mentors. For the last 2 years, FRAP alums have closed the circle by participating as mentors. This cohort activity also involves the senior mentor students and FRAP faculty, enabling the development of a cohesive interdisciplinary STEM community. After completing FRAP, many students choose to stay and continue working in faculty labs as research students but are also more competitively positioned for teaching assistant jobs, as well as external internship positions at other institutions." Programs such as this are designed to bring at-risk students into the community at the start of their careers while at the same time offering academic and multileveled mentoring support.

TEACHER CHARACTERISTICS AND STYLES

One important variable in the academic success of all students is the skill of the teacher. Canning et al. examined the outcomes of students enrolled in the STEM classes of faculty classified as growth mindset or fixed mindset in relation to ability. A growth mindset is a mental attitude or belief that intelligence is malleable and can be honed with practice. A fixed mindset is associated with the belief that intelligence is fixed and cannot be learned. These authors found that racial achievement gaps were twice as high in the cohort of students enrolled in a class with a professor who was classified as fixed mindset. The relationship between student achievement and faculty mindset suggests that the beliefs of the teacher may have important implications for the ultimate success of underrepresented minority students.[41] Other authors have proposed that varied teaching styles may help to close achievement gaps. One study from Cornell compared traditional teaching methods to "active learning." These authors found that "active learning" methods closed the achievement gap between underrepresented and nonunderrepresented students. These authors also noted an increase in self-efficacy among all students (*Figure 11.2*).[42,43]

Other authors discuss concepts related to affective learning (self-efficacy, sense of belonging, and science identity) that may have a significant impact on underrepresented students persisting in STEM majors. They suggest a number of ways college biology instructors can assess these characteristics in students and adjust teaching methods to help develop these traits. By building self-confidence, helping students feel a part of the community, and helping students think of themselves (and be thought of) as scientists, small adjustments in teaching can pay large dividends.[44] Other groups have suggested that the ethnicity of the teacher can also influence academic performance. In one study, the racial achievement gap fell by 50% when students were taught by an underrepresented minority faculty member.[45]

Psychological Interventions

Light-touch interventions may be beneficial for some students. In one study, 7686 students of a large Midwestern university were randomly assigned to online growth-mindset intervention, social belonging intervention, or a comparison group. Latino students who participated in the growth-mindset arm experienced a 0.4-point increase in GPA. This represented 72% of the gap between Latino and white students. These authors concluded that light-touch interventions might be specifically helpful for improving academic outcomes of underrepresented students.[46] Fink et al. demonstrated similar findings with a chemistry-specific growth-mindset intervention among first-year college students enrolled in General Chemistry. This program encouraged students to view intelligence as a flexible characteristic that can be enhanced with practice and dedication rather than as a fixed entity assigned at

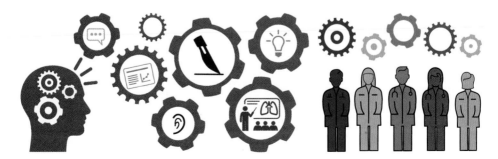

Figure 11.2 Characteristics of effective teachers.

birth. These authors reported eliminating the racial achievement gap after controlling for differences in preparation.[47] The success of this type of approach has also been demonstrated in other disciplines including biology.[48,49]

There is some evidence that underprepared students can be brought up to speed quickly if provided the resources. For example, Fischer et al. report that a 3-week online preparatory course allowed students to fare better in organic chemistry.[50] Results were particularly strong for historically at-risk groups, where the online course seemed to have increased grades by about one-third of a letter grade.

More Study

There is a need for rigorous statistical measures to identify factors that may help underrepresented groups to thrive in STEM disciplines.[12] That is, while a number of different institutions have tried, and are trying programs to improve success for underrepresented groups, there is a need for more detailed studies on how programs work, which elements of programs are most effective, and what factors may work most efficiently in concert. This is particularly important (not to mention challenging) as many programs are multifaceted and have both tangible and intangible elements that are not easily measured. By using a factor analysis statistical technique and surveys, this approach seeks to identify the role that elements of affective learning have in program success.

Student Affinity Groups

Because a sense of belonging is important for persistence of premedical students, groups such as the Student National Medical Organization that provide support for medical and premedical students of color can be instrumental in supporting undergraduate students. Student groups such as XCHROM that support women and students of color in the sciences have the potential to help at-risk students identify themselves as scientists within the community.

CONCLUSION

There are a number of structural and academic obstacles to increasing the number of physicians for underrepresented minority groups. Ultimately these challenges culminate in an academic achievement gap that begins in elementary school and can persist as higher educational levels are attained. A lower proportion of underrepresented minority students are prepared for STEM majors when starting college in comparison with white students. This emphasizes the importance of early, quality, scientific education for underrepresented groups as they are moving through their early school years. There is a growing understanding of how underprepared and underrepresented groups of students can be supported as they enter their college years. Programs that offer strong mentoring and defined structures have demonstrated success in closing the academic achievement gap. It appears that modules which emphasize a values-based or growth-mindset approach to intelligence are able to achieve success. These challenges appear to be ideal "laboratories" for institutions that serve underrepresented communities to create partnerships that are designed to address the social and environmental factors that contribute to the academic achievement gap.

REFERENCES

1. Grogan-Kaylor A, Woolley ME. The social ecology of race and ethnicity school achievement gaps: economic, neighborhood, school, and family factors. *J Hum Behav Social Environ.* 2010;20(7):875-896.

2. Mandell B. Racial Ratification and Global Warming: Truly Inconvenient Truth. *B.C. Third World L.J.* 2008;28:289-344.

3. Badger E. 2014. Housing segregation is holding back the promise of Brown v. Board of Education. https://wwwwashingtonpostcom/news/wonk/wp/2014/05/15/housing-segregation-is-holding-back-the-promise-of-brown-v-board-of-education/?utm_term=58bafaf31460.

4. Mundy AC. 2014. Transitioning from elementary school to middle school: The ecology of black males' behavior. Available from ProQuest Dissertations & Theses Global Retrieved from http://ezproxystthomasedu/login?url=http://searchproquestcom/docview/1551595454?acc ountid=14756.

5. Bailey ZD, Krieger N, Agenor M, Graves J, Linos N, Bassett MT. Structural racism and health inequities in the USA: evidence and interventions. *Lancet.* 2017;389(10077):1453-1463.

6. Dehon E, Weiss N, Jones J, Faulconer W, Hinton E, Sterling S. A systematic review of the impact of physician implicit racial bias on clinical decision making. *Acad Emerg Med.* 2017;24(8):895-904.

7. Sellers SL, Cunningham BA, Bonham VL. Physician knowledge of human genetic variation, beliefs about race and genetics, and use of race in clinical decision-making. *J Racial Ethnic Health Disparities.* 2019;6(1):110-116.

8. http://www.aamcdiversityfactsandfigures.org/section-ii-current-status-of-us-physician-workforce/index.html.

9. U.S. Census Bureau http://quickfacts.census.gov/qfd/states/00000.html. Accessed September 11.

10. Laveist TA, Nuru-Jeter A. Is doctor-patient race concordance associated with greater satisfaction with care? *J Health Social Behav.* 2002;43(3):296-306.

11. National Science Foundation, National Center for Science and Engineering Statistics. *Women, Minorities, and Persons With Disabilities in Science and Engineering: 2017.* Special Report NSF 17-310. Arlington, VA; 2017. Available at www.nsf.gov/statistics/wmpd/.

12. Byars-Winston A, Rogers J, Branchaw J, Pribbenow C, Hanke R, Pfund C. New measures assessing Predictors of academic persistence for historically underrepresented racial/ethnic undergraduates in science. *CBE Life Sci Educ.* 2016;15(3):ar32.

13. Alsan C, Garrick O, Graziani C. *Does Diversity Matter for Health? Experimental Evidence from Oakland,* NBER Working Paper 24787; 2019.

14. https://www.aamc.org/download/321442/data/factstablea1.pdf.

15. https://www.aamc.org/download/485288/data/factstablea14_3.pdf.

16. Morgan HK, Haggins A, Lypson ML, Ross P. The importance of the premedical experience in diversifying the health care workforce. *Acad Med.* 2016;91(11):1488-1491.

17. Powis DA, Bristow T. Top school marks don't necessarily make top medical students. *Med J Aust.* 1997;166(11):613.

18. Marley J, Carman I. Selecting medical students: a case report of the need for change. *Med Educ.* 1999;33(6):455-459.

19. Nicholson S, Cleland JA. "It's making contacts": notions of social capital and implications for widening access to medical education. *Adv Health Sci Educ.* 2017;22(2):477-490.

20. https://www.aamc.org/download/321498/data/factstablea18.pdf.

21. Olszewski-Kubilius P, Steenbergen-Hu S, Thomson D, Rosen R. Minority achievement gaps in STEM: findings of a longitudinal study of Project excite. *Gift Child Q.* 2017;61(1):20-39.

22. Lee S-Y, Olszewski-Kubilius P, Peternel G. The efficacy of academic acceleration for gifted minority students. *Gift Child Q.* 2010;54(3):189-208.

23. Rampey BD, Dion GS, Donahue PL. *NAEP 2008; Trends in Academic Progress (NCES 2009-479).* Washington, DC: National Center for Education Statistics, I. o.; Education Sciences, U. S. D. o. E.; 2009.

24. Hemphill FC, Vanneman A. Achievement Gaps: How Hispanic and White Students in Public Schools Perform in Mathematics and Reading on the National Assessment of Educational Progress, U.S. Department of Education NCES 2011-459, Washington, 2011.

25. https://nces.ed.gov/programs/coe/indicator_coi.asp.

26. McManus IC, Richards P, Winder BC, Sproston KA. Final examination performance of medical students from ethnic minorities. *Med Educ.* 1996;30(3):195-200.

27. Wass V, Roberts C, Hoogenboom R, Jones R, Van der Vleuten C. Effect of ethnicity on performance in a final objective structured clinical examination: qualitative and quantitative study. *BMJ.* 2003;326(7393):800-803.

28. Esmail A, Roberts C. Academic performance of ethnic minority candidates and discrimination in the MRCGP examinations between 2010 and 2012: analysis of data. *BMJ.* 2013;347.

29. Vaughan S, Sanders T, Crossley N, O'Neill P, Wass V. Bridging the gap: the roles of social capital and ethnicity in medical student achievement. *Med Educ.* 2015;49(1):114-123.

30. Woolf K, McManus IC, Potts HWW, Dacre J. The mediators of minority ethnic underperformance in final medical school examinations. *Br J Educ Psychol.* 2013;83(1):135-159.

31. Eschenbach EA, Virnoche M, Cashman EM, Lord SM, Camacho MM. *Proven practices that can reduce stereotype threat in engineering education: a literature review.* In: *2014 IEEE Frontiers in Education Conference.* Madrid, Spain: IEEE; 2014:140-148.

32. Grace MK. Subjective social status and premedical students' attitudes towards medical school. *Soc Sci Med.* 2017;184:84-98.

33. Greenhalgh T, Seyan K, Boynton P. "Not a university type": focus group study of social class, ethnic, and sex differences in school pupils' perceptions about medical school. *BMJ.* 2004;328(7455):1541-1544A.

34. Kaplan RM, Satterfield JM, Kington RS. Building a better physician – the case for the new MCAT. *New Engl J Med.* 2012;366(14):1265-1268.

35. Barr DA, Matsui J, Wanat SF, Gonzalez ME. Chemistry courses as the turning point for premedical students. *Adv Health Sci Educ.* 2010;15(1):45-54.

36. Lovecchio K, Dundes L. Premed survival. *Acad Med.* 2002;77(7):719-724.

37. Thurmond VB, Cregler LL. Why students drop out of the pipeline to health professions careers. *Acad Med.* 1999;74(4):448-451.

38. Toven-Lindsey B, Levis-Fitzgerald M, Barber PH, Hasson T. Increasing persistence in undergraduate science majors: a model for institutional support of underrepresented students. *CBE Life Sci Educ.* 2015;14(2):ar12.

39. Goonewardene A, Offutt C, Whitling J, Woodhouse D. An interdisciplinary approach to success for underrepresented students in STEM. *J Coll Sci Teach.* 2016;45(4):59-67.

40. Ballen CJ, Mason NA. Longitudinal analysis of a diversity support program in biology: a national call for further assessment. *Bioscience.* 2017;67(4):366-372.

41. Canning EA, Muenks K, Green DJ, Murphy MC. STEM faculty who believe ability is fixed have larger racial achievement gaps and inspire less student motivation in their classes. *Sci Adv.* 2019;5(2).

42. Ballen CJ, Wieman C, Salehi S, Searle JB, Zamudio KR. Enhancing diversity in undergraduate science: self-efficacy drives performance gains with active learning. *CBE Life Sci Educ.* 2017;16(4).

43. Snyder JJ, Sloane JD, Dunk RDP, Wiles JR. Peer-led team learning helps minority students succeed. *PLoS Biol.* 2016;14(3):e1002398.

44. Trujillo G, Tanner KD. Considering the role of affect in learning: monitoring students' self-efficacy, sense of belonging, and science identity. *CBE Life Sci Educ.* 2014;13(1):6-15.

45. Fairlie RW, Hoffmann F, Oreopoulos P. A community college instructor like me: race and ethnicity interactions in the classroom. *Am Econ Rev.* 2014;104(8):2567-2591.

46. Broda M, Yun J, Schneider B, Yeager DS, Walton GM, Diemer M. Reducing inequality in academic success for incoming college students: a randomized trial of growth mindset and belonging interventions. *J Res Educ Eff.* 2018;11(3):317-338.

47. Fink A, Cahill MJ, McDaniel MA, Hoffman A, Frey RF. Improving general chemistry performance through a growth mindset intervention: selective effects on underrepresented minorities. *Chem Educ Res Pract.* 2018;19(3):783-806.

48. Harackiewicz JM, Canning EA, Tibbetts Y, et al. Closing the social class achievement gap for first-generation students in undergraduate biology. *J Educ Psychol.* 2014;106(2):375-389.

49. Harackiewicz JM, Canning EA, Tibbetts Y, Priniski SJ, Hyde JS. Closing achievement gaps with a utility-value intervention: disentangling race and social class. *J Pers Social Psychol.* 2016;111(5):745-765.

50. Fischer C, Zhou N, Rodriguez F, Warschauer M, King S. Improving college student success in organic chemistry: impact of an online preparatory course. *J Chem Educ.* 2019;96(5):857-864.

12

The Preclinical Years

Michael Englesbe
Christopher J. Sonnenday

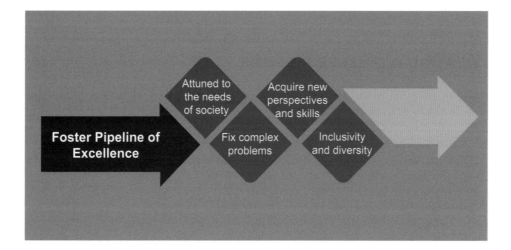

Students entering medical school demand a diverse and inclusive community. Diversity and inclusion have been a social norm within their lives. They have witnessed a black president in the United States as well as female world leaders. Many have traveled extensively, and all are in touch with broad communities through technology. Students view diversity well beyond just race; they view it as the complex milieu of backgrounds, experiences, and perspectives within a team. Thoughtful leaders call this "cognitive diversity."

Preclinical students have been educated in teams and are well aware that diversity is a key aspect for successful teams. Students enter medical school with an expectation that their differences will be appreciated and celebrated. They do not expect to have to hide these differences. They expect to be heard.

Entry into medical school is more competitive than ever. Acceptance rates at many medical schools are less than 5%, and the majority of students who apply to medical school are not admitted to any schools.[1] It is increasingly rare for medical students to enter medical school immediately upon completion of an undergraduate degree. For example, at the University of Michigan, less than 20% of students enter immediately following college. Students expect to take several "gap years" to solidify their personal narrative and decision-making. The average student has 3 years of professional experience. During this time, students most commonly work in biomedical research, technology, service organizations, or entrepreneurial endeavors. These organizations frequently have very informal and flat organizational structures. Young students are used to calling the professors and their bosses by their first name, they are used to freely voicing their opinions and beliefs, and they have an expectation that they'll be treated with civility and judged by their thoughts and actions.

The educational experience is more student-centered than in previous generations. Students are taught to consider their unique gifts. They are purpose-driven, seeking meaningful work that is impactful beyond themselves. Entry into competitive medical schools requires that students demonstrate self-reflection. Students have experience identifying their strengths and communicating their core values. Students expect to do meaningful work. They are keenly aware of the importance of belonging within a community. They have specific skills on how to act within a community and with this, value inclusion. Students aspire to deeply improve the world. They are committed to being "givers," focusing on their contributions. The medical school admissions team at most institutions has deep experience in building a talented and diverse class.

CREATING A DIVERSE PIPELINE

Students demand more than ever; surgery must meet these demands or the discipline will not flourish. More importantly, the field will fail to meet the growing needs of society. Students are better suited to serve as surgeons than ever. They have had deeper and more diverse experiences, are more focused on service, understand technology, and are willing to work hard (when there is a reason). Attracting them to surgery requires that surgical culture and curricula are respectful of their previous experiences.

Intentional effort is needed to engage preclinical students in surgery. Early exposure to surgeons can have a profound impact on career choice. Within this context, students need to be able to see themselves as able to thrive within surgery. Preclinical students are likely to value diversity and inclusion more than older members of clinical care teams.

EXPOSING PREMEDICAL STUDENTS TO THE SURGICAL COMMUNITY

Cultivating engagement in surgery by preclinical medical students requires an intentional curriculum. The curriculum should create an approachable opportunity for students with a passion for surgery. A small and diverse cohort of faculty should be given responsibility (and credit) to run this group. The operations of this group need to be supported by administrative staff, and departmental leadership should generously fund this effort. A diverse and excellent group of senior students should set the agenda and organize and lead activities. These activities should include opportunities for networking, outreach, and research.

Diverse student leadership is key to the success of these efforts. Current upper-level students will be most attentive to the needs of preclinical medical students. Discretionary time during the preclinical curriculum can be relatively scarce for some students, and the opportunities must be designed to optimize

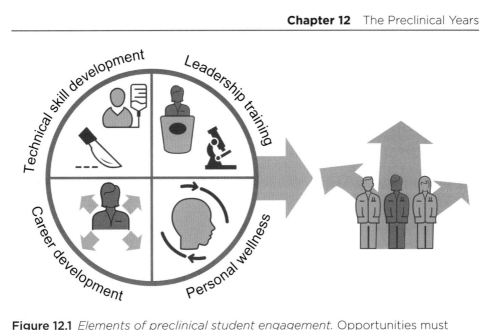

Figure 12.1 *Elements of preclinical student engagement.* Opportunities must be designed to optimize student engagement that integrates the day-to-day demands of preclinical medical school curriculum. The program should include opportunities for technical skill development, **leadership training**, and **research**. Trainees and faculty should talk frankly about career development and **personal wellness**.

student engagement and thus integrate with the day-to-day demands of the preclinical medical school curriculum. The program should include opportunities for technical skill development, leadership training, and research. Trainees and faculty should talk frankly about career development and personal wellness. Preclinical students are as interested in what the attending surgeon did on the weekend as they are with what the attending surgeon did in the operating room or clinic on Monday (*Figure 12.1*).

A SUCCESSFUL PRECLINICAL CURRICULUM

Engage With High School Students

The Doctors of Tomorrow program (University of Michigan, 2019) inspires and prepares high school students from underrepresented communities to successfully pursue careers in health care in order to increase diversity among medical professionals. The students are carefully selected from a magnet high school in Detroit, Michigan. Students come to the University of Michigan for a longitudinal program of clinical immersion, academic preparation, and leadership development coupled with continued engagement and mentorship throughout high school and beyond. The program creates an educational experience where all participants are actively engaged in developing and promoting cultural awareness to reduce bias in the medical field. This program is overseen by a surgeon. All members of the department can participate in this program, creating a virtuous community of impact and inclusion. These talented young students come to the clinic, they spend time in the simulation lab, and they become familiar with surgical staff and equipment. They are exposed to nurses, house officers, and surgeons. They are able to ask questions about all aspects of a surgeon's life. This program has significant spillover benefits for participants, solidifying the mission around education, diversity, and service. This program was initially funded by the Department of Surgery but is now sustained through philanthropy.

Engage With Undergraduate Students

The most efficient way for surgeons to engage undergraduate students is to participate in the medical school admissions process. The admissions team is uniquely skilled at recruiting a diverse and excellent cohort of young people. Surgeons can learn from engagement with the admissions team and bring this knowledge to related efforts (residency selection, faculty recruitment) within the Department of Surgery. The medical school interview day should include exposure to surgery. For example, students who interview at Michigan participate in a surgery simulation center event on the day of their interview. A diverse group represents the Department of Surgery in this event so that all applicants can begin to see themselves as surgeons. Prematriculation (the summer before medical school) students are able to use small grants to fund research with a diverse selection of surgeons and surgical trainees. This program links students with surgeons even before they begin classes. Surgeons must be willing to engage; this requires leadership and alignment of departmental priorities.

Surgery Olympics

Preclinical students have a grinding schedule. Many schools have consolidated the preclinical phase of the medical school curriculum into a single year. Students are busy and have less opportunity to do impactful work like research or community service. As a consequence, careful planning is needed to optimize opportunities for students. At Michigan, the Surgery Olympics program occurs during the relatively "slow" final month of the first-year curriculum and during the 6-week summer break. A team of five students is linked with a senior surgical resident and a surgical faculty member. Intentional efforts are made to create diverse teams. Each team does a group project (quality improvement, research, etc.) and practices surgical skills. Teams compete in surgical skills and oral presentations at the end of the program. The final event is done with the entire department, and intentional efforts are made to foster inclusion and fun. Students are able to engage with surgeons and do meaningful work, which is a powerful force to build momentum for a career in surgery.

Careful consideration is required to assure a productive team project. Small case series requiring data collection, a small audit-based quality-improvement project, or review articles are well suited. Some "first author deliverable" should be considered for each student including local, regional, and national presentations and publications. An example of a good project is an investigation of the relationship between the number of opioid pills prescribed and consumed following laparoscopic cholecystectomy at our institution. The resident did the survey and institutional review board work before the students began the program. Students attended the clinic and operating room to understand the clinical context. The team (including the faculty and resident) drafted the paper introduction during a 1-hour session, where the hypothesis was declared. Each student was responsible for collecting data from 50 patients over a specific time period. Each student analyzed the data from the cohort of 250 patients and presented their findings to the resident. The resident harmonized these efforts and helped the students prepare the data for the faculty. Once the analysis was finalized, the data display and an outline of the discussion were established during a 1-hour seminar with the faculty. Each student was assigned a portion of the writing. The resident and faculty edited the manuscript. The group created a poster and a slide deck for presentation. A strategy was made to submit the work to maximize opportunities for first authorship. This included local quality-improvement venues, educational sessions, and local, regional, and national meetings. Navigating attribution of credit is a fundamental skill for academics and should be part of the curriculum. One student from this project wrote numerous papers on this topic, received several grants, and matched into a surgical training program.

The Michigan Journal of Medicine

This journal is a peer-reviewed, student-led forum to bring high-quality scientific and clinical research generated by the members of the University of Michigan to the scientific community at large. Students occupy all editorial leadership roles for the journal and supply all content. The journal editorial work is conducted under the guidance of faculty at the University of Michigan Medical School. The journal was started within the Department of Surgery and is now integrated into the curriculum with a surgeon faculty mentor. Students receive medical school credit for their work on the journal. Students learn organizational skills, leadership, and academic communication skills. This is a natural opportunity for submission of work done within the numerous department career development programs for students. Preclinical students are deeply involved in the peer-review process.

Informal Dinners at Faculty Homes

Frequent events for preclinical students in faculty homes are powerful, likely the most memorable career development activity for preclinical students. Student leadership should set the agenda and make the arrangements. The hosting faculty should represent the diversity of the students. Not all faculty are well suited to host these events, and departmental leadership should have some role in the process. Faculty must be prepared for informality and personal questions, and should be willing to share stories. Faculty should discuss the importance of a diverse, equitable, and inclusive workforce as necessary to optimally meet the needs of society.

Teaching in the Preclinical Curriculum

Historically, surgeons have had little involvement in the preclinical education of students. Surgeons must engage to facilitate early exposure for students. Preclinical education has moved from lecture-based to small-group, problem-based sessions. Surgical problems are well suited for teaching foundational scientific and clinical knowledge. Departmental leadership should make efforts to understand the details of the curriculum and enable surgeons to teach. At our institution, surgery is deeply engrained in all aspects of the curriculum.

Introduction to the Patient

Preclinical students best represent the diversity of our professional community (they are not initiated in our systems). Working with these young, engaged students offers a critical opportunity for faculty to stay rooted and open to the energy, curiosity, and heterogeneity of preclinical medical students. These students are introduced to clinical skills and patient care during the first weeks following matriculation at most medical schools. For example, at our institution students have two 4-hour sessions every week (appropriately called the "Doctoring Program") where they achieve competencies in clinical skills such as physical examination, history taking, communication, and medical humanism. These small groups (10 students and 2 faculty) stay together all 4 years of medical school. When this course was started, 130 faculty applied for 30 spots to be part of this course. The course required faculty to devote two half-days per week. Engaging with preclinical students is actually critical to foster their interest in surgery, and support from leadership is necessary.

Team Action Projects in Surgery

Surgical house officers must complete a quality-improvement project; this is a requirement from the Accreditation Council for Graduate Medical Education. This requirement can be integrated into the training program through "Team Action Projects" (*Figure 12.2*). Surgical house officers learn core skills in leadership, management, and quality improvement while running the project. The project ideas come from the house officer. The projects are completed during the academic development time (i.e., while off clinical duties). The house officers work with the faculty member and are assigned a team of both senior and preclinical medical students. The students are given specific tasks, usually clinical auditing or data collection. The preclinical medical students work closely with the surgical house officer and the senior medical students (who are interested in surgery). This creates an impactful community; the preclinical students feel like they are part of "real work," helping to improve care. These improvement projects serve missions of the department including education, quality improvement, clinical excellence, and leadership development. The program is an operational arm of a 2-year leadership development program for house officers that includes competencies in communication, management, inclusion, and quality improvement. It is remarkable how many of the teams stay linked long term and how the projects feed larger-scale institutional efforts.

The Michigan Women's Surgical Collaborative

This program employs research and outreach to identify factors that hamper the success of women in surgery and find solutions that will break through these barriers. This collaborative fosters a culture that actively supports women and helps them attain their career goals. This national program focuses on surgeons, faculty, and house officers. Nonetheless, the spillover impact on medical students is profound. Empowering women is critical to reduce disparities in care, improve outcomes,

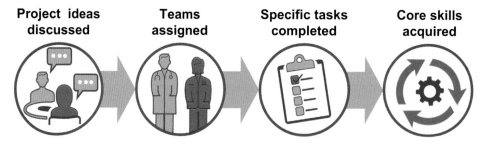

| Project ideas discussed | Teams assigned | Specific tasks completed | Core skills acquired |

Figure 12.2 *Team Action Projects in Surgery.* Surgical house officers learn core skills in leadership, management, and quality improvement while running the project. The project ideas come from the house officer. The house officers work with the faculty member and are assigned a team of both senior and preclinical medical students. The students are given specific tasks, usually clinical auditing or data collection. These improvement projects serve missions of the department including education, quality improvement, clinical excellence, and leadership development.

foster innovation, and attract excellence into the field of surgery. Exposing preclinical students (male and female) to these efforts builds foundational strength for this movement.

Surgical Stereotypes

Preclinical medical students must be exposed to surgical students, house officers, and faculty who represent the best of the surgical community. We are all well aware of surgical stereotypes, and breaking these biases can be challenging. Effective strategies to manage surgical stereotypes include the following.

Countering Stereotypes Directly

One needs to ask preclinical medical students what they care about and what they think about surgeons. More specifically, ask them which negative surgical stereotypes concern them. Talk frankly about the surgical stereotypes and present individuals who represent a counter to this stereotype. For example, one negative stereotype about surgeons could be that they are so career-driven that they neglect other aspects of their lives. This stereotype can be best managed by having a diverse group of senior medical students, surgical trainees, and surgeons talk about their lives. They must make themselves vulnerable and share stories of failures as well as successes. This strategy will have a powerful impact on cultivating the pipeline of excellent students interested in surgery. Even a small number of surgeons who "play into the worst" of the surgical stereotype can devastate efforts to recruit the best into surgery. These individuals should be carefully managed by departmental leadership.

Viewing Stereotypes as Opportunities

Empower preclinical students who do not fit within the stereotypes. Create a surgical community where students who think, look, or feel differently than "the successful surgeon" appreciate the differences as unique strengths. Improving the field of surgery is best informed by individuals with a diverse set of experiences and skills. There are many examples of successful surgeons who have created impactful careers because they thought about things differently. There is a growing appreciation and robust opportunities for young surgeons with deep interest in the humanities, ethics, population health, technology, and discovery. All of these fields are wide-open opportunities for surgeons.

CONCLUSION

With the platform they have, surgeons must foster a pipeline of excellence within surgery. Aspiring young surgeons must be attuned to the needs of society and able to fix the complex problems of the future. New perspectives and new skills are mandatory to meet these needs. We must understand this new generation of young surgeons and adapt surgical education and care to their needs. Fundamental to this change is fostering an inclusive and diverse pipeline.

REFERENCE

1. American Association of Medical Colleges —FACTS Applicants and Matriculants, 2019.

13

The Clerkship Experience

Rishindra M. Reddy

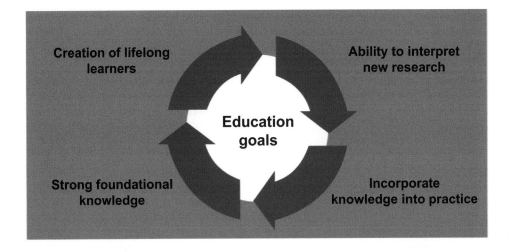

The preparation of medical students to become physicians is changing dramatically as medical schools recognize that they cannot cover all of the current practice of medicine as medical knowledge increases exponentially. Educational goals are shifting to the creation of lifelong learners who have strong foundational knowledge, the ability to interpret new research, and the tools to incorporate new knowledge into practice. The new physician may not have the same grounding in anatomy as generations past but will be better prepared to learn on the go as new medical treatments and techniques are developed. The core clerkship experience for many schools has shifted to the second year of medical school, allowing for a broader, more diverse curriculum during the third and fourth years. Changing educational formats require educators to reflect on the core goals and function of the Surgery Clerkship within an Academic Surgery program and to examine how diversity, equity, and inclusion can impact the surgical exposure of future physicians.

GOALS OF A SURGICAL CLERKSHIP

The traditional goals of the surgery clerkship are (1) teaching students about surgical diseases and surgical management, (2) teaching technical skills related to surgery (tying, suturing), (3) teaching students how to communicate with patients and other physicians, and (4) recruiting future generations to the field (*Figure 13.1*). While these goals apply to all core clerkships, surgery tends to provide the most exposure to technical skills development and to acute patient scenarios—e.g., how to recognize a sick patient. These goals have not changed as curricula have been modified, but when building a clerkship experience for the future, one can emphasize certain aspects to improve a student's experience and future practice.

Traditional patient care has focused on specific diseases without explicitly recognizing that different populations may have different treatment needs relative to the majority population. The social determinants of health (socioeconomic status, education, etc.) have been increasingly recognized to affect a host of illnesses. Access to cancer surgery has been well documented to be reduced in patients with lower financial means and in underrepresented minorities. A lack of insurance status has been associated with increased mortality after pediatric trauma.[1] Understanding health disparities that occur currently in the health system is critical to training future physicians. Prior curricula taught students about screening for breast or colon cancer but failed to highlight the poor rates of screening in African-American populations. Cardiovascular care for everyone is important, but knowing that women are much less likely to receive appropriate intervention should become a standard part of new curricula.

A focus on underserved populations with regard to surgical diseases helps the learner understand how surgical treatments can have a broader impact for more people. For example, women with Medicaid or of Hispanic status are less likely to

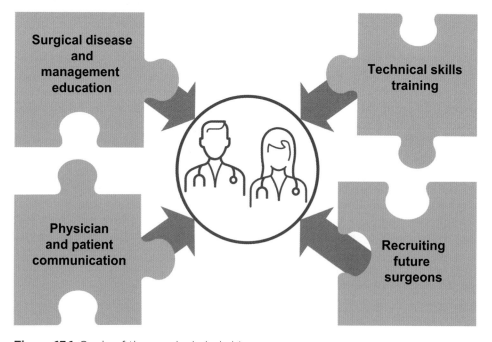

Figure 13.1 Goals of the surgical clerkship.

receive a minimally invasive hysterectomy for benign disease.[2] As another example, African-American race is associated with higher rates of limb amputation.[3]

Communication skills are a hallmark of the LCME and ACGME training paradigms. In the past, the surgery clerkship focused on how surgeons communicate with patients, but in the future, surgeons will need to teach students, residents, and faculty how to better communicate with each other as well as with patients as they encounter a more diverse population. The majority of graduating medical students in the United States have been female for over 15 years. Schools are actively recruiting a more diverse candidate pool so that graduates will better reflect the population of this country. With each new generation comes new expectations, and current students want clearer communication from their colleagues. For example, the frequency of transgender people within the population is estimated to be 2%, and understanding how people prefer to be addressed is something novel to many workplaces and can be especially challenging in more traditional arenas, such as surgery.

Learning technical skills like suturing has been a critical role of the surgery clerkship and will continue to be so in the future. Often, faculty recognize technical skill and may boost a student's evaluation based on technical ability. However, as surgeons encounter students with broader backgrounds, can they still expect everyone to perform, let alone master, these skills? Can a student have one arm and successfully complete a surgical clerkship? They likely cannot be a surgeon in the current environment, but they can definitely be a successful physician in a variety of different fields. Should their inability to perform a two-handed knot limit their success on a clerkship? As educators, surgeons will need to recognize that this is not a limitation of the learner, and that they will have to create alternative experiences to assess students for grading purposes.

As future generations of surgeons are recruited, the discipline must also monitor internal biases of what a surgeon "looks" like. Surgical trainees are still predominantly male with limited minority representation compared with other fields. Surgeons need to recruit students from all backgrounds and recognize that many students may not consider a field where there is limited representation by faculty with a similar background. The onus is on the faculty to connect with a broader group of students and to help them overcome their biases toward surgeons and to a career in surgery.

CLERKSHIP STRUCTURE

Surgical clerkships have changed in length and structure as other specialties have needed time within the core year (emergency medicine, for example) and as surgical subspecialties have formed separate departments. In the past, many surgery clerkships were 3 months with most now being 6 to 8 weeks and some programs having only 1 month. Students were assigned to services with limited input from the students themselves. Clinical lectures were given by surgeons when they were available but often with last minute cancellations. Morning rounds were focused on getting through in time to get to the OR with a focus on the learners being resident-dependent. The traditional operating room model was for students to be present, but not heard, and to cut suture when asked. Clinic time was an opportunity for students to see patients, but the clinical demands often outweighed the educational goals as students felt rushed compared with other clinical situations. Feedback to students was minimal and given with an opaque grading process including subjective oral exam assessment.

The clerkship has to change to survive and the way things "were done as we've always done them" will not suffice in the future. Rotations assignments should be made taking into account student preference and needs. Placing future pediatricians on a pediatric surgery service can be a boost to future careers. Understanding that some students may have limitations that could prevent them from standing for 6 to 8 hours straight will allow for better student assignments and better team functions. Assuring that faculty are present for lectures and engaged is critical to teaching the next generation. Utilizing a flipped classroom approach with more student engagement is critical. The flipped classroom approach reverses the traditional lecture followed by homework model by using preclass videos and instruction, with in-class work centered on interactions with the instructor and active learning by the trainees. Evidence of the success of this model is substantial,[4] but faculty development is needed to accomplish this as asking faculty to change without providing them with the tools to do so is bound for failure.

The goal of improving the student experience on rounds, in the operating room, and in clinic is often viewed poorly by surgical residents and faculty. Residents and faculty often feel overwhelmed by trying to implement changes and may need education in how to accomplish this. Minor changes are often all that is needed to dramatically improve the educational atmosphere and student's experience, which can also help the team. In our institution, one faculty was highlighted for shaking everyone's hand at the end of surgery and debriefing in the process. This simple process of engaging the residents, students, and OR staff creates a more open environment allowing for greater comfort in being able to ask questions. Another faculty was noted for asking students at the start of the day what their learning goals were. Again, this made students much more comfortable to engage early and often. Clear communication at the start of rounds, in an operation, or in clinic can clarify the leader's expectations, and allowing a moment for questions or comments can give students the chance to have greater input and sense of control of their daily routine. Regular communication can help overcome misperceptions or biases that all have and also allow for a better understanding of what learners need.

Communication can also take the form of feedback, both to the students and to the faculty or residents. There has been a clear shift over the past few decades away from giving students meaningful feedback, as this can be misconstrued as mistreatment. Feedback is critical to learning and to teaching but must be given with more context to the learner than was done in the past. Surgeons must also be able to receive feedback about their own teaching styles and be open to changing teaching style as needed. Millennials are often viewed as being too sensitive to receive feedback, but this same concern can be applied to surgical faculty who struggle to take an honest appraisal of their teaching skills and ability to teach all learners. Going forward, developing the skills to give and receive quality feedback will be a cornerstone of the educational and performance evaluation processes.

FUTURE WORK TO IMPROVE THE CLERKSHIP

Changes to improve the quality of teaching for medical students will not occur easily. Surgical culture has a significant amount of inertia with sometimes too much deference to the past and former giants within the field. While honoring history is critical, recognizing and implementing change is no different than learning minimally invasive techniques or advanced endoscopy. Faculty development is essential to help surgeons learn how to be better teachers and to reach a broader audience. Residents need to be a part of this process with their own curriculum on how to improve communication skills to create a more inclusive setting. A new requirement for medical school accreditation requires a resident-as-teachers program for all residents involved in teaching students. In our institution, surgeons have used this as an opportunity to help create a curriculum and teaching materials for the residents to facilitate their teaching efforts.

Areas to focus a development plan include an understanding of health disparities, creation of interactive didactic lessons, and antibias training as it relates to colleagues, patients, students, and new recruits to the field of surgery. Leadership training, as a form of faculty development, now includes components of unconscious bias that can greatly increase emotional awareness in the learner. Our institution has made STRIDE training (Strategies and Tactics for Recruiting to Improve Diversity and Excellence) mandatory for all faculty, which has had a broader impact beyond recruiting by increasing awareness of underrepresented populations. A focus on health disparities does not detract from the care of the majority but allows one to be more empathetic to underserved groups and to be a better physician by being able to understand and troubleshoot underlying barriers to care. Examples abound in the health literature with clear benefits to the broader health system by understanding why disparities can occur.

Learning how to improve teaching sessions should be a goal for anyone within academic medicine. There are many observations that show the traditional 45- to 60-minute lecture loses most audience members within minutes. Developing a lesson plan that includes prework and an interactive session with active audience participation and thinking can improve lesson retention and lesson effectiveness. Increased student engagement will improve communication and outreach to a broader student audience. Faculty must be willing to also hear feedback on their own skills as teachers and to not ignore this feedback. While the process of learning how to do this can be hard, it can be accomplished with practice, with huge dividends in student satisfaction. Antibias training is not only about diversity and inclusion but also about being a better doctor and a better person. This type of education can be transformative if done with deep introspection and reflectiveness. The ability to connect with a more diverse group of people will make the recruitment of future surgeons much easier.

REFERENCES

1. Jones RE, Babb J, Gee KM, Beres AL. An investigation of social determinants of health and outcomes in pediatric nonaccidental trauma. *Pediatr Surg Int.* 2019;35(8):869-877. doi:10.1007/s00383-019-04491-4.
2. Price JT, Zimmerman LD, Koelper NC, Sammel MD, Lee S, Butts SF. Social determinants of access to minimally invasive hysterectomy: reevaluating the relationship between race and route of hysterectomy for benign disease. *Am J Obstet Gynecol.* 2017;217(5):572.e1-572.e10.
3. Feinglass J, Abadin S, Thompson J, Pearce WH. A census-based analysis of racial disparities in lower extremity amputation rates in Northern Illinois, 1987-2004. *J Vasc Surg.* 2008;47(5):1001-1007; discussion 1007.
4. Szparagowski R. *The Effectiveness of the Flipped Classroom.* Honors Projects; 2014:127. Available at https://scholarworks.bgsu.edu/honorsprojects/127. Accessed July 1, 2019.

14

Diversity Outreach

Marion C. W. Henry
Erika Adams Newman

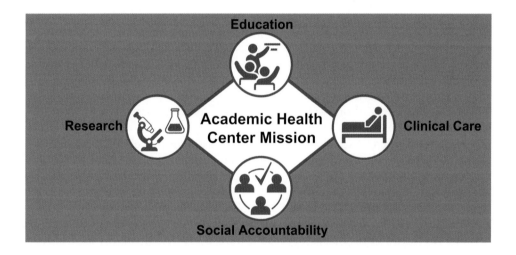

The practice of medicine provides an opportunity for positive interventions that advance the overall well-being of our communities. This requires commitment and outreach not limited to physical ailments of patients, but rather a holistic approach to addressing comprehensive needs in the community as a whole. Imagine if physicians and surgeons would leverage their professional stature and abilities for complex problem-solving to also address the most pressing social and advocacy issues of our patients such as generational poverty. Imagine further if Academic Medicine would expand the tripartite mission to encompass the social context of well-being as a critical component of health maintenance and quality outcomes. If we consider such outreach a critical aspect of our responsibility as physicians, we broaden our impact to improve health and the socioeconomic status of undeserved communities. Partnerships with community agencies, professional organizations, public health officials, and school systems provide a realistic framework for action-based expansion of resources, advocacy, and community-based programmatic development.

AMERICAN POVERTY

The depth of poverty in America is rising and exceeds that of all other industrialized countries, with the largest overall level of inequities of modern societies.[1] The rate of American childhood poverty has been linked to poor population health and long-standing economic disparities.[2] The most recent US Census Bureau data found that children are the poorest age group, accounting for almost one-third of people living below poverty lines (https://www.census.gov/topics/income-poverty/poverty.html). This is defined as an annual income below approximately $25,485 for a family of four and extreme poverty below approximately $12,500.[3] This is an urgent crisis to address because poverty in children is associated with broad deficits in physical and mental health, academic achievement gaps, and higher rates of social or behavioral dysfunction.[4] Such gaps are even more pronounced in deep poverty, with families trapped for long periods from early childhood into adulthood. Children of color and ethnic minorities disproportionately make up nearly three-quarters of all poor children in the United States. Rigorous research has also found statistical relationships between children growing up in poverty to adult earnings, the propensity to commit crimes, and poor overall health.[4] Aggregate costs to the US economy for childhood poverty is averaged at $500 billion/year, nearly 4% of the GDP.[5] Multiple studies have demonstrated that poverty affects student achievement at all levels, and the US Department of Education found that poor students score below norms in all grades and that schools with high percentages of poor children have worse achievement scores in all subjects.[6]

Many negative health outcomes have been related to poverty. The rates of low-birth-weight and infant mortality are all significantly higher in children born into poverty in the United States.[7] Even more striking is that one in eight US households report being food insecure (limited or uncertain availability of adequate food), and this affects infant feeding practices, toddler and childhood obesity, and depressive symptoms among parents.[8] Children born into poverty are also more likely to experience injuries related to trauma and accidents, and neighborhood-level socioeconomic characteristics are associated with pediatric injuries.[9] Recently connections between these and other health disparities have been closely related to neighborhoods with high rates of poverty and crime.[10] For example, certain neighborhoods in Chicago, IL, with the highest rates of violent crime also have the highest rates of infant mortality.[11] Likewise, with the highest homicide rate in the Midwest, Cincinnati also carries the highest infant mortality rate in the state of Ohio. Violent crime and health disparities in birth weight, infant mortality, obesity, and asthma cluster to segregated poor neighborhoods. Recent research around health disparities has shifted to addressing differences in socioeconomic status and the links between poverty, neighborhood segregation, and health outcomes.[12]

The Harlem Children's Zone Project is a successful national outreach model of a holistic approach to breaking the effects of generational poverty through innovative programming (https://hcz.org/). The goals of the program are to provide full support for children to and from college with education, family support, and health initiatives for 100 blocks of neighborhoods in central Harlem, NY. The ultimate goal of the program is for children to attain college graduation. The comprehensive project has made incredible progress toward neighborhood transformation with results that include 97% college acceptance rate across programs, 9000 youth across Harlem participating in health and fitness programs, keeping over 1000 families intact and avoiding foster care, and currently serving over 14,000 children and just as many adults. The program has received many accolades and has been described as one of the most comprehensive and successful broad antipoverty efforts to date in the United States. The nonprofit organization raises approximately $4500 per person served from private and public charity; according to the organization's CEO:

> We spend $167,000 on an inmate in Rikers (jail). We find the money to scale that and we find the money to replicate all of that…I'm telling you if you gave me half of that for a third-grader, I could do what I needed to do to give them and their family what they needed.
>
> Anne Williams-Isom, CEO, The Harlem Children's Zone Project, from *The Economist*, 9/29/19.

The success of the Harlem Children's Zone Project led to the establishment of Promise Neighborhoods, which is the legislative authority of the Fund for Improvement of Education Program for nonprofit organizations, institutions of higher education, and Indian tribes to develop educational initiatives and strong systems of family. Promise Neighborhoods is aimed at poverty reduction and education reform that are based on and maintained by the collective strength of individuals in communities, philanthropy, and universities. Promise Neighborhoods illustrates the potential of strong collaborations and partnerships between institutions and community organizations to create impactful outreach.

The Project on Human Development in Chicago Neighborhoods was an interdisciplinary study on how child and adolescent development are affected by neighborhood and family structure (https://www.icpsr.umich.edu/icpsrweb/PHDCN/about.jsp). The project studied pathways to and from poverty that included crime, violence, substance abuse, social behaviors, and health. The authors provided insight into Chicago's neighborhoods over time, following over 6000 children and the circumstances of their lives that might lead to antisocial behaviors.[13] The findings were compelling in that nearly all health disparities in a modern city can be traced regionally to communities, socioeconomic status, and neighborhood well-being. Many such segregated neighborhoods and communities are home to vibrant and successful academic medical centers.[13]

Given this, meaningful outreach efforts on poverty reduction and neighborhood support can be viewed as a public health opportunity and responsibility of Academic Medicine.

ACADEMIC HEALTH CENTERS: SOCIAL ACCOUNTABILITY

Academic Health Centers (AHCs) have traditionally had a three-part mission of education of the future healthcare workforce, biomedical and clinical research, and high-quality clinical care.[14,15] Despite advances, the US population continues to struggle with shorter life expectancy and poorer health compared with other countries internationally.[16,17] Increasingly, research is demonstrating that "the conditions in which people are born, grow, work, live, and age" influence health outcomes far more than medical care.[18] Despite the impact of these social determinants of health (SDOH) on individual and population outcomes, the US healthcare system continues to pour disproportionate resources into medicine rather than health.[18,19] The lack of a more organized approach to addressing the main driver of health status, SDOH, has led to underwhelming impacts on improvements in the US health system. Major determinants of health are 50% social and behavioral; 10% environmental; 15% genetic; and only 25% related to medical care received (*Figure 14.1*). Thus, the overwhelming preponderance

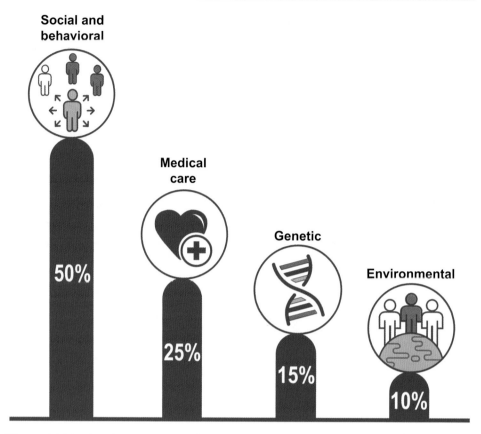

Figure 14.1 Major determinants of health.

of U.S. health status is not related to medical care but rather to environmental and social determinants of health (SDOH).[15,20,21] Therefore, in order to make real progress in health improvements, it is time for AHCs to expand their mission to include addressing social determinants of health and health inequities through social accountability.[14]

Social accountability requires AHCs to move from establishing awareness and intentions to addressing a community's or society's needs and to producing outcomes for which success is measured by community impact.[15] Who is better equipped than AHCs to undertake the scope of this mission?

AHCs are the organizations within the healthcare delivery system that "are well equipped to (1) enable collaborative identification of community or population health needs; (2) facilitate identification and understanding of underlying causes, mediating factors, and mechanisms of action leading to population health challenges; and (3) participate in the design and implementation of requisite innovations and strategic interventions to meet these challenges."[15] They have the capacity and experience to lead and coordinate a broader team with key nonhealthcare community stakeholders to develop innovative solutions and community interventions and to evaluate the impact in targeted populations. Furthermore, 75% of AHCs are located in underserved communities, and they have the capacity, opportunity, and obligation to serve the public good in these communities by addressing health equity and the elimination of health disparities.[15] Academic health centers frequently care for disadvantaged populations and witness the health effects of lack of access to housing, healthy food, living wages, and safe working conditions.[22] They hold a special place in these communities that obligates their participation. There is a societal expectation of health professionals from the general public to work and contribute in this area.[15] Additionally, there is an obligation that stems from financial benefits that AHCs receive in the form of federal funds. When considering the unmet health needs of our society, the funding advantages, societal obligations, and healthcare assets that AHCs have, there is a real obligation and opportunity for AHCs to lead in addressing these unmet needs and improve our national health status.[15]

Adopting a fourth mission for AHCs, that of social accountability, would move AHCs to producing outcomes for which success is measured by community impact. One proposed method through which AHCs can assume this national role in collaborating with communities and address this fourth mission of social accountability involves a four-point strategy as described by Park et al.[14]:

1. Cocreate more equitable and inclusive practices for healthcare workforce recruitment and promotion

There are major disparities in health outcomes and quality of care for minority patients.[23,24] Increasing the diversity of the workforce could provide more effective and equitable care delivery through improved engagement and improved abilities to problem solve, provide care, educate, and generate research representative of a diverse population.[25-29]

2. Implement curricula focused on equity as a core component of health professions education

Curricula that emphasize SDOH need to raise awareness AND empower learners to take ownership of influencing these areas.[30,31] A curriculum about inequity-responsive care[32] would demonstrate to healthcare professionals their own societal power and privilege and would "emphasize the responsibility to educate, research, and provide care in ways that interrupt this cycle and support disproportionately impacted communities."[14,32,33]

3. Offer opportunities for our workforce to partner with communities to develop equity-promoting skills

The vast majority of medical care is delivered in community-based settings.[34] Therefore, partnerships between AHCs and community-based primary care settings are critical in order to develop, lead, and test innovative programs to address health inequities.[35] "Building sustainable partnerships between AHCs, community health centers, and community-based organizations is a critical strategy for bidirectional learning in an academic-community health system".[14]

4. Develop community-based research agendas that support community-based efforts to address inequities

AHCs need to expand beyond the traditional role of clinical trials confined to the academic facility and shift toward a community-partnered participatory research (CPPR) approach.[36] By hiring researchers proficient in these methods, creating promotion tracks that account for community-based research, and advocating for increased research funding for this work, AHCs can promote and encourage CPPR initiatives.

This four-part proposal takes advantage of all aspects of an academic medical center. Integral to this success is the leadership of healthcare professionals who can be the critical advocates to speak out against the aforementioned barriers that impede AHC participation in equity work.

Integrating health equity into health quality improvement efforts is a form of advocacy that reduces disparities.[37] Leadership and advocacy are becoming key skills for all physicians, especially as demands on physicians increasingly include tasks around coordination of care and the role of social determinants of health becomes clearer.[22] While advocacy has been defined as an action by a physician to promote social, economic, educational, and political changes that ameliorate threats to human health[38] and is increasingly recognized as part of every physician's responsibility based on its inclusion in many professional charters,[39-43] not all agree that a physician is obliged to take on a public, political stance as part of their professional duties.[44]

Breaking advocacy down may help differentiate roles that can then be better understood. Advocacy occurs on a spectrum that includes legislative, administrative, clinical, and patient-centered endeavors.[45] Separating advocacy into two subroles of agency and activism helps differentiate the activities and thus the obligations of physicians.[46] An agent acts on behalf of the patient—helps them navigate through the health system. An activist acts at a systemic level. Dobson describes activism as "a quality of legacy; it extends beyond the improved health of an individual patient and, in fact, would ideally extend and persist beyond the efforts of the individual physician. Engaging in activism is about changing the system."[46] In understanding the two roles of advocacy this way, the agent role remains the duty of all physicians, while the activist role might become its own medical specialty whereby a subset of individuals would be entrusted, empowered, and educated to perform activist activities on the profession's behalf.[46]

Appropriately incorporating advocacy education into medical training will be essential to enabling healthcare professionals to respond effectively to external challenges. Although trainees show dedication to addressing public health challenges, they often lack a knowledge and approach to investigating and addressing them. Thus, the AHC carries the obligation to develop formal training programs in advocacy at the undergraduate and graduate medical education levels. Such training programs are a successful way to raise knowledge and skills about community engagement and the role of the physician advocate in using professional expertise to promote solutions to health concerns. The goal of such a health advocacy curriculum would be to develop a cadre of physician advocates who are committed to and skilled in working with communities in collaborative ways and effectively serve in an activist role.[47,48]

Over 150 years ago, Rudolph Virchow asserted that "physicians are the natural attorneys of the poor, and social problems fall to a large extent within their jurisdiction."[49] With growing support, today this notion of a physician advocate needs to become primary to the professional concept of medicine. AHCs can lead the way in developing leaders in this specialty area.

REFERENCES

1. Smeeding TM. Public policy, economic inequality, and poverty: the United States in comparative perspective. *Soc Sci Q.* 2005;86:955-983. doi:10.1111/j.0038-4941.2005.00331.x.
2. Drake B, Rank MR. The racial divide among American children in poverty: reassessing the importance of neighborhood. *Child Youth Serv Rev.* 2009;31:1264-1271. doi:10.1016/j.childyouth.2009.05.012.

3. Short KS. Child poverty: definition and measurement. *Acad Pediatr.* 2016;16:S46-S51. doi:10.1016/j.acap.2015.11.005.

4. Chetty R, Hendren N, Jones MR, Porter SR. *Race and economic opportunity in the United States: an intergenerational perspective. National Bureau of Economic Research Working Paper Series.* 2018. doi:10.3386/w24441.

5. Holzer H, Schanzenbach DW, Duncan GJ, Ludwig J. The economic costs of poverty in the United States: Subsequent effects of children growing up poor. IRP Publications (discussion papers, special reports, and the newsletter Focus) are available on the Internet. The IRP web site can be accessed following address: http://www.irp.wisc.edu.

6. Lacour M, Tissington LD. The effects of poverty on academic achievement. *Educ Res Rev.* 2011;6(7):522-527.

7. Moore KA, Redd Z, Burkhauser M, Mbwana K. Children in poverty: trends, consequences and policy options. *Child Trends Res Brief.* 2009:1-12. Data from the US Census Bureau Database. Available at www.childtrends.org.

8. Bronte-Tinkew J, Zaslow M, Capps R, Trends AHC. Food insecurity and overweight among infants and toddlers: new insights into a troubling linkage. *Child Trends Res Brief.* 2007:1-6. Data from the US Census Bureau Database. Available at www.childtrends.org.

9. Veras Y, Rogers ML, Smego R, Zonfrillo MR, Mello MJ, Vivier PM. Neighborhood risk factors for pediatric fall-related injuries: a retrospective analysis of a statewide hospital network. *Acad Pediatr.* 2019;19:677-683. doi:10.1016/j.acap.2018.11.012.

10. Sampson RJ. The neighborhood context of well-being. *Perspect Biol Med.* 2003;46:S53-S64. doi:10.1353/pbm.2003.0073.

11. McClaine RJ, Garcia VF. Unnatural causes: social determinants of child health and well-being. *Arch Pediatr Adolesc Med.* 2011;165:476. doi:10.1001/archpediatrics.2011.48.

12. Laveist TA. Racial segregation and longevity among African Americans: an individual-level analysis. *Health Serv Res.* 2003;38:1719-1734. doi:10.1111/j.1475-6773.2003.00199.x.

13. Sampson RJ. Moving and the neighborhood glass ceiling. *Science.* 2012;337:1464-1465. doi:10.1126/science.1227881.

14. Park B, Frank B, Likumahuwa-Ackman S, et al. Health equity and the tripartite mission: moving from academic health centers to academic-community health systems. *Acad Med.* 2019;94:1276-1282. doi:10.1097/ACM.0000000000002833.

15. Smitherman H, Baker R, Wilson MR. Socially accountable academic health centers: pursuing a quadripartite mission. *Acad Med.* 2019;94:176-181.

16. World Health Organization. The World Health Report 2000. Health systems: Improving performance. Available at http://www.who.int/whr/2000/en. Accessed November 12, 2019.

17. National Research Council and Institute of Medicine of the National Academies. *U.S. Health in International Perspective: Shorter Lives, Poorer Health.* Washington, DC: National Academies Press; 2013.

18. Marmot M, Friel S, Bell R, et al; for the Commission on Social Determinants of Health. Closing the gap in a generation: health equity through action on the social determinants of health. *Lancet.* 2008;372:1661-1669.

19. Bradley EH, Elkins BR, Herrin J, Elbel B. Health and social services expenditures: associations with health outcomes. *BMJ Qual Saf.* 2011;20:826-831.

20. Association of Academic Health Centers. The AAHC Social Determinants of Health Initiative. 2015. Available at http://wherehealthbegins.org/report.php. Accessed November 12, 2019.

21. O'Hara P. *Creating Social and Health Equity: Adopting an Alberta Social Determinant of Health Framework.* Edmonton, AL: Edmonton Social Planning Council; 2005. Available at http://www.who.int/social_determinants/resources/paper_ca.pdf. Accessed November 12, 2019.

22. Andrews J, Jones C, Tetrault J, et al. Advocacy training for residents: insights from Tulane's internal medicine residency program. *Acad Med.* 2019;94:204-207.

23. Trahan LC, Williamson P; for the Center for Prevention and Health Services. Eliminating racial and ethnic health disparities; a business case update for employers. 2009. Available at https://minorityhealth.hhs.gov/Assets/pdf/checked/1/Eliminating_Racial_Ethnic_Health_Disparities_A_Business_Case_Update_for_Employers.pdf. Accessed November 11, 2019.

24. Williams DR, Yu Y, Jackson JS, et al. Racial differences in physical and mental health: socioeconomic status, stress and discrimination. *J Health Psychol.* 1997;2:335-351.

25. Pololi LH, Evans AT, Gibbs BK, et al. The experience of minority faculty who are underrepresented in medicine, at 26 representative U.S. medical schools. *Acad Med.* 2013;88: 1308-1314.

26. Page SE. *The Difference: How the Power of Diversity Creates Better Groups, Firms, Schools and Societies.* Princeton, NJ: Princeton University Press; 2007.

27. Cooper LA, Roter DL, Johnson RL, et al. Patient-centered communication, ratings of care, and concordance of patient and physician race. *Ann Intern Med.* 2003;139:907-915.

28. LaVeist TA, Nuru-Jeter A, Jones KE. The association of doctor-patient race concordance with health services utilization. *J Public Health Policy.* 2003;24:312-323.

29. LaVeist TA, Nuru-Jeter A. Is doctor-patient race concordance associated with greater satisfaction with care? *J Health Soc Behav.* 2002;43:296-306.

30. Williams DR, Costa MC, Odunlami AO, et al. Moving upstream: how interventions that address the social determinants of health can improve health and reduce disparities. *J Public Health Manag Pract.* 2008;14(suppl):S8-S17.

31. Sharma M, Pinto AD, Kumagai AK. Teaching the social determinants of health: a path to equity or a road to nowhere? *Acad Med.* 2018;93:25-30.

32. Browne AJ, Varcoe CM, Wong ST, et al. Closing the health equity gap: evidence-based strategies for primary health care organizations. *Int J Equity Health.* 2012;11:59.

33. Acosta D, Ackerman-Barger K. Breaking the silence: time to talk about race and racism. *Acad Med.* 2017;92:285-288.

34. Green LA, Fryer GE Jr, Yawn BP, et al. The ecology of medical care revisited. *N Engl J Med.* 2001;334:2021-2025.

35. Kaufman A, Powell W, Alfero C, et al. Health extension in New Mexico: an academic health center and the social determinants of disease. *Ann Fam Med.* 2010;8:73-81.

36. Jones L, Wells K. Strategies for academic and clinician engagement in community-participatory partnered research. *J Am Med Assoc.* 2007;297:407-410.

37. Chin MH, Clarke AR, Nocon RS, et al. A roadmap and best practices for organizations to reduce racial and ethnic disparities in health care. *J Gen Intern Med.* 2012;27:992-1000.

38. Earnest MA, Wong SL, Federico SG. Perspective: physician advocacy: what is it and how we do it? *Acad Med.* 2010;85:63-67.

39. American Medical Association. Declaration of Professional Responsibility: Medicine's Social Contract with Humanity. Available at http://www.ama-assn.org/ama/upload/mm/369/decoprofessional.pdf. Accessed November 12, 2019.

40. American College of Surgeons. Fellowship Pledge and Code of Professional Conduct. Available at https://www.facs.org/about-acs/statements/stonprin#pledge. Accessed November 12, 2019.

41. ABIM Foundation, ACP-ASIM Foundation, European Federation of Internal Medicine. Medical Professionalism in the new millennium: a physician charter. *Ann Intern Med.* 2002;136:243-246.

42. Snyder L, Leffler C. American College of Physicians Internal Medicine Ethics Manual. 5th ed. p 159. Available at http://www.acponline.org/runing_practice/ethics/manual/ethicman5th.htm. Accessed November 12, 2019.

43. American Academy of Family Physicians. The Future of Family Medicine Project. Available at http://www.futurefamilymed.org/x24878.html. Accessed November 12, 2019.

44. Huddle TS. Perspective: medical professionalism and medical education should not involve commitments to political advocacy. *Acad Med.* 2011;86:378-383.

45. Furrow BR. The ethics of cost-containment: bureaucratic medicine and the doctor as patient – advocate. *Notre Dame J Law Ethics Public Policy.* 1988;3:187-225.

46. Dobson S, Voyer S, Regehr G. Perspective: agency and activism: rethinking health advocacy in the medical profession. *Acad Med.* 2012;87:1161-1164.

47. Belkowitz J, Sanders LM, Zhang C, et al. Teaching health advocacy to medical students: a comparison study. *J Public Health Manag Pract.* 2014;20:E10-E19.

48. Leveridge M, Beiko D, Wilson JW, et al. Health advocacy training in urology: a Canadian survey on attitudes and experience in residency. *Can Urol Assoc J.* 2007;1:363-369.

49. Ashton JR. Virchow misquoted, part-quoted and the real McCoy. *J Epidemiol Community Health.* 2006;60:671.

15

The Fourth Year

Rian M. Hasson
Andrea B. Wolffing
Sandra L. Wong

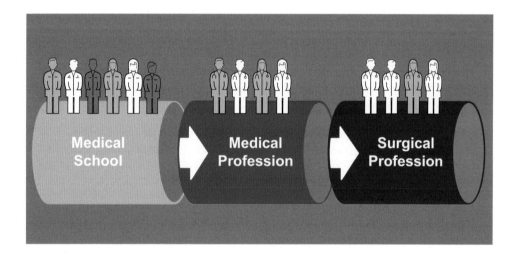

The vital importance of diversity in the surgical workforce has been covered in other chapters of this book, so the focus here will not be on the inherent business case for diversity, but rather on the needed work around the fourth clinical year of the medical school curriculum to attract and recruit talented students to careers in surgery. While many of the illustrative examples included in this chapter are focused on women and underrepresented in medicine students, the principles may be extrapolated to broader issues of diversity and inclusion in surgery.

CURRENT STATE

Many statistics portray the changing demographics of medical schools. Data from the American Association of Medical Colleges[1] show that, in 2018, numbers of female, black or African-American students, and American Indian or Alaska Native applicants and enrollees increased. In fact, more women than men enrolled overall.

The number of black or African-American men who enrolled increased by 4.6% after many years of decline or minimal growth. Medical schools are becoming more diverse.

While women now represent the majority of students enrolling in US medical schools, there are still a gap with those underrepresented in medicine (defined as those racial and ethnic populations underrepresented in the medical profession relative to their numbers in the general population[2]) and in the pipeline for surgical careers. There is more of a paucity of data around the LGBTQ + population (encompassing all members of the sexual behavior minority and gender identity minority communities) because so many choose not to disclose sexual or gender identity status.

There is underrepresentation of diverse populations in the ranks of practicing surgeons, and this perpetuates barriers to careers in surgery. Women make up less than 21% of practicing general surgeons, but a far lower proportion in subspecialties such as orthopedic surgery (5.3%) and thoracic surgery (7.0%).[3] While the overall number of women in surgery has steadily increased, their numbers in academic surgery positions and high-ranking leadership positions remain low,[4] and women constitute only 25% of assistant professors, 17% of associate professors, and 9% of full professors in the United States. As such, medical student exposure to women in surgery is sparse, and the profession is still strongly influenced by surgical stereotypes[5]:

> The "iron surgeon" powerful, invulnerable, untiring. Those trained by him pass on the mystique, transmitting from one surgical generation to the next an embodied professional ethos. The iron surgeon does battle with death, exterminates disease, declares war on softness, sloth, and error. He is technically brilliant, clinically astute, technologically sophisticated. His feelings, if he has any, are private; his inner life, if he has time for one, is unengaged by his work. The feelings of his patients are also private. Their personalities, problems, hopes, aspirations, are irrelevant. The iron surgeon's task is to excise disease. The rest is for nurses or social workers.

This picture portrays surgeons as an example of decisive, masculine perfection; it is implied that surgeons do not display weakness or emotion, nor give excess thought to communication or family issues which, if raised, are thought to be contradictory to their role. This view has discouraged those whose values or personal characteristics do not align with such an antiquated (and untrue) portrayal of a rewarding career in surgery.[6]

Applications from US medical students to general surgery programs decreased 13% in the 2 decades between 1994 and 2014,[7] though these numbers appear to have stabilized more recently. Of course, many factors impact career decisions, and not all students should consider a surgical career.[8] This is a decision that may have been solidified even before the start of the clinical curriculum.[9] When there is possible interest in the field, multiple factors contribute to perceived barriers to careers in surgery, notably including a lack of exposure to and participation in surgical procedures[10,11] and decreased access to surgical role models, gender concerns, and perceived inability to achieve work–life balance.[12] Suggestions for improvement include improved attending surgeon awareness of such stereotypes, participatory encouragement in surgery, and the sharing of "real-life" narratives to dispel the negative stereotypes influencing surgical recruitment.[6]

EXPOSURE MATTERS

While medical student exposure to interest groups typically takes place far earlier in the medical school curriculum than the senior year, the impact of exposure to and engagement in surgical experiences should be emphasized during the third- and fourth-year clerkships and elective/subintern rotations. During the fourth year, students select their rotation schedules based on specialties of interest to them as possible career choices. Electives or subinternships are unique opportunities to engage those students who have identified a potential interest in a surgical career or who have demonstrated talents or skills that would be desirable in a future surgeon.

Surgical activities such as use of surgical simulation tools (e.g., suture kits, laparoscopic box trainers) or participation in wet labs (e.g., skull base labs or bone labs), either as a component of a rotation or as a supplemental resource, may increase a student's desire to pursue a surgical residency. Many medical schools now offer "boot camp" opportunities for students who have matched into a surgical specialty in preparation for internship (typically toward the end of medical school), but consideration of such electives earlier in the senior year may influence decision-making prior to specialty selection. These popular practicum electives have an interactive focus on developing clinical and procedural skills in a structured setting. Many curricula are designed to include surgical anatomy and surgical skills (with highly sought-after opportunities to use simulation tools or work with animal or cadaver models) as well as scenario-based instruction around perioperative floor or ICU management (i.e., mock paging).

Outside of classic curriculum-based learning, unique opportunities for medical student engagement include short but high-impact activities such as the Student Surgery Leadership Weekend hosted by Michigan Medicine (www.surgeryleadershipweekend.umich.edu) and the Society of Thoracic Surgeons Looking to the Future Scholarship Program (https://www.sts.org/resources/student-resident-resources/looking-future-scholarship-program). Engagement of students and exposure to the field (including time with attending surgeons) appear to be key elements of these local and national programs, especially since such exposure goes beyond the walls of a familiar "home institution" and demonstrates the reach of a surgical career outside of a clinic or operating room.

Data suggest that both surgical residents and faculty members greatly underestimate their outsized influence on a student's ultimate decision-making around a career in surgery. A cross-sectional survey showed that over 62% of residency applicants "strongly agreed" that residents and faculty played an important role in shaping their decisions, but only 10.7% and 4.5% of residents and faculty, respectively, felt similarly about the degree of their influence.[13] For those faculty who may take an opportunity to reminisce about their own days as medical students, they may in fact recall how instrumental their resident team was to their education on any given rotation or the special sense of engagement when a faculty member made an extra effort to notice the student during a complicated case or during a busy clinic to go over a teaching point. Even simply demonstrating "joy in your work" in the form of patient care or an operative procedure can have an impact on a student otherwise inundated with patient lists and daily tasks. What many surgeons may also recall is the moment when someone indicated to them that surgery should be a career they consider. These points of contact, which can actually be quite brief, have high impact. Taking advantage of these informal opportunities matters to students and can make the difference between a student who feels like they could be a surgeon (or not).

AN INCLUSIVE EDUCATIONAL ENVIRONMENT

Diversity and Inclusion

Medical schools and healthcare institutions continue to promulgate a more diverse workforce, but parallel efforts to ensure inclusion seem to lag. A key factor needs to be accounted for: creating a work environment that does not undermine efforts to achieve diversity.

A common scenario: A student has finally made it... Made it through the first 2 years of medical training and they have completed their third-year rotations. Career paths have narrowed, life decisions are being finalized, and the students are well on their way to securing their fate in surgery. They appear "bright-eyed, bushy tailed," and ready to conquer the world. Despite the notion that surgery is a homogenous "old boys club" with grueling hours, thankless sacrifice, and minimal efforts to improve diversity and inclusion, things appear to have changed. Work hours have been reduced, there is greater emphasis on teaching and simulation, and the field is ready to welcome them with open arms. It is a new day... or is it?

While more and more improvements in diversity and inclusion efforts are being realized, students are reporting that once they matriculate, they are told to leave the unique features that they bring to the table at the entrance of the hospital.[14] Rhetorically, if our goal is to attract talented medical students, how can we be successful in this climate?

Medical schools certainly work to recruit and enroll a variety of applicants from different backgrounds, and this leads to a diverse medical school class. However, when they arrive, the hidden curriculum teaches them to obscure what makes them different. Women are taught to mind the "ambition gap" and "lean in" (but to leave gender politics in a space outside the ORs). Some are asked to unlearn accents, and LBGTQ + students mute their identities out of fear of discrimination. Trainees fraught with chronic illness or disability learn early on not to share their diagnoses, and minority students feel pressure to endure explicit racial insults in silence.[14] In the end, students and trainees are left with a charge to "fit in," where fitting in is about assessing a situation and becoming who you need to be to be accepted. Rather, the charge for leaders is to assure belonging, which doesn't change who you are and actually requires you to be who you are.[15]

The difference between fitting in and belonging often becomes clearer as a fourth-year student since it is during these more selective rotations that one becomes more acutely aware of their individualism as opposed to being just one of many third-year students rotating on a core clerkship team. Even subtle feelings of social exclusion can lead to marginalization, disengagement, and burnout. A truly inclusive educational environment still needs to be developed, and this requires work from the entire surgical team, with behaviors modeled by the attending surgeon. True inclusivity is "not having to check your identity at the door" every day at work. There is a clear need for quantitative evaluation of progress in diversity and inclusion. Having a diverse group is, in many ways, easier than having a truly inclusive group (it is, at least, easier to measure). Feeling different often translates to normalizing behaviors in order to avoid being treated differently or unfairly by others. When added to the stress and conflict associated with perceptions of not being treated fairly, some interested students may start to question their identity as a future surgeon.

ROLE MODELS AND MENTORS

By conveying a sense of enjoyment and interest to potential students, practicing surgeons can attract the talented students to be the future of their profession. Quite often, well-intentioned or off-handed advice detracts from a desire to ultimately pursue a career in surgery. A recent survey study revealed that up to 75% of students reported "verbal discouragement" from pursuing a career in surgery.[16] This subtle "gatekeeper" role deserves attention. A gatekeeper can be loosely defined as a person or group who controls access to something. In this context, a gatekeeper can be viewed as "holding the keys" to a career in surgery or deciding who does or does not have access to a community or identity. Because of the underrepresentation of women and minorities in surgery, relative indifference to recruiting a diverse workforce is a potential gatekeeper issue.

Intentional actions around advising interested students require upfront preparation. Becoming well informed about the resources that are available for women and minorities in surgery will increase the effectiveness of potential advisors to those applying for surgical residency. The Association of American Medical Colleges (www.aamc.org) has a wealth of information about seminars, classes, and online webinars on topics such as inclusivity, diversity, and gender bias. The American College of Surgeons (www.facs.org) has several diversity resources listed on its website with topics ranging from cultural competency to implicit bias. Similarly, the Society of Black Academic Surgeons (https://www.sbas.net/) has a wealth of resources available, ranging from job listings to video seminars to scholarships for diversity fellowships and clerkships. By becoming educated on the challenges students will face, advisors can help them along their career path, with a goal of creating a more diverse community of surgeons. Commitment to diversity and inclusion needs to be an intentional and shared goal—programs and actions must be by design.

Intentional and strategic actions on the part of individual programs and professional societies are needed and can increase exposure to subspecialty fields. For example, the Society of Vascular Surgery Medical Student Vascular Annual Travel Scholarship (https://vascular.org/career-tools-training/svs-diversity-medical-student-vascular-annual-meeting-travel-scholarship) is an example of a longitudinal one-on-one mentorship program meant to foster meaningful and productive relationships between the underrepresented in medicine students/scholarship recipients and minority vascular surgeon SVS members.

Many individual residency programs now sponsor visiting elective programs for students underrepresented in medicine to give eligible fourth-year students clinical and research training opportunities at tertiary academic medical departments. The sponsoring departments help develop a pipeline of underrepresented in medicine students to recruit and retain in their field. Within the field of Otolaryngology/Head and Neck Surgery, experience with such a program for underrepresented students appears to have yielded successful research collaborations and increased interest in the field even based on 3-month–mentored research rotations and 1-month clerkships.[17] Engagement in research is an ideal way to foster a mentor–mentee relationship. Though time for a longitudinal research project may be limited during a student's fourth year, even a small role in such work can engage a student and pique interest in an academic career. Certainly, students are more likely to choose a specialty if they can see themselves having a career within that field.

Mentorship is more effective when it starts with an understanding of the mentee's past experiences and current challenges. Effective mentorship starts by recognizing one's own implicit biases in order to increase awareness. By recognizing the challenges that underrepresented minority students face, one can also work with the residency program to monitor and address biases. Similarly, change should happen at the faculty level, with deliberate efforts to recruit and retain a diverse faculty who can be role models and mentors. However, medical school and health system leaders must be mindful that diversity and inclusion cannot solely be the job of women or minority faculty members. The role of allies and supporters is supremely important since underrepresented faculty members disproportionately assume the burden of diversity work in many invisible forms (the so-called "minority tax") with much uncompensated and underrecognized time spent advising, mentoring, and counseling. Benefits in the form of student and mentee success are truly rewarding but lead to "diversity fatigue"[18] on the part of those who shoulder the work.

Women especially are more likely to choose a surgical career if they have opportunities to interact with strong, positive female role models and mentors during their training. Interestingly, the "if you can see it, you can be it" social media campaign ignited in 2017. The Twitter-based #ilooklikeasurgeon that "went viral" quickly became a rallying cry for women based on a woman in scrubs featured on the cover of *The New Yorker* and the ensuing #NYerORCoverChallenge that brought awareness that surgeons have more than one stereotypical "look." More importantly, it allowed an open conversation about issues that women and minorities have long understood: those not fitting the dated surgical mold are less likely to be recognized as part of the surgical field (*Figure 15.1*).

While local advising and mentoring has an immediate impact, at medical schools or hospital programs where there may be a lack of female leadership or representation, organizations like the Association of Women Surgeons (https://www.womensurgeons.org/) and social media movements like #HowIBecameAWomanInSurgery have been able to serve as a guide and a support for students interested in surgery as a potential career.

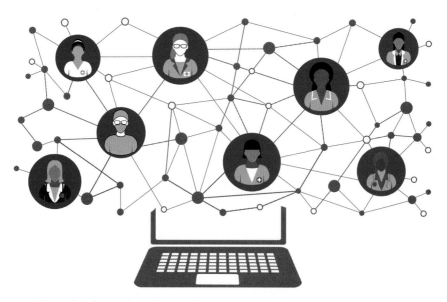

Figure 15.1 Role of social media in changing perceptions of women in surgery.

PLATFORMS FOR SUPPORT AND ADVANCEMENT

Physicians who are identified as black, Hispanic, or Native American continue to be underrepresented in surgery. In a study based on in-depth, qualitative interviews with underrepresented minority residents (n.b., not in surgery), three overarching themes emerged: a daily barrage of microaggressions and bias, minority residents tasked as race/ethnicity ambassadors, and challenges negotiating professional and personal identity while struggling to "fit in." Stories about bias and subtle racism abound. One resident revealed that he had frequently been mistaken for "transport help." Another resident was mistaken for a janitor despite wearing a white coat and stethoscope.[19] These encounters are altogether too common and not well understood by those who do not experience them. The biases are multidimensional and covert, adding to the challenges of implementing alternative interventions to combat not just social isolation and inadequate mentorship but to reconcile professional and personal identities. Actions taken by surgical leaders to acknowledge these issues are certainly a starting point and a way to build inclusivity in the field.

News stories have emerged about the increasing awareness of sexual harassment in the workplace. A report published by the National Academies of Sciences, Engineering, and Medicine (NASEM) in 2018[20] revealed that women in medicine are much more likely than their peers in engineering and sciences to be sexually harassed. Female medical students who have experienced harassment are more likely to perform worse on examinations, earn lower grades, or leave their profession altogether. LGBTQ + students and women of color fare even worse due to an added frequency of harassment. The field of surgery is not immune, and a zero tolerance of harassment must be part of the surgical culture.

COMMITMENT TO DIVERSITY AND INCLUSION AS A SHARED GOAL

The silent witness phenomenon, when discriminatory or insensitive actions or statements are witnessed but not addressed, detracts from inclusion efforts in and out of the operating room. A safe reporting environment is essential, as many victims of harassment have cited fear of retaliation as a reason for delayed reporting or simply not reporting at all. Bystander training is based on principles of action and empowerment, providing tools to a person who observes a problem, or potential problem, conflict, or an unacceptable behavior to influence the outcome of the situation. At moments when bias manifests, bystanders can speak out in response to those all too common, "Did they really just say that?!" moments.

Raising awareness and creating a platform to have difficult conversations is the first step to achieving diversity and inclusion. Engaging support from all parties is a critical next step. For example, one of the keys is not just improving diversity but assuring inclusion including engaging allies. For example, gaining support from male colleagues became a #HeForShe campaign designed for men to show their support. From this, #BlackMenInMedicine and #BlackWomenInMedicine, promoting racial diversity, along with hashtags such as #HijabInTheOR, were created to increase awareness.

With increasing interest in support for other identity groups, there has been recent growth in professional societies such as the Society of Asian Academic

Surgeons (www.asiansurgeon.org) and the Latino Surgical Society (https://latino-surgicalsociety.org/) in addition the Society of Black Academic Surgeons that was formed over 30 years ago.

In addition to supporting the advancement of their respective memberships, these groups have generally supported interested students in their career endeavors, including providing resources for research and academic development.

Many students who consider careers in surgery may ultimately choose other specialties due to perceived barriers. Efforts are needed to address concerns about work hours and time for outside interests, including time for family aspirations (including time to have a child during residency or considerations of age for childbearing). Many of the perceived barriers to a career in surgery may have a gender basis, especially around marriage and childbearing.[16] The issue of childbearing during residency deserves attention. Familial goals are often felt to be incongruent with career goals in surgery given the relatively long length of training that tends to overlap with a woman's fertility years and limited flexibility to have and care for a child due to ill-defined parental leave policies and rigors of a surgeon's schedule.

NUTS AND BOLTS: THE APPLICATION PROCESS

Student advisors, associate deans, and program directors are key stakeholders in the ongoing engagement, recruitment, and retention of fourth-year students interested in careers in surgery.

The American College of Surgeons provides resources for medical students (https://www.facs.org/education/resources/medical-students), as do many medical school student affairs offices. Advising includes a dedicated review of the student's portfolio and application. Many women and underrepresented in medicine applicants may require more attention during this process so that their applications are given the appropriate encouragement, especially if there is possible uncertainty in such a career choice. Personal statements may need additional rounds of review and editing to ensure that they "ring true." Practice/mock interviews, while difficult to coordinate, are extraordinarily helpful to all students as they prepare for visits to unfamiliar institutions for interviews.

Those who are asked to provide letters of support should know best practices for letter writing. There is evidence to support biases between letters for men and women,[21,22] especially in terms of word count (longer letters for men) and so-called "achievement" or "standout" adjectives for men compared with "caring" words for women. One useful one-page reminder/resource is available through the University of Arizona Commission on the Status of Women,[23] and it covers such topics as adjectives to avoid (e.g., caring, compassionate, warm) and adjectives to include (e.g., accomplished, skilled, independent) when writing letters to recommend a woman. While less studied, it is highly plausible that similar biases apply when writing letters for Asian, black, and Hispanic students who face their own racial and ethnic stereotypes.

Attention to implicit bias training is an important component of the selection process, including review of applications and interviews. Consideration for mandatory training should be given, especially so that those involved in the selection process better understand and manage their own potential biases. This may be hard and uncomfortable to do but represents a major opportunity to avoid making decisions based on opinions we've formed about different groups or sets of people (often without realizing we are doing it). The main pitfall in selecting and recruiting a diverse class of residents includes "confirmation bias," which is the tendency to pay attention to, remember, and seek out information that confirms a belief we already have as well as the tendency to ignore, explain away, or forget information that conflicts with it. This encompasses a tendency to like people who are similar to themselves or to only recruit and hire people who are similar to (or the same as) those who are already there.

SUMMARY

In terms of "showing a path forward" to ensure a diverse pipeline of surgeons to care for future generations, intentional and strategic efforts to attract and recruit talented medical students are paramount. Outreach and demonstration efforts to increase the number of women and underrepresented in medicine students in surgical fields are just the beginning. Necessary next steps include continued work to promote a culture of inclusive education and an inclusive profession.

REFERENCES

1. Kalter L. *Medical Schools Are Becoming More Diverse.* AAMC News. December 7, 2018. https://news.aamc.org/medical-education/article/medical-schools-are-becoming-more-diverse/.
2. AAMC. Underrepresented in medicine definition. Available at https://www.aamc.org/what-we-do/mission-areas/diversity-inclusion/underrepresented-in-medicine.
3. AAMC. *Number and Percentage of Active Physicians by Sex and Specialty.* 2017. Available at https://www.aamc.org/data-reports/workforce/interactive-data/active-physicians-sex-and-specialty-2017.
4. Webster F, Rice K, Christian J, et al. The erasure of gender in academic surgery: a qualitative study. *Am J Surg.* 2016;212:559-565.
5. Cassell J. The woman in the surgeon's body: understanding difference. *Am Anthrop.* 1996;98:41-53.
6. Hill EJR, Bowman KA, Stalmeijer RE, Solomon Y, Dornan T. Can I cut it? Medical Students' perceptions of surgeons and surgical careers. *Am J Surg.* 2015;208:860-867.
7. Are C, Stoddard H, Carpenter LA, et al. Trends in the match rate and composition of candidates matching into categorical general surgery residency positions in the United States. *Am J Surg.* 2017;213:187-194.
8. Tambyraja AL, McCrea CA, Parks RW, et al. Attitudes of medical students toward careers in general surgery. *World J Surg.* 2008;32:960-963.
9. Cleland J, Johnston PW, French FH, et al. Associations between medical school and career preferences in Year 1 medical students in Scotland. *Med Educ.* 2012;46:473-484.
10. Maiorova T, Stevens F, Scherpbier A, et al. The impact of clerkships on students' specialty preferences: what do undergraduates learn for their profession? *Med Educ.* 2008;42:554-562.
11. Marshall DC, Salciccioli JS, Walton SJ, et al. Medical student experience in surgery influences their career choices: a systemic review of the literature. *J Surg Educ.* 2015;72:438-445.
12. Are C, Stoddard JA, O'Holleran B, et al. A multinational perspective on "lifestyle" and other perceptions of contemporary medical students about general surgery. *Ann Surg.* 2012;256:378-386.
13. Quillin RC, Pritts TA, Davis BR, et al. Surgeons underestimate their influence on medical students entering surgery. *J Surg Res.* 2012;177:201-206.
14. Tsai J. *Diversity and Inclusion in Medical Schools: The Reality.* Scientific American Voices blog. July 12, 2018. Available at https://blogs.scientificamerican.com/voices/diversity-and-inclusion-in-medical-schools-the-reality/.
15. Brown B. *The Gifts of Imperfection.* Center City, MN: Hazelden Publishing; 2010.
16. Giantini Larsen AM, Pories S, Parangi S, Robertson FC. Barriers to pursuing a career in surgery: an institutional survey of Harvard Medical School students. *Ann Surg.* 2019. Epub ahead of print.

17. Nellis JC, Eisele DW, Francis HW, et al. Impact of a mentored student clerkship on under-represented minority diversity in otolaryngology-head and neck surgery. *Laryngoscope.* 2016;126:2684-2688.

18. Lam MB. Diversity fatigue is real. *The Chronicle of Higher Education.* September 23, 2018. https://www.chronicle.com/article/Diversity-Fatigue-Is-Real/244564.

19. Osseo-Asare A, Balasuriya L, Hout SJ, et al. Minority resident physicians' views on the role of race/ethnicity in their training experiences in the workplace. *JAMA Netw Open.* 2018;1(5):e182723. doi:10.1001/jamanetworkopen.2018.2723.

20. National Academies of Sciences, Engineering, and Medicine. *Sexual Harassment of Women: Climate, Culture, and Consequences in Academic Sciences, Engineering, and Medicine.* Washington, DC: National Academies Press; 2018. Available at (https://www.nap.edu/catalog/24994/sexual-harassment-of-women-climate-culture-and-consequences-in-academic).

21. Turrentine FE, Dreisbach CN, St Ivany AR, et al. Influence of gender on surgical residency applicants' recommendation letters. *J Am Coll Surg.* 2019;228:356-365.

22. Madera JM, Hebl MR, Martin RC. Gender and letters of recommendation for academia: agentic and communal differences. *J Appl Psychol.* 2009;94:1591-1599.

23. University of Arizona Commission on the Status of Women. Available at https://csw.arizona.edu/sites/default/files/avoiding_gender_bias_in_letter_of_reference_writing.pdf.

Part 3

DEVELOPING TALENT IN SURGERY RESIDENTS

16

Sustaining a Creative Residency Culture

Joceline V. Vu
Calista M. Harbaugh
Kyle H. Sheetz
Arielle E. Kanters
Sarah P. Shubeck

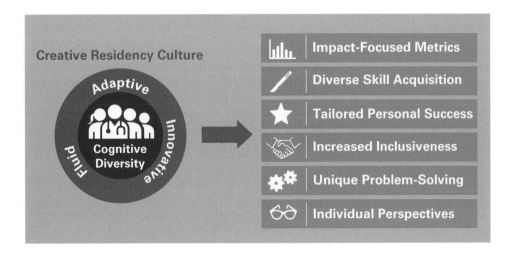

WHAT IS A CREATIVE RESIDENCY CULTURE?

A creative residency culture is many things—adaptive, fluid, innovative—but at its core, it is focused on developing a cohesive group of cognitively diverse individuals. Rather than using traditional metrics (e.g., test scores, case logs, or academic publications), creative residency programs measure success by a resident's impact on clinical care, scientific advancement, and society. These programs foster diverse skill acquisition and encourage residents to define their personal success in the context of their individual strengths, values, and goals. In doing so, residents develop the requisite leadership, academic, clinical, and personal skills to progress into roles with increasing responsibility. Creative programs empower residents to utilize their unique perspectives as they engage in solving the complex problems facing health care today. This chapter will discuss the rationale for developing a creative culture in surgical residency, the elements necessary to maintain this culture, potential threats to sustainability, and examples of what can be achieved.

CREATIVITY AND COGNITIVE DIVERSITY

A creative culture is one that values, recruits, and intentionally develops cognitive diversity (*Figure 16.1*). As discussed in Chapter 1, cognitively diverse teams offer a competitive advantage. Corporations with the highest levels of ethnic and cultural diversity outperform those with the lowest and consistently generate greater profitability and long-term value.[1-3] This competitive advantage arises in part from an increase in creativity—input from multiple perspectives fosters new and innovative ideas, and diverse skill sets allow those ideas to become reality.[4] However, increasing cognitive diversity alone may not yield benefits unless the environment promotes inclusion and values each individual's contributions.[5] This environment is the creative culture that is essential to success. In surgical residency, a creative culture promotes clinical, professional, and academic success.

To achieve a creative culture in surgical residency, one must recognize three key facts. First, the surgeon's primary responsibility is to the patient. Because residents care for a diverse population of patients with varying social and cultural needs, today's surgical residents must function beyond clinical and technical expertise to provide optimal care. They must also recognize the human experience of being a patient. While each resident brings their own limited personal experiences to the patient care environment, a cognitively diverse group that shares their experience offers a greater breadth of understanding of human needs. For example, residents may learn from other residents who themselves live with chronic medical conditions or who have had an operation. A creative residency fosters an appreciation for these different perspectives and provides the psychological safety and open-minded platforms through which residents can share their experiences.

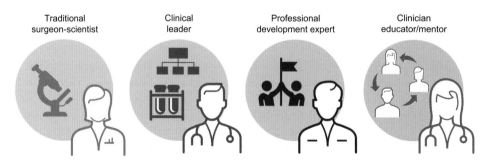

| Traditional surgeon-scientist | Clinical leader | Professional development expert | Clinician educator/mentor |

Figure 16.1 Uphold diverse phenotypes of excellence in the department.

Surgeons no longer occupy a narrow clinical domain—instead, they are expected to rise to influential roles in healthcare systems, address deficits in health policy, and work toward advancements in science. To do so, surgeons need to learn how modern economic and political forces intersect with the delivery of health care as well as with the broader strategic goals of health systems. Surgeons must be cognizant of the healthcare needs of the communities they serve and recognize opportunities to drive local and national change. These powerful lessons become only more challenging to learn as surgeons move further into their careers. Therefore, creative programs are needed to encourage resident participation early on to facilitate their commitment to the greater healthcare community after completion of training.

Clinical subspecialization has flourished to care for patients with complex problems, and integrated training programs have emerged to promote early subspecialization. These programs create microcosms of multidisciplinary clinical teams within a single department. Similarly, promoting expertise in the basic sciences, health services, social sciences, business, education, innovation, and other diverse fields fosters cognitive diversity within a department. Residents in a creative culture are encouraged to pursue training in nonclinical areas of interest and develop diverse skill sets to more effectively contribute to their department, institution, and national societies. They will begin to think about their accomplishments in terms of impact, rather than checkboxes for advancement, and they will carry this mental model forward throughout their surgical career.

NECESSARY ELEMENTS TO SUSTAIN A CREATIVE CULTURE

Valuing a creative culture is closely tied to creation of an inclusive environment that relies on departmental support for its success. In fact, the costs of creativity are not in provision of funding or protection for trainees to pursue advanced degrees or research. The elements that sustain creativity are not material—they are cultural. Thus, creating a creative residency culture should not be viewed as a luxury for well-resourced programs but rather as essential in the surgical field's response to the trajectory of modern health care. A creative residency culture relies on a different type of capital, derived from the empowerment of residents to drive their own growth, openness from departmental leadership to challenging new ideas, and promotion of cross-disciplinary engagement (*Figure 16.2*).

Empowerment of Residents to Drive Their Own Growth

A creative culture cannot be top-down. Instead, the department leadership should support the resident community in developing their own culture. Specifically, the program must support an inclusive environment that amplifies each resident's unique contribution to the program. This is accomplished by recognizing and celebrating many different examples of excellence, including dedication to patient care, contributions to organizational initiatives, service to the community, and non-traditional avenues of academic pursuit in education, wellness, or the social sciences. The surgical hierarchy remains a strong influence, and residents will value

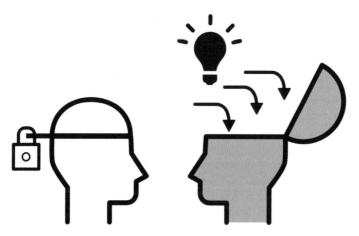

Figure 16.2 Be open to challenging the status quo.

the same phenotypes that are upheld as examples of success by departmental leadership. Recognition of diverse achievements encourages residents to explore new interests, take risks, and define their own success.

A residency program can train residents in skills that will maximize their opportunities within the creative environment, such as nontechnical and interpersonal skills. These domains are as valuable as clinical and technical training given surgeons' leadership roles in a multidisciplinary healthcare environment. Mental models can give residents frameworks for improving skills in communication, collaboration, leadership, finance, or strategy. Mental models drive behavioral change, and repeated behaviors result in skill development. These skill sets can be intentionally practiced and developed in training programs to best equip future surgical leaders.

Residents should be encouraged to take ownership of growing and sustaining a creative culture. Through thoughtful self-reflection, surgical trainees will become aware of their strengths and personal vision, identify opportunities for continued nontechnical growth, and find opportunities that align with their career goals and passions.

Openness to New Ideas From Departmental Leadership and Residents

Programs that wish to sustain a creative culture must recognize that the desired outcome will be "innovative new ideas." These ideas may radically challenge the status quo. They may even propose that the values on which our profession was built no longer align with the needs of today's patients and workforce. To sustain a creative culture, both program leaders and residents must learn how to respond to such ideas from a place of curiosity and openness rather than negativity and defensiveness. Not every new idea will be feasible or appropriate, but consideration and evaluation of new ideas require departmental leaders and residents to view their interaction as a partnership rather than a hierarchical relationship.

Residents should not expect that challenging new ideas will immediately be embraced by program leadership. Rather than abandoning new ideas that meet resistance, residents should learn to explore why ideas are rejected or efforts are discouraged. In doing so, residents learn resilience and may gain a deeper under-standing of others' perspectives, motivations, and constraints. They will learn to approach problems from a system-based approach, which may hone their ideas so that they are more likely to succeed. These are critical opportunities for the residents to become more effective as future leaders.

Promotion of Cross-Disciplinary Engagement

Surgical residency programs should strive to be well connected within their institution and encourage residents to seek academic, mentorship, and leadership opportunities outside of their surgical department. Mentorship by nonsurgical faculty may provide exposure to innovative research, diverse perspectives for multidisciplinary care, or expertise in external sectors of health care. Surgical mentors should encourage residents to explore their interests and help guide their mentees to cross-disciplinary collaboration (*Figure 16.3*).

THREATS TO SUSTAINABILITY OF A CREATIVE RESIDENCY CULTURE

Surgical residency training has not traditionally been viewed as a creative time in one's professional development. The significant physical and mental demands on surgical trainees have been well described in the literature. For example, it is estimated that 69% of surgical trainees experience burnout at some point during their residency.[6] These demands threaten the sustainability of a creative residency culture and necessitate intentional and longitudinal attention. A program must be cognizant that residents be provided with adequate time outside of work to care for their wellness and basic needs. This commitment is essential. Well-being—from a physical and emotional standpoint—is fundamental for a resident to be engaged in their own development. Residents overly burdened by clinical or academic service will not have discretionary motivation to realize their creative potential.

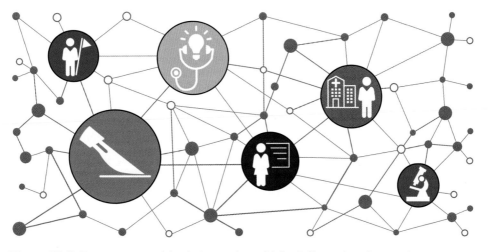

Figure 16.3 Encourage residents to seek multidisciplinary involvement.

There are numerous competing interests for residents' time even within the hospital. For example, residents frequently attempt to balance the demands of clinical service work and educational requirements with their own wellness and personal needs. Further, residency programs may place emphasis on meeting measurable requirements—often without fully considering how much time each requirement truly deserves. For example, programs may require that a considerable amount of time be allocated toward the American Board of Surgery In-Service Training Exam (ABSITE). While this may be an important strategy to encourage continuous learning habits, there are very little data that ABSITE scores are reliable metrics for long-term success or even effective tools to identify residents with additional educational needs.[7,8]

The traditional approach to skill acquisition and development has a tendency to fit residents into specific phenotypes. The "triple-threat" surgeon—an excellent clinician, surgeon-scientist, and educator—is often upheld as the marker for professional achievement. However, this archetype ignores the fact that many residents do not share the same career goals as those who have historically ascended into leadership roles in surgery. Forcing someone into a traditional role may suppress different talents or passions that would otherwise allow them to excel personally and contribute to the program's culture or vision. This is perhaps most evident when residents discover that they lack a passion for research. Continuing along this path may limit their ability to evolve into a leader.

EXAMPLES OF CREATIVITY IN RESIDENCY

Developing a Resident Leadership Development Program

Effective healthcare leadership is integral for patient safety and provider well-being.[9,10] Leadership skills are particularly important for surgical residents, who are on the frontline of patient care, lead complex multidisciplinary teams in the operating room and on the wards, and report disproportionately high levels of burnout.[6] Although leadership can be learned and practiced systematically, programs that teach these skills are generally only offered at the faculty level. As a result, residents navigate the labyrinth of leadership development through ad hoc experiences and self-directed approaches.

To address this gap, a group of residents proposed a Resident Leadership Development program to a faculty mentor. They were then guided to a qualitative methodologic expert who encouraged them to conduct an exploratory needs assessment to define the gap in leadership training for residents. After completing the needs assessment, the residents worked with program leadership to implement the program. This process required several iterations of program redesign, working with educators, department leaders, faculty surgeons, and residents to fit within the constraints of residency. By empowering residents to drive this grassroots effort, the residents developed their communication, collaboration, and leadership skills.

Creation of Lactation Guidelines

There are significant barriers to physicians reaching their breastfeeding goals, including inadequate time for milk expression, limited flexibility in work hours, and insufficient access to private lactation spaces. These barriers contribute to

58% of surgical trainees failing to meet their personal lactation goals, with rates of continued lactation at 6 months less than that of the general US population.[11-13] Given the growing population of women in surgical training programs and the increased attention to wellness and environment in medical training, improving lactation support for surgeons is critical to providing an inclusive environment for all trainees.

In the context of their own experiences, two current surgical residents wrote and presented a policy in support of lactating trainees to the residency and departmental leadership.[14] This document identified the challenges lactating trainees face, clarified the balance of health needs with educational and clinical requirements, and recognized departmental support for lactating residents. This creative effort initiated by residents and supported by department leadership led to the development of the first institutional lactation policy for medical trainees, resulting in departmental culture change and facilitating similar programs across specialties within the institution and nationally.

REFERENCES

1. Hunt V, Layton D, Prince S. *Why Diversity Matters*. New York, NY: McKinsey & Company; 2015.
2. Hunt V, Prince S, Dixon-Fryle S, Yee L. *Delivering Through Diversity*. New York, NY: McKinsey & Company; 2018.
3. Herring C. Does diversity pay? Race, gender, and the business case for diversity. *Am Sociol Rev.* 2009;74:208-224.
4. Lamb BW, Brown KF, Nagpal K, Vincent C, Green JS, Sevdalis N. Quality of care management decisions by multidisciplinary cancer teams: a systematic review. *Ann Surg Oncol.* 2011;18(8):2116-2125.
5. Page SE. *The Diversity Bonus: How Great Teams Pay Off in the Knowledge Economy*. Princeton, NJ: Princeton University Press; 2017.
6. Elmore LC, Jeffe DB, Jin L, Awad MM, Turnbull IR. National survey of burnout among US general surgery residents. *J Am Coll Surg.* 2016;223(3):440-451.
7. Ray JJ, Sznol JA, Teisch LF, et al. Association between American Board of Surgery In-Training Examination scores and resident performance. *JAMA Surg.* 2016;151(1):26-31.
8. Jones AT, Biester TW, Buyske J, Lewis FR, Malangoni MA. Using the American Board of Surgery In-Training Examination to predict board certification: a cautionary study. *J Surg Educ.* 2014;71(6):e144-e148.
9. Wong CA, Cummings GG, Ducharme L. The relationship between nursing leadership and patient outcomes: a systematic review update. *J Nurs Manag.* 2013;21(5):709-724.
10. Curry LA, Spatz E, Cherlin E, et al. What distinguishes top-performing hospitals in acute myocardial infarction mortality rates? A qualitative study. *Ann Intern Med.* 2011;154(6):384-390.
11. Rangel EL, Smink DS, Castillo-Angeles M, et al. Pregnancy and motherhood during surgical training. *JAMA Surg.* 2018;153(7):644-652.
12. Gupta A, Meriwether K, Hewlett G. Impact of training specialty on breastfeeding among resident physicians: a national survey. *Breastfeed Med.* 2019;14(1):46-56.
13. Breastfeeding Report Card United States, 2018. 2019. Available at https://www.cdc.gov/breastfeeding/data/reportcard.htm. Accessed June 15, 2019..
14. Livingston-Rosanoff D, Shubeck SP, Kanters AE, Dossett LA, Minter RM, Wilke LG. Got milk? Design and implementation of a lactation support program for surgeons. *Ann Surg.* 2019;270(1):31-32.

17

Teaching by Residents During Contemporary Surgical Training

Patrick Georgoff
Paul G. Gauger

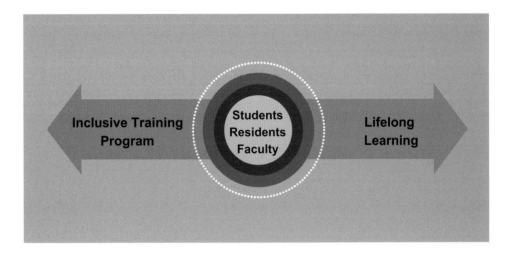

The past 2 decades have seen significant shifts and disruption in surgical residency education. From the proper perspective, it is clear that much of this change has actually been in the form of disruptive innovation and improvement. Perhaps there has never been a better time to be a surgical resident. As contemporary American Surgery has begun to examine and redesign training deliberately for a more successful future, the current surgical residency experience has undoubtedly improved the focus on the learner at all levels. Opportunities to develop as an educator are now available to most surgical residents, and those destined to make the biggest future impact embrace them.

RESIDENCY PROGRAM CULTURE AND EDUCATIONAL PRIORITIES

Success for the academic surgical training programs of the future requires an intentional pursuit of cognitive diversity for both learners and teachers, the use of creative educational and assessment methods, and the support of effective educational teams to promote continuous learning at all levels. When surgical training programs embrace these values rather than relying on the assumed by-products of a busy clinical program or faculty expertise, the benefits to the program culture extend far beyond the learners themselves. For teaching to become a cultural priority for busy residents during training, there must be legitimate and visible role modeling of such behavior from faculty. Without positive role modeling, expectations and encouragement will not be enough. It is also important for residents to observe faculty advancing in their careers in recognition of educational contributions in order to engender trust in the larger system and the extra effort that improvement requires. With these influences, residents will be more likely to pay forward the sorts of behaviors that benefitted them in their own development.

Medical students—especially those pursuing surgical careers—derive great benefit from excellent resident teaching. Peer residents benefit from each other's elevated expectations of deliberate learning and dynamic refinement of knowledge. The program improves as excellent applicants are drawn to a supportive learning environment and the opportunity to develop themselves as educators. In a learning culture centered on residents and students, faculty surgeons benefit from healthy challenges to their viewpoints or traditions and the inspiration to continue to develop themselves as lifelong learners. As a complex organization begins to view itself as a system that needs to continuously "learn" from the outcomes of its processes in order to improve them, it is easy to understand how the profession of surgery and future surgical patients benefit from a healthcare system led by facile learners and dedicated educators at all levels.

MOTIVATIONS TO PRIORITIZE RESIDENT TEACHING

From the perspective of program and department leadership, creating a culture that prioritizes resident teaching can pay notable dividends. It is worthwhile to understand the motivators to do so. There are external expectations for residents to develop these skills delineated in the Accreditation Council for Graduate Medical Education (ACGME) Common Program Requirements. As an aspect of their interpersonal and communication skills, the resident must demonstrate competence in educating patients, families, students, residents, and other healthcare professionals.[1] In the first version of the milestones, teaching was considered an important developmental domain of Practice-Based Learning and Improvement. In the second version of the milestones, because of the focus on development of a surgeon to serve their patient in a complex healthcare system, teaching skills are not evaluated distinctly but instead integrated into many of highest level anchors of competencies such as Practice-Based Learning and Improvement and Interpersonal and Communication Skills in terms of coaching, role modeling, and enhancing team performance.[2] The Liaison Committee on Medical Education clearly delineates in its standards for medical student education that residents who supervise medical students must be prepared for their roles in teaching and assessment and that the medical school must provide resources to enhance residents' skills in these regards.[3]

Even if not driven by external requirements, most academic training programs that have the goal of creating academic surgical faculty would choose to develop and evaluate resident teaching of medical students. This is often encouraged by integrating residents into the medical student evaluations of their educators (traditionally the faculty). Formative and summative feedback about teaching evaluations can occur as part of the end-of-rotation evaluations or during the semiannual reviews with the program director.

However, the most effective and desirable motivators should be internal to the program and be totally apparent in the values and daily decisions of the leadership. This can be best illustrated when considering the converse when teaching is not a top-tier priority (which can easily become the default condition without deliberate attention). In most current medical school curricula, students typically have less exposure to Surgery than in years past as a function of the exponential expansion of specialty scientific knowledge and the unique needs of training physicians for the needs and complexities of contemporary medical practice. Even during clerkship rotations, students are often required to be in formal educational sessions such as lectures, seminars, etc. instead of the practical learning environment of the operating room or surgical clinic. Add to that the increasing time and productivity demands on faculty, and it is easy to understand how teaching of medical students can be marginalized unless it is expected, encouraged, and recognized. As residents are among the most influential medical student teachers in the current environment, efforts to support their success can have a major ripple effect. Therefore, the motivation for residents to teach effectively can become a feature of program culture that becomes propagated by each new class of outstanding resident teachers. From a recruitment perspective, it can be very effective to consider teaching experience and skill as a critical attribute to be sought and evaluated during the resident selection process. At least one interviewer should explore the applicants' self-assessment of their skills and attitudes in this domain if the cultural expectations are to be sustained. The program must be built around the right sort of attitudes and talents to foster this within the culture, and recruiting residents for whom this is not a priority can impede group progress in an insidious way—particularly in terms of the supportive learning environment. Group accountability can be fostered by peer evaluation of teaching in the workplace—particularly during patient rounds and in the operating room.

GENERATIONAL SEGMENTATION AND EDUCATIONAL INTERACTIONS

As the traditional lines between a teacher and learner have blurred significantly, it is important to acknowledge evolving characteristics and expectations of different team members to design for educational success and sustainability. Each new generation of surgeons shares a common history and frame of reference that is unique from those that came before, and the concepts of generational segmentation can be useful in adapting to the needs of current learners[4] (*Figure 17.1*). The majority of current surgical trainees and medical students are members of Generation Y. Also referred to as Millennials, most were born between 1985 and 2005. In general terms, Millennials have been deeply influenced by the rise of the Internet, smartphone technology, reality television, social media, school shootings, the great recession, 9/11, and global terrorism. Collectively, Millennials have been described as self-confident, civic-minded, achievement-oriented, and

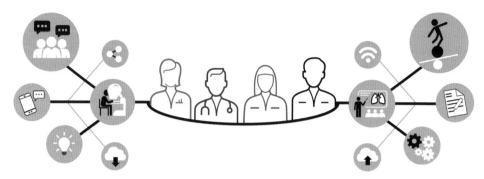

Figure 17.1 Generational segmentation.

technologically savvy but also as self-centered and entitled. An important characteristic is that Millennials crave feedback and may feel somewhat uncomfortable without it.

Practicing surgeons are most likely to be Baby Boomers (born approximately 1945-1964) or members of Generation X (born approximately 1965-1984). Just like Generation Y, these generations were influenced by a common history. They also share common characteristics, some of which can clash with Millennial values. While this divergence is not unique to the field of surgery, it is particularly relevant because of the high-stakes nature of surgical education and the intimacy of the interaction between surgeons and trainees. For relationships between surgeons and trainees to be optimized, both parties must recognize the inherent conflicts between generations and work to create interactions that highlight the positive attributes of each group. To add this layer of understanding to interactions requires both learners and teachers to realize these attributes may be as much cultural phenomena as they are individual. Embracing and understanding these differences can elevate the performance of the entire educational team. Accomplishing this can be a very practical expression of the current goals of cognitive diversity and inclusion within a traditionally hierarchical structure. When all parties can realize that students, residents, and faculty are fundamentally similar in goals and values but simply exist on different phases of the developmental and experiential spectrum, it can be potentially liberating to the inherited culture and can foster innovation and open communication. To do so effectively requires flattening the hierarchy or at least making the communication within it more fluid.

The following generalized observations may be helpful in designing surgical education for Millennial trainees—primarily surgical residents and medical students:

1. **Millennials are digital natives.** Millennials literally grew up with the Internet. They are hyperconnected, adapt easily to new technology, and rely almost exclusively on digital resources to learn. Textbooks have been replaced with smartphone apps, podcasts, Twitter, online question banks, and comprehensive resources like UpToDate®. While the magnitude of resources available may be staggering, Millennials are particularly adept at finding and applying information quickly. Millennials also use text messaging as a primary means of communication, often favoring text messages over paging, phone calls, or emails. Social media platforms are increasingly used for learning and dissemination of knowledge. In addition, Millennials often look to innovate. They are often comfortable taking on the role of entrepreneurs and have grown up in an age of quality improvement and "big data."

2. **Millennials learn differently.** They prefer experiential learning (e.g., case-based presentations and simulation) and relaxed/informal learning environments. They also work well in groups and *expect* to spend their professional lives working in highly integrated teams.

3. **Millennials want feedback (and lots of it).** Millennials are goal-oriented, and they want to know how they are progressing when it comes to achieving their goals. While feedback is a relatively simple concept, the delivery of frequent high-quality feedback is actually quite challenging. Without an explicit process for doing so and in the absence of any education in feedback practices, many traditional surgeon educators fall short of feedback expectations, often giving feedback that is neither specific nor actionable. Additionally, learners who want feedback may not actively seek it out or may purposefully avoid it if they feel it might be negative. Even when feedback is given, learners may not recognize it, which leads to frustration for the teacher and learner alike.[5]

4. **Millennials prioritize work–life balance.** This priority is part of a larger cultural shift in surgical training and perhaps American society at large. Millennial trainees expect some influence upon their work–life balance and feel compelled to push this agenda forward. They openly discuss topics like burnout, personal wellness, and family. Seeking out work–life balance should not be confused with a lack of commitment, and dedicated surgical trainees should be supported in their efforts to preserve a healthy future for the profession. This characteristic creates an important opportunity for a forward-looking department to improve the overall culture by making sure these opportunities and enhancements are available to all.

THE INFLUENCE OF COGNITIVE DIVERSITY

Inclusion efforts can help to counteract traditional hierarchies and alliances that are often perpetuated by the phenomenon of homophily (we tend to seek out those who are like us). Intentionally building a diverse program culture of people with different backgrounds, experiences, and perspectives also helps to introduce and foster cognitive diversity. Academic Surgery is evolving to embrace diversity as a bonus in solving complex problems. While care of the surgical patient is increasingly based on pathways, guidelines, and best evidence, innovation and discovery in surgery are prototypically complex problems that can benefit from cognitive diversity. This principle requires thoughtful implementation of expectations around team learning and teaching. If the goal is rote transfer of surgical traditions and routines, cognitive diversity may be of limited incremental benefit. Fortunately, that is rarely the goal in contemporary training. However, if the goal is to challenge assumptions and create new knowledge and understanding, the benefit of cognitive diversity is much more apparent. To embrace diversity allows evolution of traditional surgical teaching to better meet the goals of the future for patients and the profession.

CREATING AND RECOGNIZING OPPORTUNITIES FOR RESIDENT TEACHING

For refinement of teaching skills, residents must be provided practical opportunities to practice those skills, seek feedback on their effectiveness, and even make mistakes. Typical examples of these opportunities include traditional ward teaching on rounds, preoperative discussions and goal setting (e.g., scrub sink discussions), and intraoperative teaching. This last opportunity can be particularly rich if faculty members share some of their intraoperative teaching and feedback responsibilities with a capable resident. As the resident explains the anatomy, decision-making, or technical maneuvers to the student, the faculty member is able to add context or experiential information to help the student cement their knowledge. Additionally, this allows the faculty member to assess the resident's teaching ability and provide feedback to them after the case or in the moment.

As a generality, surgical trainees have a tremendous influence on medical students, and the influence of residents likely exceeds that of the faculty surgeons.[6,7] Medical students have identified the most desirable behaviors of residents in the workplace that led to their being considered highly effective teachers. In one multi-institutional qualitative study, the themes commonly identified (in order) included role modeling, focusing on teaching, creating a safe learning environment, providing experiential learning opportunities, giving feedback, setting expectations, and stimulating learning[8]. It is notable that these are not necessarily the same behaviors demonstrated by faculty in more formal teaching roles. Some practical tips for surgical residents looking to enhance their teaching skills and improve the overall educational environment of their program include (*Figure 17.2*):

1. **Recognize teachable moments.** Surgical residents are extremely busy, and many feel that they cannot find time to teach. Fortunately, dedicated blocks of time set aside for teaching are not required to be an effective educator. Like faculty, the key is for residents to recognize the large number of teachable moments each day that can be either taken or missed. The best way for one to recognize these teachable moments is to imagine oneself in the shoes of the learner. This can be a particular challenge on a team with diversity of previous experiences and

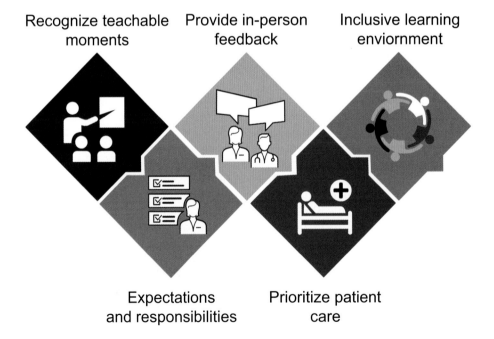

Recognize teachable moments   Provide in-person feedback   Inclusive learning enviornment

Expectations and responsibilities   Prioritize patient care

Figure 17.2 Enhancing the educational environment.

differences in specific knowledge. If residents can appreciate (or better yet ask) what students know or don't know, they will better be able to harness that opportunity. This requires constant reevaluation of the learner and the context in which they are learning. Teachable moments can and should be brief. Teachable moments are most effective when captured at the moment they arise, not later. For example, a third-year medical student may be presenting their patient on morning rounds who has a new ileostomy with high output. The student may mention this finding but may not articulate a plan to address it. Recognizing a teachable moment, the chief resident can take a minute to explain why new ileostomy output is often high, articulate the risks of dehydration, and outline a step-wise approach to managing high ostomy output.

2. **Set clear expectations and level-appropriate responsibilities.** In order to succeed, medical students and residents need to understand expectations. How are expectations set? Resident educators must be highly specific when discussing expectations and associated responsibilities—especially as they relate to performance in the operating room, clinic, and on the ward. This can be accomplished with a clearly worded email and/or in-person discussion at the beginning of each rotation and by providing regular feedback regarding how these expectations are being met or not. Again, resident educators should be specific. What exactly are you going to ask of a student who scrubs into a case? Do you want them to know the indications for surgery? Anatomy? Key operative steps? What fundamental technical skills will you expect them to have or to develop? For residents, setting expectations requires a rough understanding of that individual student's previous experience and level of knowledge and skill that can only be gained by asking. A particularly effective way of asking this is to inquire about how they hope to improve during the rotation.

3. **Provide frequent, timely, in-person feedback.** Feedback is defined as specific information that describes a learner's performance in a given activity that is shared with the intent of improving on that performance.[9] Despite its importance, feedback is often limited in quantity and quality.[10] The delivery of frequent and high-quality feedback is actually quite challenging. Without an explicit process for doing so and in the absence of any formal education about it, many clinical educators fall short of feedback goals, often not giving feedback at all or giving feedback that is neither specific nor actionable.[11] Despite these challenges, resident educators can provide effective feedback, which may be immediate or delayed. Immediate feedback is particularly useful because the learner's performance just occurred and is still fresh in their mind (e.g., immediately following a case or after an oral presentation in clinic). Feedback should be honest but constructive and must include actionable items for the student or resident to improve upon. This can be challenging but with practice becomes routine. By providing easy access, quick turnaround, and specificity for what the student seeks to learn about their performance, ubiquitous cell phone technology is helping to decrease the burden associated with frequent and timely feedback.[12]

4. **Create a supportive and inclusive learning environment.** A supportive and inclusive learning environment has long been recognized as ideal, and there continues to be a great deal of focus on this issue at a national level since the detrimental effects of nonsupportive environment are well understood.[13] Unfortunately, surgical services are often implicated as not upholding this ideal and interventions to address this have started to gain traction.[14] By virtue of their close working

relationships with students, residents are one of the prime influences on the quality of the learning environment and the support and psychological safety that a student perceives. How can resident educators create this type of environment? The most important step is ensuring every team member is valued and respected, which is in exact alignment with the pursuit of diverse and inclusive educational programs. One particularly valuable approach is to limit hierarchy (at least in the traditional culture of surgical training) while preserving respect for seniority and defined leadership roles. A supportive environment is also one in which every team member is important. In the clinical environment, team members achieve a sense of value when they contribute to the work being performed. This requires integration of all team members into day-to-day patient care activities. For medical students, this might mean performing dressing changes on morning rounds, assessing patients independently in clinic, and being given the opportunity to participate in the operating room (e.g., perform the incision, fire the stapler, and close skin). Sometimes, based on the nature of the task at hand, medical students are not able to safely contribute in such tangible ways. This does not mean they should be excluded. Instead, an effort should be made to include them through verbal engagement: explain what one is doing and why, ask them questions, and recognize their presence by engagement.

5. **Prioritize patient care above all else.** Role modeling is a powerful educational tool.[15] Student learners adopt, through conscious and unconscious mechanisms, the knowledge, values, and skills of the resident educators with whom they work. Residents should seek to internalize the significant responsibility inherent in this relationship. When resident educators demonstrate compassionate patient-centered care, learners are more likely to follow suit.

Less obvious opportunities for resident-led teaching include thoughtful and mentored integration into the formal teaching curriculum of the program. Traditionally, teaching conferences have involved a faculty surgeon teaching as a "sage on the stage" to seated residents about their particular area of expertise. If teaching teams are established as a single resident and a single faculty member far in advance of the scheduled session, the resident will be prepared to be the primary teacher with the faculty there as a "guide on the side" to stoke discussion, add context, and assess the knowledge level of the group as part of program improvement efforts. The team should determine four to five clear learning objectives for the session and circulate these in advance to involved resident and student learners along with any supplemental material. Audience response systems such as quiz questions and a case-based format increase the effectiveness of the session. This format has the added benefit of establishing resident accountability and influence on the quality of their education. For this format to be fully effective, the resident must receive written feedback from peers and mentoring faculty about content and communication soon after the session. Similar success can be had by placing capable residents in roles as seminar or curriculum leaders with appropriate oversight from expert faculty. Examples include curricula in areas such as surgical ethics and leadership development. These areas may stretch the concept as the teacher as expert, but with appropriate faculty guidance and involvement in the planning and execution, these educational experiences can be remarkably valuable and practical as they tend to be more grounded in the particular needs of resident learners while remaining very beneficial for engaged medical students.

PREPARING RESIDENTS TO BE EDUCATORS

Setting high expectations and creating opportunities are insufficient without preparing residents to excel as teachers. Although most residents have been learning as adults for many years, few have had the opportunity to reflect on the principles of andragogy (adult learning) and how they may differ from the pedagogical approach that formed the basis of their education as a child. Although there are course offerings at national meetings or online, a minority of training programs have developed Resident-as-Teacher or Resident-as-Educator courses to supplement their residency curriculum.[16,17] In general, these curricula may improve resident self-assessed teaching behaviors and teaching confidence and may be linked to improved student evaluations.[18] One example of topics included in a Resident-as-Educators course is shown in *Table 17.1.* These longitudinal educational initiatives or fellowships are occasionally sponsored at the institutional level. One such example is the CoMET program (Community of Medical Educators in Training) at the University of Michigan, which concentrates both on teaching residents to teach as well as inspiring achievable curriculum development.

WHEN A RESIDENT STRUGGLES AS AN EDUCATOR

When residents are deliberately put in teaching roles, some may not succeed initially. Especially if they have had negative experiences in the past when they were the learner, it becomes easy to propagate that as "normal." The most common stumbling point may be in creating a supportive learning environment or maintaining

Table 17.1 Example Topics for a Residents-as-Educators Curriculum at the University of Michigan

Topic Examples
• Deliberate Teaching/Teaching On-the-Fly
• Entrustment in the Operating Room
• Making Conferences Effective
• Modifying Teaching Styles
• Intraoperative Teaching, Learning, and Interactions
• Setting Examples
• Use of Strategic Questioning
• Giving Feedback
• Teaching When Time Is Limited
• Teaching Technical Skills
• Small-Group Teaching

respectful communication styles. When a resident has a pattern of negative teaching evaluations, it is important not to accept the issue and the resident should not be allowed to avoid teaching responsibilities or they will fail to improve. Especially when this translates to a decrement in milestone ratings and the resident starts to separate negatively in performance compared with their peers or compared with clear expectations, targeted intervention is needed. One option is to have a faculty educator embedded along with the resident when they are asked to deliberately teach medical students (e.g., a "chalk talk") or to accompany them on rounds. Using the principles above, the faculty can then meet with the resident privately to give them specific and actionable feedback. It is important to repeatedly assess them in the act of teaching after that to make sure improvements are occurring.[19]

EVALUATION AND RECOGNITION OF RESIDENT TEACHING PERFORMANCE

To accomplish sustainable change in the educational expectations of residents as educators, feedback to them about their performance is critically important. If at all possible, medical students should be asked to evaluate individual residents (not just faculty) as teachers. Instructions to student evaluators should be aimed at also eliciting rich feedback about communication styles and creation of a supportive learning environment. These evaluations should be provided in an anonymous aggregated form as frequently as is feasible. Just as it is important for aspiring resident teachers to see faculty teachers recognized for their educational skills, it is effective to create a culture of recognition for resident teachers as well. Department- or program-level awards for effective teaching are recommended and Medical School awards for residents providing exceptional clinical teaching or creating exemplary learning environments can be very inspiring. Truly exceptional resident teachers should be nominated by their program leaders for national awards such as those offered by the Association of Surgical Education or the American College of Surgeons.

Surgical residents have great influence on the experiential learning of medical students and their perceptions of surgeons and the discipline of Surgery. With proper preparation, deliberate and spontaneous opportunities, and evaluation and recognition of the development of resident teaching skills, the benefits reach far beyond just the learner. Especially in an inclusive training program, culture that embraces diversity of thought and experience, the educational environment continues to improve along the full spectrum of lifelong learning for students, residents, and faculty.

ACKNOWLEDGMENTS

The authors gratefully acknowledge Gurjit Sandhu, PhD, for her development and implementation of the Residents-as-Educators curriculum for the University of Michigan Surgery Program and for sharing the outline in *Table 17.1*.

REFERENCES

1. ACGME Common Program Requirements 2019. Available at https://www.acgme.org/What-We-Do/Accreditation/Common-Program-Requirements. Accessed January 9, 2020.
2. ACGME Accreditation Website 2019. Available at https://www.acgme.org/what-we-do/Accreditation/Milestones/Milestones-by-specialty. Accessed January 9, 2020.

3. LCME Publications 2019. Available at http://lcme.org/publications/. Accessed January 9, 2020.
4. Busari JO. The discourse of generational segmentation and the implications for postgraduate medical education. *Perspect Med Educ.* 2013;2:340-348.
5. Dedhia PH, Barrett M, Ives G, et al. Intraoperative feedback: a video-based analysis of faculty and resident perceptions. *J Surg Educ.* 2019;76:906-915.
6. Pelletier M, Belliveau P. Role of surgical residents in undergraduate surgical education. *Can J Surg.* 1999;42:451-456.
7. Whittaker LD Jr, Estes NC, Ash J, Meyer LE. The value of resident teaching to improve student perceptions of surgery clerkships and surgical career choices. *Am J Surg.* 2006;191:320-324.
8. Karani R, Fromme HB, Cayea D, Muller D, Schwartz A, Harris IB. How medical students learn from residents in the workplace: a qualitative study. *Acad Med.* 2014;89:490-496.
9. Ende J. Feedback in clinical medical education. *J Am Med Assoc.* 1983;250:777-781.
10. Bing-You RG, Trowbridge RL. Why medical educators may be failing at feedback. *J Am Med Assoc.* 2009;302:1330-1331.
11. Anderson PA. Giving feedback on clinical skills: are we starving our young?. *J Grad Med Educ.* 2012;4:154-158.
12. Barrett M, Georgoff P, Matusko N, et al. The effects of feedback fatigue and sex disparities in medical student feedback assessed using a minute feedback system. *J Surg Educ.* 2018;75:1245-1249.
13. AAMC Medical School Graduation Report 2017. Available at https://www.aamc.org/system/files/reports/1/2017/gqallschoolsummaryreport.pdf. Accessed January 9, 2020.
14. Lau JN, Mazer LM, Liebert CA, Bereknyei Merrell S, Lin DT, Harris I. A mixed-methods analysis of a novel mistreatment program for the surgery core clerkship. *Acad Med.* 2017;92:1028-1034.
15. Cruess SR, Cruess RL, Steinert Y. Role modelling–making the most of a powerful teaching strategy. *Br Med J.* 2008;336:718-721.
16. Geary A, Hess DT, Pernar LIM. Resident-as-teacher programs in general surgery residency – a review of published curricula. *Am J Surg.* 2019;217:209-213.
17. Geary AD, Hess DT, Pernar LIM. Resident-as-Teacher programs in general surgery residency: context and characterization. *J Surg Educ.* 2019;76(5):1205-1210.
18. Wamsley MA, Julian KA, Wipf JE. A literature review of "resident-as-teacher" curricula: do teaching courses make a difference?. *J Gen Intern Med.* 2004;19:574-581.
19. Magas CW, Wancata LM, Gauger PG, et al. How general surgery milestones and the clinical competency committee can be successfully leveraged to address gaps in assessment. *Int J Health Sci.* 2016;4:1-4.

18

Contemporary Delivery of Surgical Education

Gurjit Sandhu
Gifty Kwakye
Rebecca Minter

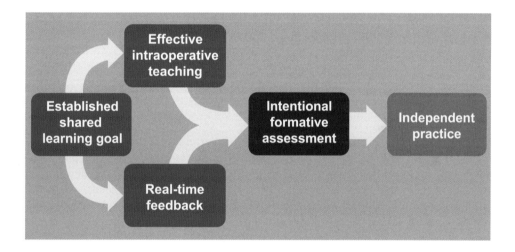

HOW DO FACULTY ENTRUST A TRAINEE?

It is 7:40 AM on a Friday and the OR is already running 10 minutes late with the first patient not in the room yet. This is the first of four complex cases Dr. Smith has scheduled that day, with the last one tentatively slated to be done by 4 PM so she can make it to a meeting at 5. It's almost 8 when the "room ready" page goes out and the Anesthesia team roles the patient into the room. Also walks in the PGY 2 on the service who apologizes for not being there earlier and explains that due to an emergency, the chief resident initially assigned had been pulled for coverage elsewhere. When asked if she'd ever assisted with an abdominoperineal resection for rectal cancer before, her answer is no.

However, she is eager to learn and assist however necessary. Dr. Smith appreciates her enthusiasm but realizes this could impact her intended pace for the day. Prior to scrubbing in, she calls her administrative assistant to cancel the 5 PM meeting.

THE PARAGON TRIPLE-THREAT SURGEON

Most enter academia drawn by the opportunity to practice clinically, conduct research, and be involved in teaching learners across all stages—the heroic "Triple-Threat" surgeon.[1,2] In an attempt to provide a more in-depth definition of what this entails, Rosengart and his team studied the curriculum-vitae and self-descriptive vignettes of seven surgeons considered giants in the field.[3] Seven key attributes discovered were

1. identifies complex clinical problems ignored or thought unsolvable by others,

2. becomes an expert,

3. innovates to advance treatment,

4. observes outcomes to further improve and innovate,

5. disseminates knowledge and expertise,

6. asks important questions to further improve care, and

7. trains the next generation of surgeons and scientists.

Of all these, Sir William Osler, who is credited for the Triple Threat concept, considered the training of students "by far the most useful and important work I have been called upon to do."[1,2]

Unfortunately, due to increased productivity pressures, demands to improve efficiency, and shifting expectations regarding supervision and the participation of learners, most faculty are faced with a myriad of daunting challenges. An unintended consequence is that the teaching mission has been relegated to the background or completely discarded. It is no surprise then that residents are graduating without the necessary skills to succeed in independent practice and that more are seeking additional fellowship training.[4,5] The degree of unpreparedness reported in several studies is alarming.[5-7] For instance, Mattar et al.[7] surveyed fellowship program directors regarding performance of new fellows. They found that 66% were unable to operate unsupervised for 30 minutes of a complex case and 26% could not recognize anatomical planes. This is not a judgment of the quality of contemporary trainees, but rather a system of training which has failed them.

The detrimental impact of this failed system on the ability to provide quality patient care and to educate future generations of surgeons has created a sense of urgency among governing bodies and training programs, leading to calls to revive the teaching mission.[5,8] More funding has also been allocated to research to help understand how to teach and motivate both learners and faculty more effectively. As a result, concepts such as "Autonomy" and "Entrustability" have surfaced and assessment tools, such as the System for Improving and Measuring Procedural Learning (SIMPL) smartphone application, have been adopted by many programs.[9-11]

The Conflict With Intraoperative Teaching

Despite these efforts, teaching effectively and attaining the desired outcome continue to be quite challenging especially in the operating room. Faculty have to take into account a wide range of trainee ability, even among individuals at the same level, and be quick to adapt depending on a multitude of factors.[12-14] These include the complexity of the case, number and experience of support staff, and even the surgeon's own level of experience. In addition, the faculty surgeon often has had limited contact with the trainee and does not know the level of skill and experience the resident has with the planned operation.

Before an incision is made, most faculty have an operative plan in place, in addition to alternatives depending on the operative findings. They have also predetermined, to an extent, the degree of autonomy they are willing to allow the resident.[14,15] Chen et al.[14] found that this decision was influenced by five main factors (*Figure 18.1*):

1. case schedule/start time,

2. patient morbidity,

3. procedure attributes,

4. resident current competency level, and

5. trustworthiness.

The resident's current competency—consisting of their PGY level, knowledge, experience, and/or skills—was the most important factor.[14] In follow-up studies,[15,16] the investigators took a closer look at how attending surgeons determine these resident factors preoperatively as a means of gauging readiness for autonomy. Strategies used included

1. directly asking the resident about previous experience doing the same or similar case;

2. judging preparedness for a case based on knowledge, attitude, or confidence exhibited; and

3. using evidence acquired before the case from prior interactions, assessments, or the resident's reputation among peers or other faculty.

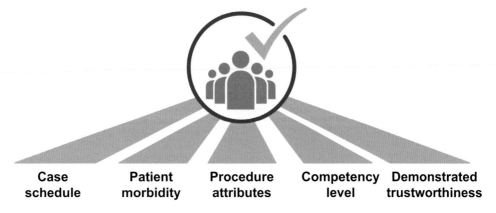

Figure 18.1 Factors determining resident intraoperative autonomy.

Of course, most if not all of these strategies lend themselves to subjective influences, which can result in mismatched intraoperative expectations. For instance, attending surgeons and residents have been found to have different learning goals and interpretations of what counts as adequate preoperative preparation for the same case.[17,18] Understandably it is also difficult to utilize these strategies when resident case assignments are changed at the very last minute, as in the scenario described above, or when faculty are less familiar with a resident.

Once the surgery begins, the amount of autonomy actually provided is strongly dependent on the attributes of the attending surgeon themselves rather than the resident.[14,19] These, as alluded to earlier, include their level of experience or comfort with a case, their preferred surgical technique, or their own beliefs regarding teaching residents in the operating room. These inherent attending attributes also influence the degree of faculty entrustment exhibited. Faculty entrustment is defined as "actions that impart trust and responsibility for patient care to the resident while providing appropriate supervision."[19] Interestingly, neither case difficulty nor faculty years of experience is associated with faculty entrustment in direct observational studies performed.[19]

Providing "teaching" in the operating room is not sufficient to ensure independent practice if it is not combined with an intentional process of assessment and feedback to residents actually participating in performing the operation. Traditionally, resident assessment has been conducted at various time intervals over the year relying on the attending surgeon's remote memory. Studies have shown, however, that evaluations completed more than 3 days after the interaction often lack granular details, especially regarding performance.[10,20] Instead, what has been found to be effective is real-time and video-based assessment with feedback pertaining to both resident technical and nontechnical skills (NOTSS—situational awareness, decision making, leadership, communication, and teamwork).[10,21,22]

HOW DO RESIDENTS DEMONSTRATE THAT THEY ARE ENTRUSTABLE?

Faculty responsibility with respect to patient care, supervisory regulations, and conditions of employment have significant bearing on surgeon actions and carry real consequences for lack of adherence.[23-25] It is thus understandable that these forces would have a constraining effect on how surgeons teach. As the surgical environment continues to change at an extraordinary pace (e.g., costs of care, operative efficiencies, patient acuity and comorbidities, virtual resources, milestones, and competencies), faculty alone cannot be responsible for the education mission.[7,26] Balancing multiple and competing responsibilities in the operating room—the dynamic high-stakes education environment unique to surgical residencies—requires an equally dynamic reimagining of teaching and learning in the operating room. Enhancing faculty–trainee intraoperative interactions to optimize learner growth is a responsibility that must also be incurred by residents. Learner responsibility is explored through resident agency in education, culture as a driver of performance, and the recognition of the important role of mentees.

Resident Agency in Education

Trust in the surgical profession is salient in the patient–physician relationship. However, trust is also seminal to faculty–resident relationships. There is substantial unspoken public trust in the faculty–resident relationship which believes the education model is preparing trainees to be competent surgeons for future patients. The discipline is in jeopardy of failing that public trust if it does not produce surgeons who are prepared for independent contemporary surgical practice. This is inclusive of safe performance of operations, but also assumes an end product that is culturally competent, possesses excellent judgment and who recognizes one's own boundaries, and will call for help when needed. Current assessment frameworks do not effectively assess the readiness of a learner to meet these needs of the public and future patients. Often assessments are distant and depersonalized—ability assessed along a Likert scale at the end of a month-long rotation. Actively integrating "trust" into teaching and learning interactions and assessment brings the magnitude of developing trustworthy competent surgeons to the fore of surgeon education.[27] Asking a faculty member if they would "trust this resident to perform this operation on their loved one independently" reframes the assessment of competence and readiness for practice in a powerful way.

When asked about trusting learners, surgeons describe having a gut feeling about the resident which leads them to advance more or scale back the degree of autonomous opportunities they extend to the trainee. ten Cate unpacks that gut feeling and describes engendering trust on the basis of four conditions: ability, integrity, reliability, and humility (*Figure 18.2*).[28] Ability is the demonstration of competence as reflected in established milestones. Integrity refers to goodwill and truth-telling. Reliability is observable through predictability of behaviors. Finally, humility is acting with modesty and restraint. Because of the privileged nature of their relationships with patients, surgeons are primed to think and respond to indications of trust. By intentionally orienting themselves according to each condition of trust, residents increase the potential for having their competence received by faculty as trustworthy for greater responsibility.[29]

Encouraging residents to emphasize behaviors associated with each of these conditions of trust has the potential to more directly fit the trust framework upon which faculty make education entrustment decisions.[30] For example, resident ability can be demonstrated through refining technical skills. In response to faculty feedback, residents who practice outside of the operating room (e.g., simulation center) sharpen their maneuvers, which is subsequently apparent in the operating room. An illustration of how resident integrity can be damaged would be when a resident states that they have checked on a patient, and they actually have just looked at the vitals and labs in the computer. Although the patient may be doing well on the ward,

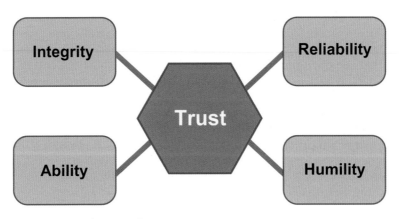

Figure 18.2 Four conditions of trust.

the impact of a resident not following through with their responsibility to examine a patient compounded by an inaccurate statement to faculty will invariably affect future trust in the operating room. Behaviors such as being present for Morbidity and Mortality rounds (whether or not one is presenting a case) and returning pages in a timely manner contribute to perceptions of resident reliability. Finally, humility necessitates confidence in reimagining the education process and contributing to a shared mental model with faculty. Humility requires the confidence to work consciously and safely to the edge of one's abilities, accompanied by the self-awareness on the part of the resident to articulate they are now struggling or need help to advance to the next step. While residents may see this as an admission of lack of expertise, faculty are more likely to perceive this as a trainee who knows their limits and can be trusted to ask for help. Entrustment of residents, that is, trust associated with sharing responsibility for patient care, is established within and outside the operating room.[31] As residents demonstrate that they are entrustable, worthy of entrustment, faculty are encouraged to provide trainees with gradually more autonomy within a safely supervised education environment.[32,33]

In order to receive learner-specific targeted teaching, residents must be active agents in establishing educational moments that accelerate them toward their goals. Even if there is limited time to meet a patient or read deeply about the disease, every operation is an educational opportunity and an incremental step in growth.[34] As adult learners who have strived for a hard-earned position in surgical residency, residents have sufficient personal, professional, and educational experiences to assess their learning needs and set realistic goals.[35] While goals are negotiable with faculty, it is essential that learners demonstrate they are invested in driving their learning forward. It is not an option to arrive at an operation, an educational opportunity, without an educational goal in mind. If a PGY2 resident finds herself involved in an abdominoperineal resection case and has never participated in this type of operation before, it is helpful for the trainee to state that they have not participated in this specific surgery before, but it is additionally important to bring related experiences, such as mobilizing the right colon laparoscopically for a cecal mass or maturing an ostomy, to the attention of the faculty member. Providing the surgeon with evidence about abilities and experiences, in addition to demonstrating integrity and humility, lends itself to developing trust and contributing to reasonable shared goal setting.

The Briefing–Intraoperative Teaching–Debriefing (BID) model offers a concrete strategy for establishing an intraoperative education goal.[36] Roberts and colleagues developed BID as a model for deliberate teaching in the operating room. Briefing occurs prior to the operation and is when faculty and resident establish a learning goal for the operation. The onus begins with the resident identifying an area of growth, which is then adjusted with the faculty member for appropriateness. Intraoperative teaching then focuses with more intentionality and frequency on the preestablished learning goal. While other coaching and instruction will still occur during the operation, the shared goal is prioritized. At the end of the case, debriefing circles back to the shared goal and begins with the resident reflecting on their performance, followed by encouragement and correction by the faculty, and ending with a shared sense of next steps for growth or a goal for the learner.

Entrustable Professional Activities (EPAs) are another approach that prioritizes learner-centered education. EPAs merge workplace-based assessment (comprehensive assessment of performance that occurs during actual practice) with assessment of competence.[37-39] Each EPA reflects an essential activity of a discipline that an individual can be trusted to perform without supervision in a given health care context, once sufficient competence has been demonstrated. The appeal of an

EPA-based assessment is its anchor in the principles of entrustment and graduated independence, core concepts embedded in the current approach to resident education.[12,13,24,32] Via EPA-based assessments, residents receive detailed, tangible, and contextualized feedback. Also, faculty members can extract iterative data from EPAs to determine the level of resident entrustment necessary for independent patient care.

Residency redesign to shift toward learner-centered frameworks—such as BID and EPAs—will require active implementation of faculty and resident development. The goal of professional development would be to establish shared mental models among faculty and residents about expectations for assessment processes and practices, adoption of real-time assessments, and advancing a road map for a learner-driven approach for achieving competency. For the resident to have agency in the education process, by being invited to drive their learning forward and co-create intraoperative teaching goals, a reframing of educational interactions in surgery residencies is needed.[40] Consideration of restructuring residency is also necessary as we shift to a learner-driven assessment framework grounded in trust. If residents and faculty do not have sufficient exposure to working together, as can occur with the current state of shorter rotations with more faculty, it is difficult to know if a trainee possesses the four conditions of trust outlined in *Figure 18.1* by ten Cate.[28] Successful reframing and implementation of a new approach to resident assessment is reliant upon a culture that supports creativity in the educational process and teaching–learning interactions.

Culture Drives Performance

Before advancing new frameworks which encourage residents to be advocates for their intraoperative experiences, invite residents to be co-collaborators with establishing their educational goals, and which insist that excellent teaching and excellent patient care are not an either-or dilemma; there must be a culture that fosters this type of environment. If the discipline heeds the call that educators are also learners, then it must be willing to nurture a culture that is intentional about inviting surgeons and residents to engage in new education paradigms *together*. The premise that strong culture drives performance is widely studied and exemplified in environments which support diversity of ideas, celebrate innovation, stress shared goals, and prioritize civility.[41] A strong culture for residency education would reflect the very same conditions.

Taking up the call for innovation is not uncommon to surgery. From designing minimally invasive approaches to addressing the opioid crisis, surgeons and residents are unabashed in their creativity. That same energy is necessary for fostering a creative culture of education. Surgery residencies have had a long reputation of adhering to hierarchies when it comes to teaching and learning. Innovations, such as the Surgical Safety Checklist and competency-based education, have reshaped traditional hierarchies and had a significant effect on including diverse perspectives for betterment of patient safety. Investing in creative and inclusive cultures is essential for building on this diversity of thought and voice in surgery education.

The OpTrust Educational Bundle is a novel program for faculty and resident professional development which is grounded in principles of an inclusive culture which promotes mutual responsibility for resident training by both the resident and faculty member.[19,42,43] Three key components from the OpTrust Bundle point to success by virtue of fostering both trust and educational innovation in the surgical residency culture in order to be successful: shared mental models, motivational

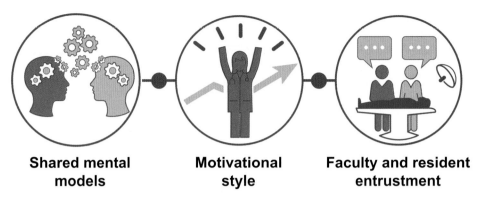

Shared mental models **Motivational style** **Faculty and resident entrustment**

Figure 18.3 Components of OpTrust bundle.

style, and direct observation of intraoperative faculty entrustment and resident entrustability behaviors (*Figure 18.3*). Shared mental models are organized knowledge structures and task demands that are similarly understood by team members.[44] Shared mental models are also about shared team outcomes. Clear and consistent messaging about the departmental educational mission and examples of observable behaviors that mirror alignment with the mission contribute to the shared mental model focused on resident development. Through OpTrust professional development, faculty entrustment and resident entrustability behaviors in the operating room are explicitly shared with surgeons and learners to facilitate transparency and mutual awareness regarding trainee readiness for additional responsibility. When faculty and residents understand intraoperative behaviors and discourse on the same channel of communication, they can more readily detect signals for entrustment and entrustability. For example, take a resident who arrives at a cholecystectomy operation with a proposal for laparoscopic operative approach and outlines safety concern. Throughout the operation, the resident asks questions that demonstrate forward thinking while carefully dissecting out the cystic duct and artery and clearing the cystic plate to identify the critical view of safety. The shared mental model for entrustment and entrustability through OpTrust empowers residents to adopt and demonstrate learner agency in their education trajectory. This advocacy for one's learning is a critical aspect of lifelong learning as well and will ensure that residents continue to learn and grow into the surgeons that their patients need.

The second component of OpTrust relevant to performance and shared mental models focuses on faculty and resident motivational style. Regulatory focus theory (RFT) is a goal pursuit theory that helps conceptualize how individuals are motivated to pursue a goal.[45-47] RFT describes individuals as either more promotion-focused or more prevention-focused. Promotion-focused individuals tend to work more quickly, feel excited and energized by success, and are willing to take risks. Prevention-focused individuals are more inclined to work with vigilance, feel quiet and calm with success, and work to ensure against errors. When faculty and resident have a shared motivational style, this feeling of flow alignment would be more apparent.[48] However, when the faculty and resident present with different motivational styles, it is easy to see how perception of the other's performance could affect entrustment and intraoperative educational opportunities. For example, a prevention-oriented faculty member who is operating with a promotion-oriented resident may perceive them to be reckless and too aggressive. They pull back on the autonomy they may have provided if they had a shared understanding of each other's perspective. Including RFT in OpTrust professional development is yet another means by which to enhance transparency and strengthen teaching and learning with a shared mental model.

The third component of OpTrust relates to a culture of inclusivity and trust. OpTrust assessment of faculty entrustment and resident entrustability relies on direct third-party observations. Trained raters (e.g., medical students, education scientists) are present in the operating room and observe teaching and learning interactions with a lens on entrustment–entrustability behaviors. The current of trust in the culture is what allows faculty and residents to include OpTrust observers in their operating rooms, be open to feedback to enhance intraoperative entrustment, and their willingness to enact the recommended strategies. From the open-ended questions that faculty ask (e.g., what do we need to be thinking about as we takedown the splenic flexure?) to the language that residents use to express awareness about their abilities (e.g., can I have a bit longer to address this problem?), there is a willingness to do things differently because there is trust in the shared goal of safe patient care while developing and graduating safe surgeons.

MENTEES AND THE DIVERSITY PROMISE

Contemporary delivery of surgical education is a reframing of relationships among faculty and residents. This is critical if we are to meet the needs of our current and future patients. The production of a surgical workforce that is prepared to deliver contemporary culturally competent surgical care is dependent upon our ability to respond and adapt our training environment and approach. As one advocates for residents to be active participants in driving their education forward, it is vital that transparency and a shared mental model for entrustment–entrustability behaviors be an explicit component of regular faculty and resident development. This education model is in keeping with the Diversity Promise for development of effective mentors for diverse and dynamic mentees as well as development of effective mentees to be sponsor-ready. A culture that nurtures an innovative and creative education environment promotes diversity of thought and a willingness to be uncomfortable in the process of moving toward a comfortable workplace dedicated to excellence in teaching, patient care, and advances in health care.

REFERENCES

1. Osler W. *The fixed period.* In: *Aequanimitas.* 6th ed. Philadelphia, PA: P. Blakiston's Son & Co; 1925.
2. Stein SL. Scholarship in academic surgery: history, challenges, and ideas for the future. *Clin Colon Rectal Surg.* 2013;26(4):207-211.
3. Rosengart TK, Mason MC, LeMaire SA, et al. The seven attributes of the academic surgeon: critical aspects of the archetype and contributions to the surgical community. *Am J Surg.* 2017;214(2):165-179.
4. Malangoni MA, Biester TW, Jones AT, Klingensmith ME, Lewis FR Jr. Operative experience of surgery residents: trends and challenges. *J Surg Educ.* 2013;70(6):783-788.
5. Bell RH Jr. Why Johnny cannot operate. *Surgery.* 2009;146(4):533-542.
6. George BC, Bohnen JD, Williams RG, et al. Readiness of US general surgery residents for independent practice. *Ann Surg.* 2017;266(4):582-594.

7. Mattar SG, Alseidi AA, Jones DB, et al. General surgery residency inadequately prepares trainees for fellowship: results of a survey of fellowship program directors. *Ann Surg.* 2013;258(3):440-449.

8. Sachdeva AK. Educational interventions aimed at the transition from surgical training to surgical practice. *Am J Surg.* 2019;217(3):406-409.

9. George BC, Teitelbaum EN, Meyerson SL, et al. Reliability, validity, and feasibility of the Zwisch scale for the assessment of intraoperative performance. *J Surg Educ.* 2014;71(6):e90-e96.

10. Bohnen JD, George BC, Williams RG, et al. The feasibility of real-time intraoperative performance assessment with SIMPL (system for improving and measuring procedural learning): early experience from a multi-institutional trial. *J Surg Educ.* 2016;73(6):e118-e130.

11. Sandhu G, Thompson-Burdine J, Matusko N, et al. Bridging the gap: the intersection of entrustability and perceived autonomy for surgical residents in the OR. *Am J Surg.* 2019;217(2):276-280.

12. Skeff KM, Stratos GA, Mygdal W, et al. Faculty development. A resource for clinical teachers. *J Gen Intern Med.* 1997;12 suppl 2:S56-S63.

13. Sprake C, Cantillon P, Metcalf J, Spencer J. Teaching in an ambulatory care setting. *Br Med J.* 2008;337:a1156.

14. Chen XP, Williams RG, Smink DS. Dissecting attending surgeons' operating room guidance: factors that affect guidance decision making. *J Surg Educ.* 2015;72(6):e137-e144.

15. Chen XP, Sullivan AM, Alseidi A, Kwakye G, Smink DS. Assessing residents' readiness for or autonomy: a qualitative descriptive study of expert surgical teachers' best practices. *J Surg Educ.* 2017;74(6):e15-e21.

16. Chen XP, Sullivan AM, Smink DS, et al. Resident autonomy in the operating room: how faculty assess real-time entrustability. *Ann Surg.* 2019;269(6):1080-1086.

17. Pernar LI, Breen E, Ashley SW, Peyre SE. Preoperative learning goals set by surgical residents and faculty. *J Surg Res.* 2011;170(1):1-5.

18. Rose JS, Waibel BH, Schenarts PJ. Disparity between resident and faculty surgeons' perceptions of preoperative preparation, intraoperative teaching, and postoperative feedback. *J Surg Educ.* 2011;68(6):459-464.

19. Sandhu G, Thompson-Burdine J, Nikolian VC, et al. Association of faculty entrustment with resident autonomy in the operating room. *JAMA Surg.* 2018;153(6):518-524.

20. Williams RG, Chen XP, Sanfey H, Markwell SJ, Mellinger JD, Dunnington GL. The measured effect of delay in completing operative performance ratings on clarity and detail of ratings assigned. *J Surg Educ.* 2014;71(6):e132-e138.

21. Yule S, Paterson-Brown S. Surgeons' non-technical skills. *Surg Clin N Am.* 2012;92(1):37-50.

22. Hu YY, Mazer LM, Yule SJ, et al. Complementing operating room teaching with video-based coaching. *JAMA Surg.* 2017;152(4):318-325.

23. Kempenich JW, Willis RE, Rakosi R, Wiersch J, Schenarts PJ. How do perceptions of autonomy differ in general surgery training between faculty, senior residents, hospital administrators, and the general public? A multi-institutional study. *J Surg Educ.* 2015;72(6):e193-e201.

24. Teman NR, Gauger PG, Mullan PB, Tarpley JL, Minter RM. Entrustment of general surgery residents in the operating room: factors contributing to provision of resident autonomy. *J Am Coll Surg.* 2014;219(4):778-787.

25. Sandhu G, Magas CP, Robinson AB, Scally CP, Minter RM. Progressive entrustment to achieve resident autonomy in the operating room: a national qualitative study with general surgery faculty and residents. *Ann Surg.* 2016;265(6):1134.

26. Frisse ME. The business of trust. *Acad Med.* 2016;91(4):462-464.

27. Salim SY, Govaerts M, White J. The construction of surgical trust: how surgeons judge residents' readiness for operative independence. *Ann Surg.* 2020;271(2):391-398. doi:10.1097/SLA.0000000000003125.

28. ten Cate O. Entrustment as assessment: recognizing the ability, the right, and the duty to act. *J Grad Med Educ.* 2016;8(2):261-262.

29. Kennedy TJ, Regehr G, Baker GR, Lingard L. Point-of-care assessment of medical trainee competence for independent clinical work. *Acad Med.* 2008;83(10):S89-S92.

30. Sagasser MH, Kramer AW, Fluit CR, van Weel C, van der Vleuten CP. Self-entrustment: how trainees' self-regulated learning supports participation in the workplace. *Adv Health Sci Educ.* 2017;22(4):931-949.

31. ten Cate O, Hart D, Ankel F, et al. Entrustment decision making in clinical training. *Acad Med.* 2016;91(2):191.
32. Mellinger JD, Williams RG, Sanfey H, et al. Teaching and assessing operative skills: from theory to practice. *Curr Probl Surg.* 2017;54(2):44-81.
33. Rekman J, Gofton W, Dudek N, Gofton T, Hamstra SJ. Entrustability scales: outlining their usefulness for competency-based clinical assessment. *Acad Med.* 2016;91(2):186-190.
34. Polavarapu HV, Kulaylat AN, Sun S, Hamed O. 100 Years of surgical education: the past, present, and future. *Bull Am Coll Surg.* 2013;98(7):22-27.
35. Mezirow J. A critical theory of adult learning and education. *Adult Educ.* 1981;32(1):3-24.
36. Roberts NK, Williams RG, Kim MJ, Dunnington GL. The briefing, intraoperative teaching, debriefing model for teaching in the operating room. *J Am Coll Surg.* 2009;208(2):299-303.
37. Norcini J, Burch V. Workplace-based assessment as an educational tool: AMEE Guide No. 31. *Med Teach.* 2007;29(9):855-871.
38. ten Cate O. Entrustability of professional activities and competency-based training. *Med Educ.* 2005;39(12):1176-1177.
39. ten Cate O. Nuts and bolts of entrustable professional activities. *J Grad Med Educ.* 2013;5(1):157-158.
40. Peters H, Holzhausen Y, Boscardin C, ten Cate O, Chen HC. Twelve tips for the implementation of EPAs for assessment and entrustment decisions. *Med Teach.* 2017;39(8):802-807.
41. Pless N, Maak T. Building an inclusive diversity culture: principles, processes and practice. *J Bus Ethics.* 2004;54(2):129-147.
42. Sandhu G, Nikolian VC, Magas CP, et al. OpTrust: validity of a tool assessing intraoperative entrustment behaviors. *Ann Surg.* 2018;267(4):670-676.
43. Nikolian VC, Sutzko DC, Georgoff PE, et al. Improving the feasibility and utility of OpTrust—a tool assessing intraoperative entrustment. *Am J Surg.* 2018;216(1):13-18.
44. Mathieu JE, Heffner TS, Goodwin GF, Salas E, Cannon-Bowers JA. The influence of shared mental models on team process and performance. *J Appl Psychol.* 2000;85(2):273.
45. Higgins ET. Beyond pleasure and pain. *Am Psychol.* 1997;52(12):1280-1300.
46. Crowe E, Higgins ET. Regulatory focus and strategic inclinations: promotion and prevention in decision-making. *Organ Behav Hum Decis Process.* 1997;69(2):117-132.
47. Higgins ET, Friedman RS, Harlow RE, Idson LC, Ayduk ON, Taylor A. Achievement orientations from subjective histories of success: promotion pride versus prevention pride. *Eur J Soc Psychol.* 2001;31(1):3-23.
48. Sutzko DC, Boniakowski AE, Nikolian VC, et al. Alignment of personality is associated with increased intraoperative entrustment. *Ann Surg.* 2019;270(6):1058-1064.

19

Teaching in the Operating Room

Brian George

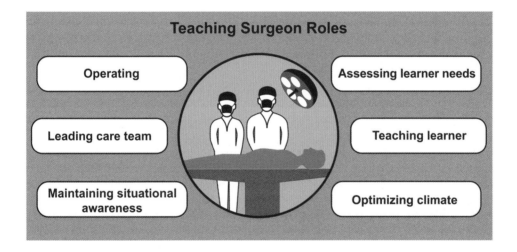

Teaching Surgeon Roles

Operating

Leading care team

Maintaining situational awareness

Assessing learner needs

Teaching learner

Optimizing climate

THE COMPLEXITY OF TEACHING IN THE OR

Teaching in the operating room is one of the most difficult activities undertaken by human beings. It requires the teaching surgeon to perform at the highest level in multiple complex roles simultaneously. While performing (or supervising the performance of) the technical steps of an operation, attending surgeons must also lead the team to execute the broader operative plan and maintain the situational awareness needed to identify when the original plan must change.[1] As if that weren't enough, teaching faculty are expected to identify, in real time, knowledge gaps to which they can teach in order to achieve the learning goals of individual trainees. This latter goal is made even more difficult when there are multiple learners and therefore multiple learning goals.

Remarkably, teaching faculty are expected to perform these instructional activities on a routine basis with little formal training.[2] Instead, most surgeons learn how to balance the competing demands of the patient, the team, and the learners through observing others and self-directed trial-and-error. Some faculty also have access to more formal didactic resources. Unfortunately, these strategies are not always successful. In those cases where faculty are not confident in their teaching skills, it can be tempting for them to minimize the time they spend teaching. This temptation is further reinforced by the fact that teaching is rarely necessary to meet the immediate needs of the current patient.

Further complicating the task, teaching in the operating room today must be different than it has been in the past. The next generation of surgeons is much more diverse than the last.[3] This diversity is clearly a strength, yet it also introduces additional challenges when teaching in the operating room. A "one size fits all" approach is now even less effective than it already has been, and more advanced techniques are needed to better individualize teaching. Unfortunately, as with other teaching skills, most faculty have not had formal training in these techniques.

In addition, bias risks compromising the education of some trainees who have not historically been well represented in surgery. For example, women are provided less autonomy by both male and female teaching faculty.[4] These effects almost certainly exist for other demographic groups. To avoid unconsciously discriminating against some learners, it is important to consciously develop a teaching framework that can be equitably applied to all learners according to their individual needs.

This chapter provides information about teaching in general while also highlighting the need to individualize the support of learners with different goals, backgrounds, and perspectives. While it is challenging to holistically integrate multiple responsibilities, doing so will bring benefits to both current and future patients.

THE BID MODEL

This chapter leverages a few existing conceptual frameworks to organize and motivate the information. The most widely known framework for teaching in the OR is the Briefing, Intraoperative teaching, and Debriefing, or BID, model.[5]

- The **Briefing** phase classically occurs while the team is at the scrub sink, where the faculty and resident can explicitly identify learning goals for the upcoming case. This is also an opportunity for faculty to define the limits of the trainee's knowledge so that intraoperative teaching can be targeted to the zone of learning that is neither too easy nor too difficult for the specific learner.

- The **Intraoperative** phase encapsulates behaviors that are typically associated with teaching in the OR, although in this model faculty teaching efforts are targeted to the goals identified during the Briefing Phase. Again, the goal is to individualize teaching to address the unique needs of learners with diverse needs and prior knowledge.

- The **Debriefing** phase occurs at the end of the case and is when faculty can provide feedback to trainees about their performance during the case, again aligned to the Briefing goals. One way for faculty to structure the Debriefing conversation is to (1) invite trainees to self-assess their performance on the identified learning goals, (2) help trainees to formulate new learning as a general principle or rule to guide future practice, (3) reinforce what was done right, and (4) correct mistakes, especially cognitive errors.

Each of these phases presents opportunities to equitably support and include diverse learners, as described below.

ESTABLISHING AND MAINTAINING CLIMATE

Importance for Learning

The most tangible aspects of an educational program are its curricula. Yet trainees are also influenced by the educational environment or "climate" of the training program.[6] For example, some programs are very authoritarian, while others may be more egalitarian. Trainees perceive these unwritten components to the curriculum differently. For some, one type of climate may be motivating while for another it may be demotivating. In general, however, a supportive climate is essential for trainees to optimize their learning (and performance).

The impact of climate on learning has been demonstrated across a range of learning domains and learning outcomes.[7] In residency programs, it has been linked to the quality of resident education,[8] performance,[9] and well-being.[10] But how does climate have these effects? One plausible mechanism may be through the stress engendered by hostile or intimidating environments.

There is a well-established relationship between psychological stress and performance, first described by Yerkes and Dodson in 1908.[11] As summarized more recently by Dobson, "A little anxiety from time to time can be beneficial to task performance... This is illustrated by the Yerkes Dodson law which states that performance is improved until an optimum level of arousal is reached."[12] Yet clearly *too* much stress diminishes performance, in part by increasing the amount of mental energy spent dealing with the emotional reaction engendered by those stimuli. This is especially true as task difficulty increases (*Figure 19.1*). As a result, managing the learning climate has a direct impact on trainees' stress and therefore their performance and learning.

Before discussing how to optimize the learning climate, one must first acknowledge that it is shaped at multiple levels. For example, a training program is situated within a hospital, a larger educational system, and a professional culture, all of which interact to create what might be usefully simplified to be the "program-level"

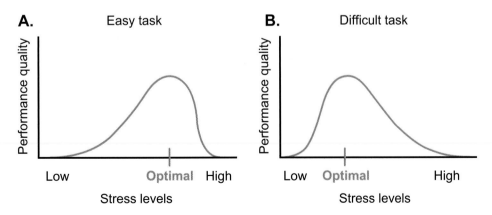

Figure 19.1 Relationship between the amount of stress and performance. Easy tasks are performed better with relatively more stress (panel A) than more difficult tasks (panel B) (Adapted from Yerkes and Dodson and Weiss KB, Bagian JP, Nasca TJ. The clinical learning environment: the foundation of graduate medical education. J Am Med Assoc. 2013;309(16):1687-1688. doi:10.1001/jama.2013.1931.)

climate. But there is also a smaller level of climate, one that can be influenced by instructors. In the wider educational literature this is referred to as the "classroom-level" climate.[7] In surgery, the operating room is a classroom, which is where trainees learn how to operate.

Approach to Establishing a Supportive Climate

Fortunately, faculty have a great deal of influence in the operating room. As such, they also have an important role to play in cultivating the operating room climate. This can be seen in the results of a student where medical students reported that attending physicians' attitudes and interactions in the OR were strongly correlated with the environment being conducive to learning.[13] Attributes such as "Attending was a positive role model" and "Attending surgeon tone" were most strongly correlated with the conduciveness of the OR environment for learning.

The climate can be established even before the team enters the operating room. The original description of the Briefing phase recommended a discussion about learning goals. This behavior also supports establishing a supportive learning climate because it is a clear signal that the trainee's needs are valued and supported. If the teaching surgeon hasn't often operated with the resident, it is also useful to set expectations not only for participation and autonomy but, importantly, for the amount of time being deliberately set aside for teaching. For medical students, an effective behavior is to learn their name—an easy but also easily overlooked intervention. Publicly introducing medical students to the OR team as one enters the theater can help put them at ease and also communicate to other team members that the student has a legitimate role and "belongs."

During the case (the "intraoperative" phase), it is important to maintain situational awareness not only of how things are going clinically but also with the team. This is especially true for learners who are uniquely vulnerable, often intimidated, and under substantial stress. For example, there is sometimes bullying of students and residents by other members of the team. These experiences diminish learning and well-being.

After the case, asking trainees how they felt the case went again signals that trainees' needs are a priority and helps establish a climate that supports their learning. Doing so for all learners demonstrates equity. This also presents an opportunity to tailor feedback according to the specific needs of diverse learners instead of teaching with a rigid, fixed approach. This can be difficult to implement in practice, especially if the instructor leaves the operating room before the trainee—one strategy is to ask the trainee to find the instructor after the patient has been dropped off in the recovery room.

Finally, the most effective leaders include and teach everyone in the team in order to optimize outcomes. They do so by communicating a motivating rationale for change and by minimizing concerns about power and status differences to promote speaking up in the service of learning.[14] These behaviors demonstrate respect for individuals and establish a climate that is conducive to high performance and learning.

In short, there are multiple ways to optimize the climate for learning. The best strategy may be to choose a few techniques and use them routinely. Doing so "the same way every time" has the added benefit of minimizing the impact of unconscious bias on the quality of support provided to different types of learners.

FEEDBACK

Effective feedback is objective and specific, engages the learner, builds trust, and invites the learner's views.[15] Furthermore, a lack of meaningful feedback causes stress and is a central contributing factor to depression.[16] Unfortunately, many clinical instructors still struggle to achieve those goals.[17]

During the Briefing phase the learner and teaching surgeon can identify specific learning goals. As suggested above, feedback in the Debriefing phase should target those goals. The key is to choose the right feedback for that trainee. For example, a trainee may be working on obtaining the critical view of safety during a laparoscopic cholecystectomy, and the instructor may have noted many areas for improvement. If they present all of those teaching points to the trainee, the trainee will struggle to integrate them all because the load of simply remembering them all will distract them from learning. It is better to choose a few points which are the highest yield and focus on them in more detail.

A typical feedback session should begin by asking the learner how they thought it went during the procedure. This can help the instructor gauge the learner's insight into their own performance and identify any other, unexpected problems. Asking a trainee for a self-evaluation helps the instructor tailor their feedback according to what the learner does and does not already know. It also helps address the diverse needs of unique learners by helping the instructor understand that trainee's frame of reference.

When providing feedback, it can be challenging to be specific. Simply saying "good job" does not constitute feedback. One strategy is to simply reflect back on the case and choose a few moments where coaching was required, and then explore those moments in more detail. As described above, it can be helpful to select those moments of the case that overlap with the goals defined during the Briefing phase.

COGNITIVE LOAD THEORY

The essence of teaching is judiciously providing learners with (1) information that is at the edge of their existing knowledge and (2) performance opportunities just beyond their comfort zone. Ideally this is done in a low-stakes environment in which the inevitable mistakes are not only permitted but even encouraged. Unfortunately, the operating room is not often this type of environment—sometimes mistakes cannot be permitted. This circumstance presents unique challenges to the teaching surgeon. It is not always appropriate to push the trainee to the edge of their abilities, yet they still need to learn. Fortunately, there is a framework—cognitive load theory[18]—that can help guide faculty when teaching in these more complex situations.

Learners in the operating room are performing a difficult task that has many facets. They are doing parts of the operation, processing information from the instructor, the team, and the patient, and—hopefully—learning. Each of these facets of the operative task has a cognitive load associated with it, yet everyone has a finite working memory with which to manage that load. It is the job of teachers to manage these cognitive loads to ensure that learning is optimized.

There are three types of cognitive load, each of which represents the different ways a person uses their working memory to learn to perform a task:

- The amount of memory required to simply perform a task is referred to as the **intrinsic cognitive load**. It represents the inherent difficulty of performing a given task and cannot be modified by the teacher. For example, cutting a suture has a lower intrinsic cognitive load than excising a mass adjacent to multiple critical structures.

- The amount of memory consumed by a task also depends on the manner in which information is presented.[19] For example, it may be easier to learn a motor skill after someone demonstrates it rather than verbally describing it. This type of cognitive load is termed **extraneous cognitive load**, and instructors should strive to minimize it in order to preserve more memory for learning.

- Learning itself requires working memory. This is, of course, the ultimate goal for instruction, and it is termed **germane cognitive load**.

One of the most important teaching strategies is to increase the space available for germane load (i.e., learning) by reducing extraneous load. This is especially true when the task is hard because there is already less working memory available due to higher intrinsic load. In these cases, any decrease in extraneous load will directly free cognitive resources for learning (*Figure 19.2*).

There are many sources of extraneous load. As described above, extraneous load can be reduced by presenting new information in a clear way. This might mean choosing the appropriate instructional method (demonstration, discussion, lecture, etc.) or breaking up a complex task into a structured sequence of smaller tasks.

Extraneous cognitive load can also be influenced by environmental factors, especially by an environment with many distractions. This will increase the extraneous cognitive load and therefore leave less room for learning (germane cognitive load). Strategies for minimizing environmental distractions include asking others to speak more softly, helping triage pages, and helping to manage interruptions from others on the team.

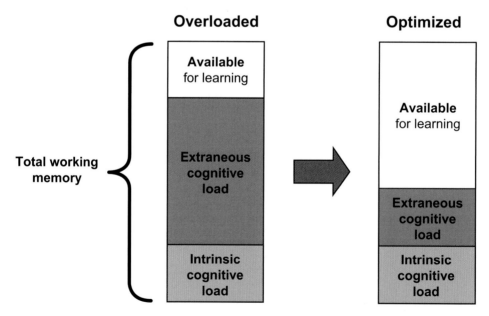

Figure 19.2 Schematic overview of working memory and how it can be filled with various types of cognitive load.

TAILORING OR TEACHING FOR DIVERSE LEARNERS

In addition to the sources of extraneous cognitive load described above, there is also extraneous cognitive load associated with psychological and emotional factors. Medical students who are in the operating room for the first time may be very nervous about offending the team, violating the sterile field, or just looking stupid. For residents, their relationship with the teaching faculty might also serve to distract them from learning. More generally, some learners may feel more "out of place" than others in the operating room. This will certainly reduce their capacity for learning (germane cognitive load) due to the extraneous cognitive load associated with that extra stress. In these cases, extra efforts must be made to ensure that everyone feels included in the team.

The principle of minimizing extraneous load also extends to optimizing the learning environment for diverse trainees, especially with respect to treatment that denigrates anyone based on their gender, race, ethnicity, sexual orientation, or other attributes. For example, sexist "jokes" can increase extraneous load for everyone in the operating room, and especially female team members. Belittling of medical students similarly causes them psychological stress—and leaves less room for learning. There is no room for these behaviors in the high-stakes environment of the operating room where both performance and learning are critically important.

As the team leader, faculty surgeons have a responsibility to address these types of behaviors. First, they can address these comments immediately and in a way that demonstrates psychological support for the learner. For example, if a medical student is being harassed by another member of the team, simply saying, loudly "We are so excited to have you here <student name>. I know a lot of this is new to you so please feel free to ask any questions you might have, and if we see anything you need to do differently, we will make sure to tell you in a way that is kind and supportive. After all, you are here to learn!"

There is also a role for teaching faculty to more explicitly establish more appropriate cultural norms when subtle methods have not been effective. For example, in addition to intervening in the moment, teaching faculty can also talk separately with those who repeatedly increase extraneous load for the learners. In aggregate, these interventions help ensure that all learners—regardless of their background—are treated well in the operating room in order to optimally support their learning.

TAILORING OR TEACHING FOR NOVICE LEARNERS

For novices in the operating room, it is important to provide them with sufficient support that they can efficiently learn in a completely new domain. There are multiple dimensions to that support, but the overarching goal is—as before—to minimize extraneous load.

For the operation as a whole, it can be very useful for them to have an outline of the procedure, ideally by writing out each big step on the whiteboard or the drapes. Depending on the case and the learner, it can be useful to have them do this themselves, before the operation begins. This can easily be integrated into the Briefing phase of the teaching case.

During the operation, it is important to choose tasks where the complexity (intrinsic load) isn't so high as to make it impossible for the trainee to have capacity to process new learning (germane load). These tasks are typically component technical skills. For example, if a learner has never driven a camera for a laparoscopic procedure, driving the camera is a perfect learning opportunity. If they have developed some expertise at driving a camera, then it is useful to add a new technical skill such as actively helping to retract. Eventually they will move into more complex technical skills as they master easier skills. The goal is to have the trainee use all of their working memory—and mostly for learning. This requires avoiding tasks that have high intrinsic and extraneous load. Of course, once there is extra capacity (because, say, they have developed expertise and the germane load of that learning is now lower), the instructor must provide them with new tasks that once again increase their germane load.

Similarly, if a learner is struggling and not making any progress, they can begin to get frustrated and anxious. At some point these feelings are not productive and simply represent extraneous load. In these circumstances there is no capacity for germane load and the trainee stops learning. Furthermore, the sense of failure can reduce their confidence and increase extraneous load for future operations as well (due to them wondering if they are "good enough" to do it the next time). Instructors should strive to recognize those moments and gently get trainees back on track. Ideally, they do so while explaining how they overcame whatever barrier was encountered by the trainee. Sometimes this will entail pointing out relevant anatomy, perceptual cues, or techniques. Once they get the trainee back on track, it is best to have the trainee resume in their original role, so they don't feel penalized by their lack of knowledge.

TAILORING OR TEACHING FOR INTERMEDIATE LEARNERS

Intermediate surgical learners are often very focused on developing their technical skills. To effectively teach these learners it is important to understand how technical skills are developed. For motor skill learning, there is a well-developed theory by Fitts and Posner that describes a progression through three phases of performance. This theory easily generalizes to technical skill learning.

- Motor skill learning begins in the **cognitive phase**, where every movement is a great effort. As an example, when learning to tie a shoe, this is where the learner is focused on each movement of both hands.

- In the **associative phase**, learners begin to link movements together. For example, the learner may know each step of tying the knot, but is working on how to do the whole task smoothly and without stumbling.

- Finally, in the **autonomous phase** the learner has mastered the skill and can do it with minimal cognitive effort. For example, most adults can simultaneously tie their shoe and hold a conversation.

The key to teaching the intermediate learner is to support the transition from the cognitive phase to the associative phase. The most important teaching behavior is to simply allow the learner to have the cognitive space to rehearse. Too much coaching can be detrimental because teaching itself can represent extraneous load. Instead, instructors must be selective about their coaching. For example, intermediate learners typically already understand the underlying principles, anatomy, and instrument handling. In that setting, teaching them more about the anatomy may actually distract them from the germane work of motor skill rehearsal. In other words, it is important to focus only on teaching which is germane to that learner in that moment.

For the instructor, it can also be very difficult to identify what type of teaching is germane and what is extraneous. As described above, it is often simply easiest to ask the trainee what they want to work on (typically during the Briefing phase) and focus teaching on those elements. If the learner suggests working on skills that are inappropriately advanced, the instructor can redirect the trainee to work on more basic skills that build to the more advanced goal.

In addition to the topics agreed upon during the Briefing phase, additional intra-operative coaching should be limited to any large or key gaps in the basic skills. This is a very challenging approach to teaching for most teaching faculty. There is no doubt that teaching the intermediate learner requires both self-discipline and flexibility on the part of the instructor. Understanding the immediate needs of the intermediate learner is key.

TAILORING OR TEACHING FOR ADVANCED LEARNERS

Advanced learners typically have a lot of spare capacity in their working memory as the germane load is markedly reduced. Furthermore, advanced trainees are moving from the associative phase of motor skill learning to the autonomous phase. As such, most teaching of advanced learners does not entail basic descriptions of anatomy or procedural steps—knowledge that the advanced learner already has. Instead, there is room in the learner's memory for teaching nontechnical skills—situational awareness, decision-making, communication and teamwork, and leadership.[1] Depending on the setting, this can also be a great opportunity to teach trainees how to teach. For example, trainees can be asked to define teaching performance goals during the Briefing phase (e.g., "I'm going to work on providing specific verbal feedback to the junior resident during the dissection"). The instructor can then provide the advanced trainee with feedback about their teaching performance during and after the case. Similar strategies apply to teaching advanced learners how to work with assistants.

As advanced learners move into the autonomous phase of motor skill learning, they should also be provided with meaningful autonomy.[20] This can be difficult to do in practice. One strategy is to ask them to start cases and call the instructor at a defined point so the instructor can check in. Alternatively, if there are other more junior learners in the operating room, the instructor can focus on those learners and leave the more advanced learner to work independently. If the instructor is trying to provide the learner with more autonomy but cannot leave the operating room, it is important to explicitly state the teaching goals with respect to trainee independence. Otherwise, some trainees are confused as to their role and how much leadership they should assert. For example, the instructor can simply say "I'm going to assist you, but I am going to be relatively silent and I want you to lead me through the case. If you have any questions, I am of course happy to help, but I will follow your lead as much as possible." Increased autonomy also provides the trainee with additional germane load, in part by asking them to manage extraneous load for themselves and the rest of the team. These are key skills not only for trainees but also practicing surgeons.

CONCLUSION

Teaching in the operating room is a complex balancing act that requires attention to the patient, the team, and the trainee. For the trainees, the most important underlying principle is to optimize the learning environment in order to minimize extraneous cognitive load. This is especially true for learners who might be more intimidated, who face discriminatory behaviors, or who are otherwise anxious about being in the operating room environment.

REFERENCES

1. Yule S, Gupta A, Gazarian D, et al. Construct and criterion validity testing of the Non-Technical Skills for Surgeons (NOTSS) behaviour assessment tool using videos of simulated operations. *BJS.* 2018;105(6):719-727. doi:10.1002/bjs.10779.
2. DaRosa DA, Roland Folse J, Sachdeva AK, Dunnington GL, Reznick R. Description and results of a needs assessment in preparation for the "surgeons as educators" course. *Am J Surg.* 1995;169(4):410-413. doi:10.1016/S0002-9610(99)80186-X.
3. Cobb AN, Kuo MC, Kuo PC. New docs on the block: a profile of applicants and subsequent PGY1 trainees of categorical general surgery programs (2013-2016). *Am J Surg.* 2019;218(1):218-224. doi:10.1016/j.amjsurg.2018.11.022.
4. Meyerson SL, Odell DD, Zwischenberger JB, et al. The effect of gender on operative autonomy in general surgery residents. *Surgery.* 2019; 166(5):738-743. doi:10.1016/j.surg.2019.06.006.
5. Roberts NK, Williams RG, Kim MJ, Dunnington GL. The briefing, intraoperative teaching, debriefing model for teaching in the operating room. *J Am Coll Surg.* 2009;208:299-303.
6. Sue Roff SM. What is educational climate? *Med Teach.* 2001;23(4):333-334. doi:10.1080/01421590120063312.
7. Fraser BJ. 5.1 science learning environments: assessment, effects and determinants. *Int Handb Sci Educ.* 1998:527-564.
8. Nasca TJ, Weiss KB, Bagian JP. Improving clinical learning environments for tomorrow's physicians. *N Engl J Med.* 2014;370(11):991-993. doi:10.1056/NEJMp1314628.
9. Weiss KB, Bagian JP, Nasca TJ. The clinical learning environment: the foundation of graduate medical education. *J Am Med Assoc.* 2013;309(16):1687-1688. doi:10.1001/jama.2013.1931.
10. Jennings ML, Slavin SJ. Resident wellness matters: optimizing resident education and wellness through the learning environment. *Acad Med.* 2015;90(9):1246. doi:10.1097/ACM.0000000000000842.
11. Yerkes RM, Dodson JD. The relation of strength of stimulus to rapidity of habit-formation. *J Comp Neurol Psychol.* 1908;18(5):459-482.
12. Dobson CB. *Stress: The Hidden Adversary.* New York: Springer Science & Business Media; 2012.
13. Schwind CJ, Boehler ML, Rogers DA, et al. Variables influencing medical student learning in the operating room. *Am J Surg.* 2004;187(2):198-200. doi:10.1016/j.amjsurg.2003.11.024.
14. Edmondson AC. Speaking up in the operating room: how team leaders promote learning in interdisciplinary action teams. *J Manag Stud.* 2003;40(6):1419-1452. doi:10.1111/1467-6486.00386.
15. Ende J. Feedback in clinical medical education. *J Am Med Assoc.* 1983;250(6):777-781. doi:10.1001/jama.1983.03340060055026.
16. Pereira-Lima K, Gupta RR, Guille C, Sen S. Residency program factors associated with depressive symptoms in internal medicine interns: a prospective cohort study. *Acad Med.* 2019;94(6):869. doi:10.1097/ACM.0000000000002567.
17. Bing-You R, Varaklis K, Hayes V, Trowbridge R, Kemp H, McKelvy D. The feedback tango: an integrative review and analysis of the content of the teacher–learner feedback exchange. *Acad Med.* 2018;93(4):657. doi:10.1097/ACM.0000000000001927.
18. Sweller J. Cognitive technology: some procedures for facilitating learning and problem solving in mathematics and science. *J Educ Psychol.* 1989;81(4):457-466. doi:10.1037/0022-0663.81.4.457.
19. Chandler P, Sweller J. Cognitive load theory and the format of instruction. *Cogn Instr.* 1991;8(4):293-332. doi:10.1207/s1532690xci0804_2.
20. Sandhu G, Teman NR, Minter RM. Training autonomous surgeons: more time or faculty development? *Ann Surg.* 2015;261(5):843-845. doi:10.1097/SLA.0000000000001058.

20

Pre- and Postoperative Teaching

Clifford S. Cho
Hari Nathan

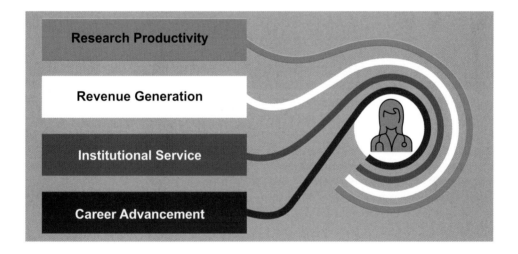

THE PROFESSIONAL IMPERATIVE OF CLINICAL TEACHING

Given the many competing demands placed on academic surgeons—research productivity, revenue generation, institutional service, and career advancement—it can be easy to overlook the fact that the task of preparing future generations of surgeons for independent practice has always been the core mission of academic surgery. Transferring clinical skills and wisdom to trainees is not only the academic surgeon's defining role but her only role that could never be fulfilled by anyone else. Despite the self-professed primacy of the training mission in many academic departments of surgery, the task of clinical teaching is often the first to be taken for granted. As it brings no professional titles or accolades to most and is usually not directly compensated financially, teaching can quickly transform from priority to burden in the mind of the academic surgeon.

The goal of this chapter is to motivate the reader to reevaluate the place clinical education has in the landscape of her many professional duties and to ask whether it may be time to rethink this. In the first segment, we will recall the experience of clinical education from the perspective of the learner. In the second, we will see how this perspective can inform the teacher's efforts to be more effective. In the final segment, we will explore how a reorientation to the professional imperative of clinical education could bring meaning and fulfillment to the academic surgeon.

THE EXPERIENCE OF SURGICAL LEARNING

Emotional and Cognitive Hyperacuity

The surgical residency is often the most intensive experience in a surgeon's life. The resident is finally invited to do what she has aspired to do for a long time—care directly for patients—and this opportunity (expectation) is at once exhilarating and harrowing. The privilege and intimacy of operating on another person become clearer than ever before; at the same time, the magnitude and complexity of responsibilities required to become a surgeon become soberingly evident. As time goes on, we may fondly recall the thrill of scrubbing a first case as primary surgeon, the anticipation of the first night on call, and the pride of successful box-checking before leaving postcall despite fatigue and a hospital system conspiring against us. Do we also recall the discomfort, if not fear, inherent in being responsible for an entire service of sick patients the first time?

This complicated mixture of excitement and trepidation creates an emotional intensity that hardwires every experience into our memories with great clarity. Compared to the hours it took to understand the cadaveric brachial plexus in medical school, the nuances of packing the hemorrhaging liver are retained immediately after one's first trauma laparotomy. Unlike nonprocedural disciplines, the inherently tactile and manually proprioceptive nature of surgery means that the essence of how we learn is no longer simply cognitive but also physical. Most medical students appropriately receive minimal exposure to performing operative techniques; as a result, residency is usually the first time one discovers that the skills acquired over decades of textbook-based learning no longer apply when acquiring the muscle memory of needle and suture placement.

THE OUTSIZED INFLUENCE OF THE FACULTY MENTOR

The system of graded responsibility means that each passing training year feels like a graduation. The experience of learning to manage the physiology of postoperative patients and distinguishing "sick" from "not sick" gives the finishing intern the confidence to manage critically ill patients in the intensive care unit in her second year. Viewed from the intern's base camp, the summit seems nearly impossible to reach—the program is long, with seemingly infinite nuances to master. Junior residents, faced with such a stark contrast between their own skills and wisdom and those of their chief residents, may feel that they might never competently lead the team, much less get to the level of the attending surgeon. (Only later does one realize that "mastery" is an illusory concept, and "finishing" really means "just getting started.")

This chasm in experiential wisdom between trainees and faculty is why residents tend to bestow respect so quickly onto their faculty surgeons and mentors; who does not recall the chairperson of surgery at the time of our residency with a sort of hero worship? Who among us could not replay from memory exact conversations we had with faculty mentors at pivotal moments of our training? Trainees view their faculty not simply as sources of wisdom but as templates by which they hope to construct their professional lives. It is a very common experience for residents to envision their future selves as an amalgamation of specific faculty mentors, noting in real time how they will someday emulate their admirable characteristics. We recall specific examples from our own training: the equanimity of one faculty during intraoperative misadventures, the humility and honesty of another when discussing his complications in conferences, the discretion of a technically gifted surgeon who frequently assisted his colleagues but never spoke of it, and the folded hands and compassionate demeanor of one when delivering difficult news to patients. (We also recall examples that we vowed *not* to emulate.) Viewed in this light, it is neither surprising nor insignificant that small gestures of interest and advocacy on the part of faculty surgeons to trainees are usually received with a disproportionate and unexpected appreciation and gratitude.

CULTIVATING A HEALTHY BALANCE OF CONFIDENCE AND INSECURITY

Despite how interminable it sometimes seems, the residency eventually comes to an end. When that happens, the transition from training to independence is a landmark milestone best navigated by those who possess an optimized balance of *confidence and insecurity*. Trainees may begin their internship with a sense that the residency process is the totality of surgical education; by the conclusion of their formal training, the healthy surgeon recognizes that she is still ascending the learning curve at a steep angle. Their ability to do this once outside the protective structure of a residency is enabled in part by a sense of confidence built from their own cumulative clinical experiences as well from the collective wisdom of their mentors. However, the safe young surgeon is also aware of her limits and blind spots, and this healthy sense of insecurity hopefully motivates her to seek out education and help when needed. Although confidence may grow and insecurity fade as experience builds and judgment matures, some degree of both is necessary to sustain a safe and effective surgeon over an entire career.

LEARNING A HABITUAL ORIENTATION AGAINST BURNOUT

In addition to acquiring cognitive knowledge and technical skills, the trainee also spends her surgical residency developing habits that will guide the rest of her professional career. Many of these habits are inculcated with great intention and effort; for example, the ethic of personally reviewing films and not simply reading radiologists' reports can become internalized after repetitive admonition and verification. Other habits are cultivated naturally, evolving through personal experience; for example, it is possible for a resident to receive excellent intensive care training with a durable antipathy for critical illness that leads her to avoid risky operations in the future.

Beyond the important dynamics of competence and safety, the surgical career is also marked by the need to continually locate and relocate meaning and fulfillment, both within and outside the hospital. We are all becoming increasingly aware of the insidious danger of burnout, which is very real during training.[1-3] The risk of burnout is like the risk of surgical complications; both are ever-present pitfalls that will accompany the surgeon throughout her career. As with surgical complications, the best hope is to avoid burnout, and the best way to avoid burnout is to implement best practices to mitigate its likelihood of occurrence. As with surgical complications, occasional encounters with burnout may be unavoidable, and the best way to handle these moments is to own strategies to understand and reverse their causes.

The healthy surgeon begins to construct these practices and strategies during residency with the same intentionality as that applied to building clinical skills. Until recently, this was a self-directed and accidental learning process, with each trainee taking on the task of (hopefully) discovering them on her own. Training programs are beginning to incorporate practices and strategies against burnout into their curricula. As is often the case in scientific studies of human experience, investigative attention to the problem of burnout is rediscovering timeless lessons. The seed of burnout often grows when the source of one's personal meaning and fulfillment becomes overwhelmed by more mundane and practical obligations. To prevent burnout, it is undoubtedly important to restrict those mundane and practical obligations; however, the practical, economic, and administrative realities of medicine, especially as a trainee, tend to tip the balance in the wrong direction. Busy schedules, financial and legal duties, and documentation inefficiencies in the life of a surgeon are unlikely to go away. Viewed in this light, an equally important strategy against burnout is to remember and fixate upon those things that offer personal significance and genuine reward: service and contribution to a greater good and the opportunity to teach those who come after us, to name but two. Unfortunately, the opportunity to lose sight of this begins in residency; fortunately, the opportunity to learn ways to retain one's focus on this can also begin in residency.

BECOMING A MORE EFFECTIVE TEACHER

The best first-grade teachers remember and understand what it was like to be a first-grader. The same is true for those of us who teach residents in their third and fourth decades of life. Consider the task of showing someone how to insert a laparoscopic port. When teaching this to a practicing surgeon wishing to learn laparoscopic liver surgery, this is a quick task of communicating port site locations for optimal operative ergonomics. When teaching this to a medical student, this is a laborious and multistep discussion in which none of the smallest details (the shape and design of the port, how to position your hands on the port, safe and unsafe places to insert a port) can be overlooked. There are many differences between these two scenarios, but the most informative difference is in the *need* the learners bring to the learning experience. For the practicing surgeon, the need is to acquire an entirely new operative skill set; if she comes away with a safe and effective roadmap of port site locations, the learning experience will have been a success. For the medical student, the need is to discover if the operating room is a place where she might eventually find career satisfaction; if she comes away engaged and interested (or not) by the thought process and physical task of port insertion, the learning experience will have been a success. To extend this

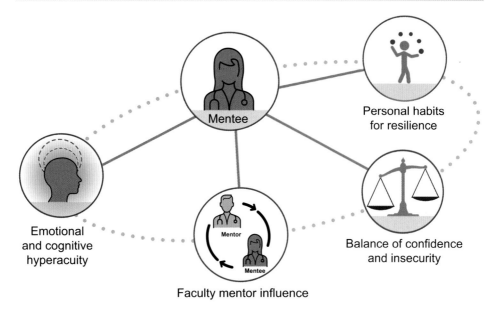

Figure 20.1 The unique experiences of a surgical residency.

illustration, if the teacher were to switch the motivations of the two learners in her teaching approach to them, the practicing surgeon would walk away from the experience offended and hurt, and the medical student would walk away from the experience confused and alienated.

As discussed in the previous section, the experience of residency is marked by an emotional and cognitive hyperacuity that accentuates one's receptivity to learning; the potential for outsized influence on the part of faculty mentors, a need to cultivate a healthy balance of confidence and insecurity, and the opportunity to build personal habits that may protect against the creeping influence of burnout (*Figure 20.1*). How can the academic surgeon use the nature of this experience to be an effective teacher?

SEIZE THE TEACHABLE MOMENT

Our surgical education occurs so gradually that it is easy to forget when it was that we learned certain things. Consider the exploratory laparotomy. The first time one witnesses the process of entering the abdominal cavity can be transformative; the second time, it is still very special, and one notices some subtleties that were obscured by the sheer wonder of the first time; by the hundredth time, excitement has been replaced by frustration that it is taking so long. For the junior resident performing the laparotomy incision, the emotional charge of the experience makes every moment memorable. The opportunity to learn and retain new knowledge may never be as strong ever again. This hyperacuity is transferable; not only the act of the incision but the many details surrounding this event—the indication for operation, the appearance of the intra-abdominal pathology on imaging, the way retraction and counter-traction facilitate the operation—become easily remembered. The senior surgeon on the other side of the table can choose to make the most of these moments—or not.

When these moments happen, it is important to acknowledge it. It does little to downplay the emotional charge that the resident is experiencing; it may be tempting to play to role of the jaded, experienced surgeon who has seen it all, but minimizing the novelty and excitement of the teachable moment not only dulls the learner's receptivity to teaching but accelerates the process of forgetting what a privilege it is to operate on another person. This process may come soon enough—and we will address the importance of fighting its inevitability later—but there is no merit in encouraging it, even subconsciously.

The teacher would do well to reserve her teaching energies for moments like this. One hundred hours of didactic teaching and slides on the subject of abdominal anatomy or disease conducted in the lecture hall, conference room, or hospital hallway may lack the cognitive impact of several minutes of practical teaching before, during, and after one's first laparotomy. The transferability of the learner's hyperacute receptivity means that the teacher can use the moments surrounding this event to impart wisdom on imaging, patient positioning, communicating with family members—any of the nearly infinite number of elements involved in caring for patients.

ACT LIKE YOU'RE BEING WATCHED

The previous section examined the outsized magnitude of modeling influence that faculty surgeons can have on trainees. Appropriate or not, this influence is an opportunity to maximize the one's impact as a surgical teacher. This impact can be positive or negative, so the teacher is obligated to maintain constant awareness of the impact her professional conduct can have on trainees. The tall pedestal on which trainees often place their teachers is also a platform from which to fall. The closeness with which residents observe us means that they will be especially quick to notice inconsistencies between what we teach and how we behave.

Fortunately for the teacher, the positive effects of laudable modeling behavior far exceed the negative impact of inconsistent or subpar behavior. The faculty surgeon who never comes in from home to see patients for urgent consultation weakens her authority to criticize residents for not personally examining patients in the middle of the night. However, the faculty surgeon who cheerfully agrees to meet the residents in the Emergency Department at 2:00 AM (and arrives well dressed and smiling) has made a seminal impact that could become an archetype of idealized surgeon behavior for the residents to remember the rest of their careers.

Thus, in exchange for the respect and authority granted by resident trainees, the faculty surgeon must always work to be at her best; this is the faculty surgeon's role in the teacher–student relationship. The best surgical educator does not shy away from this responsibility for fear of disappointing the trainee. Rather, she accepts the authority of this role and occasionally uses it to model our profession's ideals of clinical competence and genuine humanism.

FIND THE SWEET SPOT OF AUTONOMY AND GUIDANCE

As outlined in the previous section, the best thing a residency experience can do is equip the learner with a healthy balance of confidence and insecurity—enough confidence to venture into new territories of autonomy and risk and enough insecurity to seek help when needed. The exact balance that results is no doubt individualized, informed by inherent aspects of one's personality and specific moments of success and failure that occur along the way, and this balance may influence the trainee's choice of specialty and practice setting. The effective surgical educator does not attempt to externally define this for the trainee. Instead, she creates as many opportunities as possible for the trainee to calibrate her own confidence and insecurity.

The only way a surgical resident can properly advance through this maturational process is to be given opportunities to exercise autonomy while being given guidance. Simply providing opportunities for autonomy—leaving the operating room with the charge to "see how far you can get"—is insufficient. Conversely, providing suffocating guidance without any opportunity to escape the safety net of the right angle is insufficient. Any imbalance between the two can lead to misguided overconfidence or incapacitating insecurity. It is myopic to think that this sort of balance is only applicable to technical teaching in the operating room, since the vast majority of the decisions we make—decisions with direct impact on the lives of patients—are made in the clinics and hospital wards.

In truth, every clinical decision involves a willingness to stake out a position and plan (autonomy) based on accumulated clinical knowledge and experience (guidance). If we are generally more comfortable than our trainees at making clinical decisions, it is because we have had more opportunities to practice. Therefore, effective surgical teaching occurs when clinical decisions—large and small—are converted into moments of autonomy and guidance. Whenever possible, the effective surgical teacher converts clinical decisions (whether or not to operate, whether or not to transfuse, whether or not the fluid collection is sterile) into a shared endeavor with the trainee. When time limitations prevent us from inviting trainees to work through clinical decision-making on their own, it can be informative to verbally share the content and process of our cognition with the trainee—to think out loud. By hearing the rubrics and algorithms we have developed for making complex clinical decisions in the face of insufficient data, our learners may vicariously participate in the exercise of balancing autonomy and guidance.

When it comes to decision-making, the boastful surgical aphorism of "occasionally wrong but never in doubt" is both silly and dangerous. In the process of teaching, it is necessary to acknowledge that clinical decision-making is inherently imperfect. Decisions are only needed in circumstances of uncertainty, and the existence of uncertainty presupposes the possibility that decisions will occasionally be wrong. Here too, there is an opportunity to develop a proper balance of confidence with insecurity. There are so many aspects of medicine that seem rather simple—until you learn that they are not. Atelectasis is a common cause of fever—or maybe that is a myth. Beta-adrenergic blockade reduces the risk of postoperative myocardial infarction—or perhaps it does not. Wise clinical decision-making is informed by simultaneously relying on AND maintaining a healthy circumspective distance from oversimplified narratives, preliminary data, or anecdotal experiences. Uncertainty is difficult, so it is therefore tempting—but misguided—to circumvent uncertainty with simple mnemonics and decision trees. This temptation is especially acute for trainees. Therefore, it is important to model clinical decision-making in a way that rejects a dogmatic approach and acknowledges the only true certitude there is: that, despite our best efforts, we will occasionally be wrong.

MODELING HEALTHY HABITS FOR THE LONG RUN

An earlier section evaluated the insidious influence of burnout and explored the possibility that a disciplined and unwavering focus on service and contribution to a greater good can be protective. In her future career, the surgical trainee will learn—like the rest of us—that life is full of professional metrics that, although important, are unlikely to provide long-term, meaningful personal fulfillment. The surgical career requires a great deal of heavy lifting over a long period of time, and at some point along the way, the surgeon will inevitably ask whether the fruits of her labor are worth the effort she has expended thus far. The problem with professional metrics like salary, RVUs, academic titles, and research funding is that they, once achieved, are largely incapable of returning the favor of one's hard work with long-term personal fulfillment. In contrast, the continuing ability to meaningfully touch another person's life through one's surgical care can trigger a self-sustaining cascade of reward that lends meaning and significance to one's life. It is no wonder that many surgeons develop escape fantasies of leaving their jobs for a "simpler" life as a volunteer surgeon to underserved populations—often in faraway countries—as an antidote to mounting dissatisfaction with their current professional circumstances.

Research suggests that burnout occurs when discrepancies between one's efforts and one's work-related reward or gratification reaches a critical threshold. On some level, the unfortunate paradox is that there are few professions that could offer greater reward or gratification than medicine. Investigations into burnout in healthcare professions indicate that personal characteristics (characterized by parameters like grit and perseverance) strongly impact one's chances of burnout.[4,5] An analysis of emergency department trainees showed that residents with lower quantitative measurements of grit were over six times more likely to experience burnout than their cohorts.[6] Grit has been defined as "perseverance and passion for long-term goals.[7]" Research into this elusive character trait suggests that grit is not inherent or immutable but something that can be strengthened over time.[8] Viewed in this light, grit (and protecting oneself against the risk of burnout) is something that can be fortified during residency. Thus, the surgical educator should not overlook the impact she can have on her trainee's lifelong sense of personal and professional fulfillment.

Research suggests that grit is strengthened by circumstances where one is able to pursue one's interest, practice perseverance, find a higher purpose in one's work, and have hope in one's future.[9] The position that surgical educators have as role models gives them the opportunity to meaningfully impact each of these through effective teaching habits:

Pursuing One's Interest

The effective surgical educator facilitates her trainees' ability to pursue their interests by sharing her own reasons for doing what she does. We all choose our specialty and subspecialty for different reasons, and the journeys that took us to what we do now were all iterative, counterintuitive, and unique. Most of our trainees will not choose to do what we do, but sharing the details of our own career pathways and sharing a willingness to express a love for what we do may help our trainees' chances of finding what it is that they love to do.

Practicing a Discipline of Perseverance

In addition to preparing trainees for life *after* residency, the effective surgical educator also prepares trainees for life *during* residency. In truth, there is really no reason to distinguish the two, because we use the tools and wisdom gained in residency during our posttraining professional lives. Residency is often described as a marathon, and in many respects, this comparison is apt—as long as one leaves out the metaphor of the finish line. If one views residency as a challenge that must be surmounted and completed, one overlooks durability of the cognitive and behavioral disciplines gained over the course of residency. It also prolongs a mental habit of segmenting our lives into finite periods of transiency—a habit that evolved quite naturally after a lifetime segmented into discrete periods of elementary school, middle school, high school, college, and so forth. At some point, we transition from *preparing* for our lives to actually *living* our lives; when we do, we may realize that the distinctions between the two are far less clear than we had anticipated. Residents have a remarkable capacity for work and attention to detail. The resident who believes that this capacity will no longer be needed after her residency will be sorely disappointed. In contrast, the resident who intentionally builds the habits of her work ethic as a strategy for her life's work will be far better equipped for the long-term challenges and joys of her career. To that end, the effective surgical educator should work to intentionally blur the distinctions between life during and after training. By verbally reflecting on the many ways in which the lessons and disciplines learned during residency have carried over into our lives now, we have the chance to impart stamina into our trainees' preparation for their future.

Finding a Higher Purpose

Consider the differences between three surgeons asked to explain why they share emergency call coverage. The first replies that she is doing it because "they need bodies." The second answers that she is doing it because "it's my duty as a general surgeon." The third replies that she is doing it because "people occasionally get hurt, and when they do, they need help." All are technically correct, but it is easy to imagine that these three surgeons may be aligned in increasing order of personal satisfaction with their work. The transient and difficult nature of residency makes it very easy to cheapen the significance of one's work during residency—"I can do this for a few years and then I'll be done"—but doing so will paradoxically make residency more difficult and will lead to disappointment when she realizes that life after training is not that much easier. There is a tremendous amount of attention drawn to the balance of "education" and "service" in residency. However, efforts to quantify and balance these two only places them into more dramatic contradistinction, implicitly painting "education" as "good," and "service" as "bad." Lost in this arithmetic is the fact that each lends itself to the other. In some sense, the biggest difference between the two may be the fact that, whereas "education" is an inherently selfish pursuit, "service" is directed outward. A lifetime dedicated to one's own education will ultimately benefit one person, with no one else offering their thanks. A lifetime directed toward service to others will benefit a multitude of people, with many offering their thanks. The effective surgical educator seeks opportunities to elevate and magnify the reasons her trainees are doing what they are doing. Moreover, the effective surgical educator imparts habits that enable trainees to do this on their own. Trainees should be taught to inculcate the belief that the work they do is integral to the overall healing mission of our profession. Some of this may be a mental trick. Telling oneself that replacing potassium and assisting in breast biopsies is healing this world may feel shallow and disingenuous at first—but when repeated and reminded over and over again for 5 to 7 years, it becomes a part of one's truest self-definitions. Reminding and thanking trainees about the personal benefit they are imparting to their patients may ultimately strengthen the clarity and durability of their sense of calling.

Having Hope in the Future

The influence a faculty surgeon yields as a role model extends far beyond clinical and professional decision-making. Until they become independent, the lives led by faculty surgeons are often residents' sole templates for predicting their own professional satisfaction. As will be explored in the final segment of this chapter, this fact lends even more weight to the importance of an academic surgeon's sense of personal fulfillment; not only is it important to her, it is important to her trainees. Grit is comprised in very large part by a stubborn trust and faith in the expectation that good things are forthcoming, and there is no better way to build this hope in our trainees than to exemplify it for them. As with anything, this is best done in moderation and with honesty. The effective surgical educator is unafraid to share her joys and positive reinforcements with her trainees—but she does so intentionally. Superficial ebullience over one's personal good fortunes—even when communicated honestly—can come across negatively, especially to people who are not sharing in those same good fortunes. However, we all have periodic reminders of why we chose to go into surgery, and it would be a waste to not share those reminders—especially with people who may benefit from knowing that these will also happen to them someday.

In addition to the value of grit, the degree to which we shape our own satisfaction in surgery should not be understated. The power of a positive affect has been documented in multiple studies.[10] In short, the evidence suggests that happiness drives success. Of course, one may not simply will oneself to be happy, especially in the face of professional and personal pressures. However, one may start by simply contemplating how fortunate we are to be surgeons,[11] to enjoy the privilege of our patients' trust, to be able to do meaningful work with our hands, to do that work with the support of dedicated teams, and ultimately to alleviate suffering and improve health. If one is willing to impose more structure, a daily exercise of articulating one's gratitude (i.e., writing down three or so things for which one is grateful) has been shown to improve affect in clinical studies[12].

THE BIDIRECTIONAL BENEFIT OF TEACHING

The biggest hurdle to teaching is its perceived cost. Unlike other elements in our job description, the benefit of teaching often feels *unidirectional*, flowing only outward away from us. Even worse, teaching often feels like a doubly negative investment because the time commitment it demands is time taken away from other necessary pursuits (revenue generation, paperwork, family). Viewed in this light, it would seem inevitable that one's passion for or interest in teaching will eventually be extinguished—and so it often is.

The problem is that the benefits of the other professional obligations that usually take the place of teaching are no less unidirectional. In fact, the vast majority of those other obligations are far more unidirectional, and teaching can be much more fulfilling and rewarding than these other tasks, even if it is not explicitly compensated. This is a lesson that is usually learned after it is too late. At the end of the day (or more accurately, at the end of the career), it is often retrospectively appreciated that there really was no good reason to have performed the extra operation, generated the extra RVU, or received the extra academic society award—none of which end up being memorable enough to recall in much detail. In contrast, retrospective reflections on one's career and major accomplishments usually settle on patients and trainees, many of whom remain quite distinct in one's memory.[13] The intrinsic satisfaction is significant —the acknowledgment from a current or former trainee that "I did it just the way you taught me" can be even more rewarding.

As academic surgeons, our need for grit and our susceptibility to burnout are no less acute than those of our trainees. Postoperative complications occur, manuscripts and grants get rejected, salary compensation may decline, and medical documentation requirements may get worse. Like every other sentient human, we desperately need to be a part of something far more important and permanent than ourselves. Ultimately, a life spent in service is always more meaningful and easier to pursue with vigor than a life spent otherwise. In retrospect, it was likely this kind of thinking that motivated our decision to enter this profession in the first place. One of the central privileges that come with following an academic track to one's surgical career is the access to people to whom we can be of meaningful service—our trainees. If one were to believe the majority of what people say at the time of their retirement or presidential addresses, it may be true that the eventual benefit we give to them may not exceed the benefit we get in return.

REFERENCES

1. Lebareas CC, Guvva EV, Ascher NL, O'Sullivan PS, Harris HW, Epel ES. Burnout and stress among US surgery residents: psychological distress and resilience. *J Am Coll Surg.* 2018;226:80-90.
2. Lindeman B, Petrusa E, McKinley S, et al. Association of burnout with emotional intelligence and personality in surgical residents: an we predict who is most at risk?. *J Surg Educ.* 2017;74:e22-e30.
3. Shanafelt TD, Balch CM, Bechamps GJ, et al. Burnout and career satisfaction among American surgeons. *Ann Surg.* 2009;250:463-471.
4. Salles A, Lin D, Liebert C, et al. Grit as a predictor of risk of attrition in surgical residency. *Am J Surg.* 2017;213:288-291.
5. Salles A, Cohen GL, Muller CM. The relationship between grit and resident well-being. *Am J Surg.* 2014;207:251-254.
6. Dam A, Perera T, Jones M, Haughy M, Gaeta T. The relationship between grit, burnout, and well-being in emergency medicine residents. *AEM Educ Train.* 2018;3(1):14-19.
7. Duckworth AL, Peterson C, Matthews MD, Kelly DR. Grit: perseverance and passion for long-term goals. *J Pers Soc Psychol.* 2007;92:1087.
8. Duckworth AL, Quinn PD. Development and validation of the short grit scale (GRIT-S). *J Pers Assess.* 2009;91:166-174.
9. Duckworth AL, Kirby TA, Tsukuyama E, Berstein H, Ericsson KA. Deliberate practice spells success why grittier competitors triumph at the national spelling bee. *Soc Psychol Personal Sci.* 2011;2:174-181.
10. Lyubomirsky S, King L, Diener E. The benefits of frequent positive affect: does happiness lead to success?. *Psychol Bull.* 2005;131(6):803-855.
11. Sawin RS. Optimizing joy in surgery. *JAMA Surg.* 2019;154(10):893-894. doi:10.1001/jamasurg.2019.1522.
12. Wood AM, Froh JJ, Geraghty AW. Gratitude and well-being: a review and theoretical integration. *Clin Psychol Rev.* 2010;30:890-905.
13. McMasters KM. Life, surgery, and the philosophy of Dry Creek. *J Am Col Surg.* 2018;227:1-5.

21

Academic Development as a Component of Surgical Training

Lesly A. Dossett

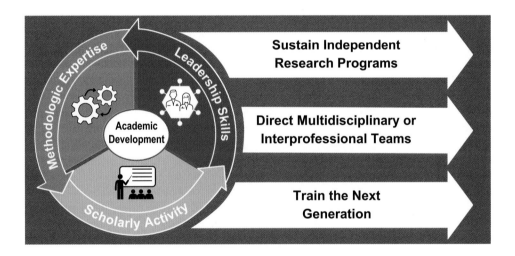

THE IMPORTANCE OF ACADEMIC DEVELOPMENT

Academic development can be defined as the time a trainee spends to purposively develop skills that are necessary for success as a surgical faculty member or health system leader. These skills may include methodologic expertise necessary to create and sustain an independent research program, leadership skills required for directing multidisciplinary or interprofessional teams, or teaching skills necessary to train the next generation of surgeons. In this chapter, we use the term *academic development time* to be synonymous with the alternate terms "research," "lab," or "professional development" time.

Whether leading a multidisciplinary or interprofessional clinical team, a research team, a training program, department, or health system, surgeons are natural and necessary leaders. Purposeful development prepares surgical trainees to step into these roles and potentially avoid learning the hard way, through failures or negative experiences. While the priority of surgical training programs will always be training excellent clinicians, the integration of academic development is a critical complement to clinical training. Particularly for trainees involved in research, learning to ask and answer important clinical questions develops the clinical knowledge base and enhances problem-solving skills. Further, development of methodologic skills allows for better understanding of clinical data and trials which ultimately enhances the clinical mission. Surgical training does not in and of itself prepare surgeons to be leaders—and some characteristics of training may even hinder professional development—a focused period in developing professional skills can greatly enhance traditional clinical training in surgery.[1]

DEDICATED TIME

Of the seven large specialties that match more than one thousand candidates in the National Residency Matching Program, General Surgery is the only specialty in which a sizable proportion interrupt their clinical training for dedicated academic development. In a national survey sent to program directors in general surgery, 35% of surgical trainees had participated in at least 1 year of research during general surgery training,[2] and this proportion is higher among academic training programs.[3] As departmental margins have tightened and more trainees are extending clinical training through fellowships, a number of studies have examined the evidence for the benefits of academic development time.

While not every trainee who participates in academic development time will ultimately achieve standing as an independently funded investigator (perhaps by some, the bar by which this time should be measured), a number of studies have documented significant return on investment for both the trainee and their institution. For example, participants in graduate medical education (GME)-sponsored academic development are more likely to have received faculty appointments and federal grants.[4] This benefit is further supported by the findings of a survey of three academic surgical organizations (Association of Academic Surgeons, Society of University Surgeons, and the American Surgical Association) demonstrating that three-quarters of the membership had performed research during residency.[5] Other possible benefits include preparation for an academic career, preparation to perform research that is not funded by the National Institutes of Health (NIH), increased chance of obtaining competitive clinical fellowships, and improved patient care skills secondary to improved critical thinking and assessment of the literature.

OPTIMAL TIMING

Dedicated academic development time is defined as a period away from clinical work which may last a few months to several years depending on the goals of the trainee and the flexibility of the training program. The advantage of dedicated time is that it allows the trainee to step away from clinical work and fully focus on academic development. This period can facilitate completion of a longitudinal research or educationally based project, or a formal degree program, such as a Master of Clinical Research or Master of Business Administration. Dedicated time has been shown to be associated with subsequent faculty appointments and external funding success.[4] There are also disadvantages of dedicated academic time. First, academic time lengthens surgical training at a time when increasing numbers of trainees are completing fellowships and facing mounting educational debt.

Dedicated time may not be feasible at every training program given needs for clinical coverage and it can be expensive. One study published in 2009 estimated the cost of dedicated research fellowships to exceed $40 million dollars nationally. Dedicated time may occur before a clinical specialty is decided upon by the trainee which can complicate the choice of mentored research.

If pursued, the ideal time for dedicated academic development is debated. Often it occurs after the second or third year of clinical training, but can also occur during fellowship training, and less often during the early faculty years. While the majority of programs requiring trainees to complete dedicated academic development time do not require trainees to seek or obtain external funding, application for funding was significantly correlated with publications during academic development time. Salary, benefits, supplies, and travels costs are most often paid out of departmental funds, institutional training grants such as the NIH T32 award, individual grants from the NIH or societies, and other sources. Traditional training paths are more likely to be funded.

Integrated time with clinical training may occur because a program cannot accommodate dedicated time or a trainee does not wish to prolong training. One advantage of integrated time is that it's more generalizable to time as a faculty member or practicing surgeon. Learning to advance research objectives in smaller increments of time while balancing clinical work is a major obstacle at the faculty level and having trainees experience this tension earlier could facilitate the development of sustainable work processes. Integrated time would also allow a focus on leadership development that was concurrent with clinical development and may be more "real life" as residents are learning to lead their own clinical teams. The disadvantages of integrated time are that it can be difficult to prioritize academic development over clinical work, particularly when residents are relied upon for service. Logistically, this form of academic development time could require more flexibility in the typical training paradigm where residents are relied upon to participate in clinical work up to 6 days per week.

ACADEMIC DEVELOPMENT PATHWAYS

Historically, academic development during surgical training was exclusively participation in basic or bench research.[3] Today, the opportunities are quite diverse, nearly limitless.

The major academic development pathways available to today's trainees include basic science research, clinical or translational research, health services research or health policy, educational research, innovation, business or administration, information technology, and global health (*Figure 21.1*). There are numerous core skills necessary for all major pathways as well as skills specific to each.

CORE ACADEMIC DEVELOPMENT SKILLS

While the paths above are diverse and broad in scope, there are several core skills that all trainees should learn during their academic development time. These include learning to ask impactful questions, problem-solving through study design, leadership skills, team building, and writing (*Figure 21.2*).

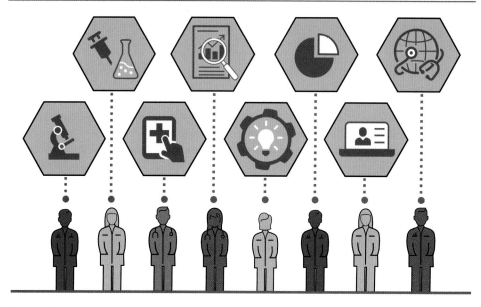

Figure 21.1 Major academic development pathways.

Asking Impactful Questions

Asking and answering impactful questions is the mechanism for advancing clinical care, healthcare delivery, and contemporary education and training. Understanding how to ask important questions in a way that they can be answered and that the answer improves health care is a skill that takes development. Initially, trainees may ask narrow questions that would have a limited impact or questions that are so broad that they cannot be answered practically. Encouraging trainees in their academic development time to think of and solve their own questions—whether these are scientific, quality-improvement, or education questions—allows them to develop their ability to ask impactful questions.

Problem-Solving Through Appropriate Study Design

Once the trainee has identified an important question or problem, understanding how to answer or solve that problem is a critical next step. Even if the trainee doesn't intend to pursue research independence, understanding how to answer questions

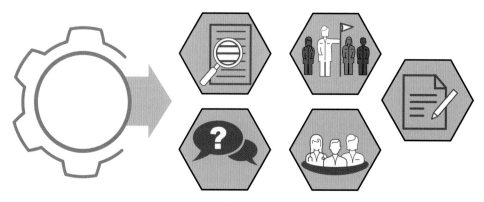

Figure 21.2 Core skills for development.

or study problems in a systematic and evidenced-based way is essential. For example, the trainee should understand the basics of study designs, hypothesis generation and testing, analysis and planning, and mitigating confounders and bias.

Writing

Writing is the currency of academic promotion, and effective written communication is a critical leadership skill. During academic development time, surgical trainees should learn to develop both their quantity and quality of writing. They should learn to effectively increase the *volume* of writing through regular work processes and the *quality* of the work through practice, feedback, and reading.

Leadership Skills

As previously mentioned, every surgeon is a leader, whether within the operating room team or clinic, or at the department, hospital, health system, or national level. Early skill development in effective leadership is critical to address changes in surgical culture. Surgery is increasingly multidisciplinary, and the authoritarian leadership style of the stereotypical surgeon is no longer embraced. While traditional leadership training during residency is informal, programs are increasingly integrating formal leadership development on topics such as conflict negotiation, giving feedback, and leading teams. These are core skills for all trainees, and academic development allows for their intentional development.

Focusing on development of these core skills is critical since many trainees may not ultimately end up on the same pathway later in their career. For example, in a survey of graduates from a single academic training program where dedicated research time was required, 100% of trainees participated in basic science training during their dedicated research fellowships. While 83% remained engaged in research 10 to 20 years after completing residency, only one-third were still engaged in basic science.[3]

Specific Skills

In addition to core skills, there are skills and special considerations that are unique to each career development path. For trainees pursuing bench or basic science academic development, special consideration should be given to the breadth and depth of exposure to various methodologic techniques, recognizing that those techniques may be outdated or obsolete by the time the trainee returns to independent research. The trainee should consider the timeframe of expected experiments and academic products and seek complimentary clinical research projects if needed to ensure continued exposure to the writing and publication process.

For clinical or translational research paths, trainees may choose to pursue specific training in clinical trial design. As many large clinical trials require long enrollment and follow-up times, the traditional 2-year period of dedicated time would not likely allow for a trainee to participate in a trial from conceptualization to publication. Instead, trainees may seek experiences on several trials that are at different phases to round out their experience. A number of professional societies offer short courses on clinical trial design, often directed at trainees.

Academic development paths focused on health services research or health policy should similarly consider the breadth and depth of exposure to methodologic techniques. Within this broad path are "big data" (large administrative databases), policy evaluation, survey, qualitative methods, and implementation science. Some of these methodologic skills can be learned through mentored research but others are often significantly facilitated with formal didactic training. For example, an understanding of basic biostatistics concepts and familiarity with at least one statistical package are necessary for success in this path.

For trainees pursuing educational research, close affiliation with the medical school or residency program can be helpful in acquiring skills and experience in curriculum development, novel methods of teaching, and trainee evaluation. Trainees may wish to develop the skills necessary for future teaching, program administration, and education research. Innovation and product development may not be a stand-alone path but could be accompanied by mentored research in a particular clinical field. In this path, the trainee may work with mentors in biomedical engineering to develop new instruments or products. Formal exposure to an innovation/entrepreneurial curriculum could facilitate success in this path. Business or healthcare administration pathways could involve formal degree granting programs or a mentored experience with hospital administration leaders. This path may look more like an internship rather than a research fellowship. Trainees interested in a global health experience typically seek out an international experience where they may practice surgery or conduct a research study.

ACADEMIC DEVELOPMENT ACTIVITIES

During academic development time, trainees are often engaged in a number of academic development activities. Ideally, trainees should seek a balanced portfolio of activities to obtain a diverse skill set and balance their productivity risk. For example, trainees should avoid solely participating in one large and major research project that may not yield an academic product in time or that is sufficiently attributed to the trainee. Instead, the trainee should seek balance, with activities that are certain to yield an objective product or accomplishment (a training degree or certificate) combined with higher risk, higher reward activities (e.g., large mentored research projects or significant curriculum development).

Formal Degree Programs

Formal degree programs are the most labor and time intensive of the possible academic development activities but also can have a high return on investment for the trainee. At many academic training programs, 1- to 3-year enrollment in a degree granting program is possible. These can range from doctorate or master's programs in disciplines such as public health, informatics, clinical investigation, business administration, or basic science disciplines. The obvious advantages of degree programs are that the trainees acquire expertise in a topical or methodologic discipline that can foster the transition to independence in the field. Additionally, the degree attests to productivity during the academic development time.

Dual-degree holders are significantly more likely to apply for and received career development awards. The completion of a degree during training has been found to be associated with the completion of more total and first author publications as compared to residents with only dedicated research time.[6] Degree completion is also significantly correlated with a first job in academia if compared to dedicated research time only. MD/PhD dual-degree holders have comprised only about

2% of medical school graduates but about one-third of physician applicants for mentored-K and R01 awards. The downsides to formal degree programs are the expense and the time required to complete coursework rather than focus entirely on research activities. Additionally, some trainees who pursue a dual degree may not go on to utilize those degrees after they return to and finish clinical training.

Workshops or Short Courses

If formal degree programs are not available or desired, multiple workshops and short courses are available through national surgical societies. For example, the Association for Academic Surgeons offers courses on the fundamentals of surgical research and grant writing. The American College of Surgeons offers courses on health services research methods, teaching as surgeons, education, and health policy. Several national cancer-based organizations offer short courses on clinical trials.

Mentored Research

Mentored research is the most common hands-on opportunity for academic development for surgical trainees. It is during mentored research that trainees can learn and practice new skills and also confirm whether or not research will be a major part of their future academic career, and if so, to what extent and in what form. Mentored research should also allow trainees to write abstracts and manuscripts and present data at national meetings.

National Meetings

Attending and presenting academic work at national meetings is an important component of academic development. Trainees can learn to prepare and deliver presentations, meet national surgical leaders, and develop skills in networking. Smaller local or regional meetings can serve similar purposes at reduced cost and disruption when travel to national meetings is not possible. National meetings are also an ideal time for sponsorship of trainees, and some national societies and organizations allow resident participation on committees.

BUILDING A MENTORSHIP TEAM

One of the more critical predictors of success during academic development time for the trainee is their mentorship team. Here mentorship team is used because rarely can one person provide necessary mentorship in all relevant domains. A mentorship team should include a diverse group of members with respect to demographics and represent the clinical and methodologic domains relevant to the trainee's chosen path.

Selection of the mentorship team should not fall entirely on the trainee. Instead, a program representative or primary mentor can help to identify or recruit mentors to provide complimentary expertise. Team members may include clinicians from outside the clinical specialty of interest or members from outside the department entirely. By gaining an early exposure to several mentors, the trainee can have diverse inputs into their development that consider a variety of opinions and perspectives. In addition, by having a number of committed members of a team, the trainee is more likely to be protected from mentorship malpractice and will have the support of other mentors if one or more mentor–mentee relationships fail.[7] The mentorship team's primary responsibility it to help the trainee establish and meet goals. Regular meetings of the mentorship team can help to establish accountability for not only the trainee but the mentors as well.

DIVERSITY AND INCLUSIVITY IN ACADEMIC DEVELOPMENT

What does diversity and inclusivity have to do with academic development? As established in earlier chapters of this book, cognitive diversity improves the performance of teams. One mechanism for improving cognitive diversity in surgery is by supporting diverse academic development paths among trainees. This requires finding creative ways to fund or prioritize diverse experiences. Dedicated academic development can also foster inclusion by inviting trainees to develop closer relationships with faculty and departmental leadership. By flattening the hierarchy of leadership, trainees in their academic development time can gain exposure to various leadership styles and perspectives that will enhance their ability to step into similar roles later in their career.

Beyond general support for diverse development paths, program leaders and faculty mentors should make certain that access to mentors and funding is equitable. When dedicated academic development time is optional, ensuring equitable access is critical. Notably, in a national survey of surgeons and GME research, there was no difference in the proportion of women or underrepresented minorities choosing to participate/not participate in research.[4] Further, as selection of primary mentors is often based on a series of informal discussions and processes, faculty leaders should ensure that selection to prestigious or funded positions is based on a clear criterion rather than personal relationships that may disadvantage underrepresented trainees. If general departmental funds are used to support academic development time for trainees, leaders should ensure that those funds are allocated in an equitable way.

REFERENCES

1. Vu JV, Harbaugh CM, Dimick JB. The need for leadership training in surgical residency. *JAMA Surg.* 2019;154(7):575-576.
2. Robertson CM, Klingensmith ME, Coopersmith CM. Prevalence and cost of full-time research fellowships during general surgery residency. *Ann Surg.* 2009;250(2):352; author reply 352.
3. Bhattacharya SD, Williams JB, de la Fuente SG, Kuo PC, Seigler HF. Does protected research time during general surgery training contribute to graduates' career choice? *Am Surg.* 2011;77(7):907-910.
4. Andriole DA, Klingensmith ME, Fields RC, Jeffe DB. Is dedicated research time during surgery residency associated with surgeons' future career paths?: A national study. *Ann Surg.* 2018. Epub ahead of print.
5. Ko CY, Whang EE, Longmire WP Jr, McFadden DW. Improving the Surgeon's participation in research: is it a problem of training or priority? *J Surg Res.* 2000;91(1):5-8.
6. Joshua Smith J, Patel RK, Chen X, Tarpley MJ, Terhune KP. Does intentional support of degree programs in general surgery residency affect research productivity or pursuit of academic surgery? *J Surg Educ.* 2014;71(4):486-491.
7. Chopra V, Edelson DP, Saint S. A piece of my mind. Mentorship malpractice. *J Am Med Assoc.* 2016;315(14):1453-1454.

22

Alumni Relationships

Thomas William Wakefield

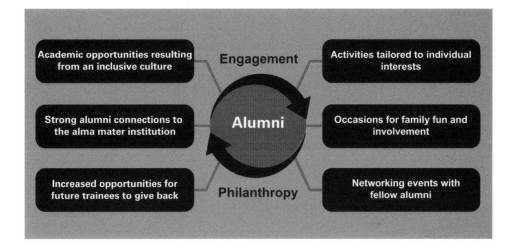

Development of strong relationships with alumni is critical to educational organizations, including academic departments of surgery. This chapter examines alumni relations from five differing perspectives, two focused on surgical alumni and three relevant to institutional needs more generally. Interviews with key individuals involved in alumni engagement provide the basis for this work.

THE FREDERICK A. COLLER SURGICAL SOCIETY

Dr. Frederick A. Coller served on the faculty of the University of Michigan (UM) from 1920 until his retirement in 1957. He was chairman of the Department of Surgery at Michigan from 1930 until 1957. While departmental chair, Coller also served as President of the American College of Surgeons in 1948. In 1946 and 1947, former residents convened to discuss ways to demonstrate appreciation for residency training.[1] Thus was born the idea of the Frederick A. Coller Surgical Society. The society was formed on October 20, 1947, commemorated in a letter to 33 former residents. In the spring of 1949, it was decided to hold an annual dinner at the time and place of the American College of Surgeons annual meeting; the first meeting of the Coller Surgical Society took place on the sixth floor of the University Club in Chicago, October 19, 1949. This was the meeting Dr. Coller was to be installed as President of the American College of Surgeons. Dr. Coller began a tradition, an annual address concerning the affairs of the Department, essentially a state of the Department address.

Subsequent dinners were held in Boston in 1950, San Francisco in 1951, New York in 1952, and Chicago in 1953. In 1954, the meeting occurred in Atlantic City, New Jersey. Until 1954, the meetings were get-togethers of surgeons, residents, and friends of Dr. Coller. At the 1954 meeting, a decision was made to start clinical meetings to occur the week before the yearly meeting of the American College of Surgeons. The first clinical meeting occurred in Ann Arbor, October 1955.

From the beginning, the Frederick A. Coller Surgical Society became a vehicle for establishing ongoing, inclusive relationships between surgeons trained by a Coller-trained surgeon. At a typical meeting, former trainees, current faculty, and current trainees (most with their spouses or significant others) exchange knowledge and cultivate friendships. From informal social gatherings to the formal scientific program to the ending banquet, the society brings together many diverse individuals who have trained at Michigan or have been trained by a Michigan-trained surgeon. The Frederick A. Coller Surgical Society has been very successful keeping the Michigan family together.

The Coller Society has given out a number of awards over the years to trainees which have spearheaded academic careers. The Jobst Award for Research in Vascular Surgery, the Resident Research Award, and the Coller tour program are three such awards. The author was fortunate to win the Jobst Travel Award as a trainee in 1982 and, during the Coller tour in 1984, was able to visit three institutions as a chief resident in General Surgery, the University of Chicago (with Chris Zarins, Bruce Gewertz, and George Block), the Mayo Clinic (with Jeb Hallet, Peter Gloviczki, and Larry Hollier), and Washington University (with Brent Allen and Greg Sicard). Friendships with these surgeons have lasted to the present time.

In the past 5 years, members of the Coller Society decided to form a Foundation, whose purpose "is to provide surgical education and conduct medical research and to implement programs to accomplish these ends." Based on donations from members of the Society, the Frederick A. Coller Foundation now presents a traveling award. The Foundation reinforces the idea that Coller Society members see real value in the Coller Surgical Society. It is a prime example of how to engage surgical alumni. Other important alumni organizations in the Departments of Surgery and Cardiac Surgery include the Reed Dingman Society in Plastic Surgery and the John Alexander Surgery in Thoracic and Cardiac Surgery.

SECTION OF VASCULAR SURGERY

The Michigan Section of Vascular Surgery has a long history of reaching out to alumni via a yearly alumni dinner at national Vascular Surgery Society meetings. James Stanley, Professor Emeritus of Surgery and the head of Vascular Surgery for 29 years, organized these dinners in the late 1970s. In 1987, when Vascular Surgery became an independent section in Surgery, the Section began to host these annual dinners.

The first formal Michigan Vascular Surgery dinner was held in Toronto, Ontario. All Vascular Surgery faculty and trainees, including the Vascular Surgery fellows and General Surgery residents interested in vascular surgery or involved in vascular research, were invited. In addition, prior faculty who had left Michigan and were at other institutions were also invited, along with surgeons from Europe and South American who had spent time in research at Michigan. Spouses were included in these dinners. In the first few years, these dinners were held in Chicago (at the top of the John Hancock Building), Manhattan (at the World Trade Center), Los Angeles (at the Hotel Bel-Air), New Orleans (at Commander's Palace), and Washington DC (the Willard Hotel).

Dinners continue today, now at national meetings of the parent organization, the Society for Vascular Surgery. After socializing, attendees are encouraged to discuss current work. Additionally, there often is a member of the University of Michigan Department of Surgery and members of the University of Michigan Samuel and Jean Frankel Cardiovascular Center Development team, who attend and make contact with alumni who may want to be more involved in supporting their surgical "alma mater." Alumni of the Section of Vascular Surgery have been very generous over the years as a result of close alumni engagement. The Section has benefitted greatly from these relationships which have led to seven endowed professorships, four endowed lectures, one endowed research fellowship, a number of other endowed educational funds, and yearly support of research laboratories.

ALUMNI ASSOCIATION OF THE UNIVERSITY OF MICHIGAN

Alumni Association of the University of Michigan (AAUM) is an affiliated organization that is legally independent of the University of Michigan. Thus, the AAUM is able to engage alumni unencumbered by transient University policies. Its members are very diverse in their education and subsequent roles in society. They represent the nation's largest university alumni organization. There are 96 domestic AAUM clubs and spirit groups, 1015 domestic volunteers, 150 international volunteers, 1424 domestic events in 2017-2018, and 200 international events with 2000 international alumni attending club events in 2017-2018. Of these events, one-half relate to watching sports and the other half to community service, education, and networking. The club model is the one that most of the campus adopts when it comes to alumni engagement.

There is a current emphasis on "online platforms" to connect alumni worldwide. These efforts include The Alumni Education Gateway and the Alumni Online Community Platform. The Alumni Education Gateway seeks to facilitate the success of all alumni by continuing to connect them back to UM resources (e.g., experts, courses and events) throughout their lifetime. The Gateway consolidates educational resources and opportunities from across the University into one location that is curated for UM alumni. AAUM works directly with campus partners to feature the most relevant and timely content for alumni. The online community platforms include *Wolverine Forum* and the *Alumni Directory*. *Wolverine Forum* allows alumni to have robust discussions around a wide variety of topics from travel experiences, to campus memories, to issues of the day. Alumni may even exchange tickets for sporting events or talk about job opportunities. The *Alumni Directory* gives access to Michigan's overall alumni base, greater than 580,000 individuals.

Younger AAUM members desire an association with an overall purpose, a purpose for them specifically, and they expect seamless technology. In view of this, AAUM strives to be an organization that will remain relevant for the next 50 years for these younger alums.

Branding of AAUM is an important part of its success. Branding begins by showing the breadth and depth of AAUM and all that it can offer to its alumni and members. AAUM has its own online "Michigan" platform. AAUM uses its online and social media presence to engage with alumni digitally, for low barrier communications.

In medicine, there are two initiatives—the first is "Find a Michigan Doctor" program, in which a member can find a Michigan-trained physician anywhere in the world. The second is an online community of physicians who communicate via Alumni online communities. This community was initiated by a group of emergency room physicians, 300-strong, who were able to share and engage via this Alumni online community. Multiple other schools, colleges, and units are following this model and partnering with AAUM.

The AAUM's LEAD scholarship program has provided a unique opportunity for underrepresented minorities to attend the University of Michigan as undergraduates and to date has a graduation rate that exceeds the overall rate of the University study body.

CAMP MICHIGANIA

Camp Michigania is owned and operated by AAUM. The camp is home for alumni camping in the summer and a variety of educational and recreational programs throughout the fall, winter, and spring.

In the summer of 1961, AAUM began its camping program with two 1-week sessions for Alumni Association members and their families at the University's Biological Station on Douglas Lake in Northern Michigan. Following the first-year success, AAUM leased the facilities of two children's camps during the postcamp seasons: Camp Charlevoix on Lake Charlevoix, and Camp Huntington/Sherwood on Walloon Lake, also in Northern Michigan. Both camps filled with alums quickly, and it was then apparent a more permanent site would be needed.

In the fall of 1962, the owners of Camp Huntington/Sherwood on Walloon Lake wished to retire and sell their camp, and AAUM purchased the camp in December 1962, after assuring the owners that it would continue to operate a camping program on the 377-acre site. In what can be called a Herculean effort, many alumni donated time and materials to renovate the camp's facilities prior to the 1963 season, in order to make them better suited for family camping. The first Memorial Day Work Weekend took place with a number of volunteers working to clean and update the camp for the approaching summer season, beginning a tradition that still occurs every year during the Memorial Day weekend.

The camping season of 1963 was made up of ten 1-week sessions. Each week was filled to capacity, averaging 50 families per week. Over the years, the popularity of alumni camping has grown steadily. The camp has been upgraded many times with more cabins outfitted for year-round use, an educational center, a new and spacious dining hall, a nature center, and a new arts and crafts facility. The camp now functions at 11 weeks, with a capacity for 100 families per week and with a wait list of over 100 families.

Following the success of Michigania on Walloon Lake, AAUM expanded in 1973 to operate an alumni camping program in upstate New York, renting the facilities of Pointe O'Pines, a private girls' camp. This program, Michigania East, can accommodate 50 families during each of its sessions.

There are very few alumni camps in the country, given that the start-up costs are prohibitive. AAUM made a bold move to buy the camps in 1963, and this investment has been returned multiple times. The activities at the Camp are outstanding, from sports such as volleyball, softball, basketball, golf chipping, tennis, and table tennis, to boating, swimming, sailing, arts and crafts, nature, and horseback riding. The camp now has activities in the fall, and special programs in the winter, especially centered around the holidays. Alumni feel like special guests at Camp Michigania.

A very important aspect of Camp Michigania is a faculty program in which UM faculty present educational topics to the campers. Each week, two UM faculty become campers and lecture their fellow campers at evening forums. The faculty program has become very popular; for the current year, there were 70 applicants for 24 spots. Hot topics which are of broad general interest are presented. These 2-hour forums frequently address the role of higher education in some of the country's most vexing social and political issues, including diversity, equity, and inclusion. Faculty forums are also an important part of the camp in the fall and winter seasons. Surgeons have been well represented in the faculty forum program, and some of the liveliest discussions have occurred around surgical issues.

UNIVERSITY OF TOLEDO ALUMNI SOCIETY

The University of Toledo (UT) Alumni Society is another example of how to engage alumni. The author graduated from UT in 1975 and the Medical College of Ohio (now the UT Medical School) in 1978. UT and the Medical College of Ohio merged on July 1, 2006. Once the medical school was part of the University, the UT Alumni Association also became responsible for the engagement of the medical community.

Among all the UT colleges that participate in alumni affairs, the medical alumni are the most engaged. In order to engage alumni, two types of events are presented. Family events such as afternoons at the theater or ice skating at a local ice rink facility are well attended and appreciated. Mixed with these family events, medical events such as continuing medical education (CME) programs that can be live-streamed, receptions at national meetings such as the American College of Surgeons annual meeting, and gatherings with current students and trainees intermixed with alumni of all ages are also well received. In the UT portfolio, the mix between family events and medical events is about half and half. Although age may play a major role in many facets of UT alumni engagement, the medical alumni (regardless of age) are more homogeneous, and they respond to emails and other traditional modes of communication in a more receptive fashion than alumni from other UT schools and colleges.

In addition to these types of programs, allowing medical alumni to give back to younger students and trainees has been very successful. For example, there is now a program for providing students with white coats and stethoscopes underwritten by alumni. Most alumni remember what it was like to be a medical student and then a resident, and they are willing, even excited, to provide improved experiences for those who follow. After every event sponsored by the UT Alumni Association, a survey is sent to the attendees to determine if the event met the expectations of those who attended, how the event could be improved in the future, and would the individual who attended plan to attend another event in the future.

The three most important aspects to engaging medical alumni, regardless of institution are: (1) diversity of programming, (2) having a way to measure effectiveness of the programming, and (3) wide engagement among students, trainees, and alumni. There are benefits to both the engaged alumni and their institution. For the individual graduate, there is the benefit of belonging to one's alma mater, access to important programs and events, and the ability to network with a wide variety of individuals from many different walks of life. Alumni engagement is an important part of institutional advancement, and in many instances, initial gifts that come after these alumni events are followed by larger and more meaningful gifts.

Alumni engagement does not come without costs. How should institutions support alumni organizations, especially as state support for higher education dwindles. There are many ways alumni organizations can be sustained, including membership dues, financial investments, and corporate partnerships. As finances become more directly focused on education, it will be important for organizations that engage alumni to be nimble and innovative in their approach to financial stability. This is especially important as alumni associations become vehicles for promoting diversity and inclusion.

Is alumni engagement pivotal for the future of higher education in the medical field? The answer is a resounding yes. Philanthropy often begins with alumni engagement, and philanthropy will become a more important part of the way medical education and surgical education will be supported in the future.

REFLECTIONS

In summary, a number of different examples exist of alumni engagement in general and surgical alumni in particular. They all have these common themes. First, alumni engagement needs to have facets that are of interest to the individual alumni involved. There is more to alumni engagement than just attending an event. Alumni want to gain from their participation and involvement, both socially and related to their careers and work life. Second, strong bonds of personal involvement and strong relationships need to be the bedrock of alumni engagement. Third, alumni want to give back to their alma maters, and alumni engagement can help them identify where opportunities exist. Alumni engagement often leads to philanthropy and ultimately, the institutions benefit. Institutions and their programs cannot be sustained without strong philanthropic support. Surgical departments, sections, and divisions are no different. Finally, alumni engagement is fun and enjoyable, is a part of a full and inclusive academic life to be cherished, and will continue to be a key part of the lifeblood of surgical departments.

REFERENCE

1. Robinson JO. *Frederick A. Coller, a Remembrance.* Detroit: Press of Thomson-Shore, Inc; 1987.

Index

Note: Page numbers followed by "f" indicate figures and "t" indicate tables.